Racial and Ethnic Differences in the Health of Older Americans

Linda G. Martin and Beth J. Soldo, Editors

WITHDRAWN

Committee on Population

Commission on Behavioral and Social Sciences and Education

National Research Council

NATIONAL ACADEMY PRESS
Washington, D.C.   1997

NATIONAL ACADEMY PRESS • 2101 Constitution Avenue, NW • Washington, D.C. 20418

NOTICE: The project that is the subject of this report was approved by the Governing Board of the National Research Council, whose members are drawn from the councils of the National Academy of Sciences, the National Academy of Engineering, and the Institute of Medicine. The members of the committee responsible for the report were chosen for their special competences and with regard for appropriate balance.
 This report has been reviewed by a group other than the authors according to procedures approved by a Report Review Committee consisting of members of the National Academy of Sciences, the National Academy of Engineering, and the Institute of Medicine.

This workshop was supported by funds from the National Institute on Aging through grant No. SES 9116694 by the National Science Foundation to the National Academy of Sciences for activities of the Committee on Population, and by Contract No. N01-0D-4-2139 between the National Academy of Sciences and the National Institute on Aging. Any opinions, findings, conclusions, or recommendations expressed in this publication are those of the author(s) and do not necessarily reflect the view of the organizations or agencies that provided support for this project.

Library of Congress Cataloging-in-Publication Data

This book is available for sale from the National Academy Press, 2101 Constitution Avenue, N.W., Box 285, Washington, D.C. 20418. Call 800-624-6242 or 202-334-3313 (in the Washington Metropolitan Area).

This report is also available on line at **http://www.nap.edu**

Printed in the United States of America
Copyright 1997 by the National Academy of Sciences. All rights reserved.

iii

CONTRIBUTORS

RONALD J. ANGEL, Department of Sociology, University of Texas at Austin

LISA F. BERKMAN, Departments of Health and Social Behavior and Epidemiology, Harvard School of Public Health, Harvard University

JIMING CHEN, Columbia University Center for Geriatrics and Gerontology in the Faculty of Medicine and New York State Psychiatric Institute

PETER CROSS, Columbia University Center for Geriatrics and Gerontology in the Faculty of Medicine and New York State Psychiatric Institute

IRMA T. ELO, Population Studies Center, University of Pennsylvania

JOSÉ J. ESCARCE, RAND, Santa Monica, CA

DAVID V. ESPINO, Department of Family Practice, University of Texas Health Science Center at San Antonio

BARRY GURLAND, Columbia University Stroud Center in the Faculty of Medicine and New York State Psychiatric Institute

ELOISE KILLEFFER, Columbia University Center for Geriatrics and Gerontology in the Faculty of Medicine and New York State Psychiatric Institute

RAYNARD S. KINGTON, RAND, Santa Monica, CA

RAFAEL LANTIGUA, Columbia University College of Physicians & Surgeons

KENNETH G. MANTON, Center for Demographic Studies, Duke University

KYRIAKOS S. MARKIDES, Center on Aging and Department of Preventive Medicine and Community Health, University of Texas Medical Branch, Galveston

LINDA G. MARTIN, RAND, Santa Monica, CA

RICHARD MAYEUX, Departments of Neurology and Psychiatry and Gertrude H. Sergievsky Center, Columbia University College of Physicians & Surgeons

JEWEL M. MULLEN, Department of Epidemiology and Public Health, School of Medicine, Yale University

JAMES V. NEEL, Department of Human Genetics (Medical School), University of Michigan

SAMUEL H. PRESTON, Population Studies Center, University of Pennsylvania

FRANK W. PUFFER, Department of Economics, Clark University

DWAYNE REED, Buck Center for Research in Aging, Novato, CA

LAURA RUDKIN, Department of Preventive Medicine and Community Health, University of Texas Medical Branch, Galveston

JAMES P. SMITH, RAND, Santa Monica, CA

BETH J. SOLDO, Department of Demography, Georgetown University

ERIC STALLARD, Center for Demographic Studies, Duke University

YAAKOV STERN, Gertrude H. Sergievsky Center, Columbia University
College of Physicians & Surgeons
DAVID WILDER, Columbia University Center for Geriatrics and Gerontology
in the Faculty of Medicine and New York State Psychiatric Institute
KATSUKIKO YANO, Honolulu Heart Program, Honolulu, HI

The National Academy of Sciences is a private, nonprofit, self-perpetuating society of distinguished scholars engaged in scientific and engineering research, dedicated to the furtherance of science and technology and to their use for the general welfare. Upon the authority of the charter granted to it by the Congress in 1863, the Academy has a mandate that requires it to advise the federal government on scientific and technical matters. Dr. Bruce M. Alberts is president of the National Academy of Sciences.

The National Academy of Engineering was established in 1964, under the charter of the National Academy of Sciences, as a parallel organization of outstanding engineers. It is autonomous in its administration and in the selection of its members, sharing with the National Academy of Sciences the responsibility for advising the federal government. The National Academy of Engineering also sponsors engineering programs aimed at meeting national needs, encourages education and research, and recognizes the superior achievements of engineers. Dr. William A. Wulf is president of the National Academy of Engineering.

The Institute of Medicine was established in 1970 by the National Academy of Sciences to secure the services of eminent members of appropriate professions in the examination of policy matters pertaining to the health of the public. The Institute acts under the responsibility given to the National Academy of Sciences by its congressional charter to be an adviser to the federal government and, upon its own initiative, to identify issues of medical care, research, and education. Dr. Kenneth I. Shine is president of the Institute of Medicine.

The National Research Council was organized by the National Academy of Sciences in 1916 to associate the broad community of science and technology with the Academy's purposes of furthering knowledge and advising the federal government. Functioning in accordance with general policies determined by the Academy, the Council has become the principal operating agency of both the National Academy of Sciences and the National Academy of Engineering in providing services to the government, the public, and the scientific and engineering communities. The Council is administered jointly by both Academies and the Institute of Medicine. Dr. Bruce M. Alberts and Dr. William A. Wulf are chairman and vice chairman, respectively, of the National Research Council.

Contents

Preface

The Committee on Population was established in 1983 to bring the knowledge and methods of the population sciences to bear on major issues of science and public policy. The committee's work has increasingly dealt with the demography and health of aging populations. Together with the Committee on National Statistics and the Division of Health Promotion and Disease Prevention of the Institute of Medicine, the committee sponsored a Workshop on Forecasting Survival, Health, and Disability in 1992. In December 1992, the committee organized a Workshop on Demography of Aging, which led to the publication of a volume of edited papers (Preston and Martin, 1995) that covered a range of topics, from household and family demography, to work and retirement, intergenerational transfers, and health. Two chapters in that volume, in particular, Medical Demography (Kenneth G. Manton and Eric Stallard) and Socioeconomic Differences in Adult Mortality and Health Status (Samuel H. Preston and Paul Taubman), pointed to the need for more in-depth analysis of racial and ethnic differences in health at older ages. This concern prompted the Committee, with funding from the National Institute on Aging (NIA), to organize a workshop, held in Washington in December 1994, at which scholars from diverse health disciplines could present and discuss analyses and reviews. This volume includes revised versions of some of the papers originally presented at the workshop. They have benefited both from the discussion at the original workshop, for which we thank all the participants, and from later review, for which we thank the generous scholars who must remain anonymous.

The committee was very fortunate to have two members, Linda Martin and Beth Soldo, who devoted time and energy to planning the workshop, guiding authors in their revisions, and editing this volume.

We want to thank our colleagues who helped develop the 1994 workshop: Ronald Abeles (NIA), Jacob Feldman (National Center for Health Statistics), Samuel Preston (the immediate past chair of the committee), Burton Singer (Princeton University), Richard Suzman (NIA), and David Willis (NIA). Thanks also are due Robert Moffitt and James Smith, members of the committee who assisted with the review of the papers. We also appreciate the contributions of Michael McGinniss and Michael Stoto. Beyond his role on the organizing group, Richard Suzman was a catalyst, both intellectually and financially, and we are grateful to him and the National Institute on Aging for their support.

Finally, the staff of the Committee on Population were essential to this endeavor. Karen Foote was diligent and thorough in handling the organization of the workshop and the review process. Joel Rosenquist ably handled all the administrative tasks for the workshop and manuscript production. John Haaga, the committee director, provided supervision throughout and critical insight in the final stages of the project. Barbara White gave a helpful and thorough copyediting of the report.

Most of all, of course, we appreciate the contributions of the authors.

Ronald Lee
Chair, Committee on Population

Racial and Ethnic Differences in the Health of Older Americans

1

Introduction

Linda G. Martin and Beth J. Soldo

Although the survival advantage of whites over blacks has generally declined over the past 30 years, there is continuing debate about differential mortality patterns by age, as well as concern about broader health disadvantages of blacks relative to whites. There is some evidence that the black mortality curve crosses over that of whites in old age—that is, that blacks have an advantage at the oldest ages—but this finding is subject to argument. Moreover, this mortality advantage, if it exists, is not necessarily associated with lower rates of morbidity and disability.

At the same time, we need to better understand the health situations of older Hispanics and Asian/Pacific Islanders, and the extent to which their immigration experiences and cultural heritages are positively or negatively related to their health outcomes. The elderly population in the United States has become more racially and ethnically diverse in recent years, and this trend is expected to continue. Projections based on recent trends in life expectancy and immigration show that the Hispanic origin and "other race" (Asian/Pacific Islanders; and American Indian, Eskimo, and Aleut) populations aged 65 and over in the United States will each increase elevenfold by the middle of the next century. The black elderly population is expected to more than triple, while the white non-Hispanic population will just double. White non-Hispanic persons were 87 percent of the population aged 65 and over in 1990, but they will be 67 percent of the much larger population aged 65 and over in the year 2050 (Hobbs, 1996).

Of course, making predictions on the basis of such projections is perilous. The Census Bureau figures cited above are middle-range projections that are based on current trends in immigration and life expectancy. Projections must also contain, if only implicitly, forecasts of how today's preteenagers, teenagers, and young adults (who will constitute the 65-and-older age group in the year 2050), and the future immigrants who will join them, will identify their race and ethnicity when they are asked these questions in the year 2050. It is likely that the race and ethnicity categories used in census and official statistics will change several times by then.

This potential for change underscores an important point for the analyses discussed here: race and ethnicity are fluid categories, whose meanings vary and are to be understood in a particular social and historical context. They are not biological taxa. In this volume we have, wherever possible, used the racial and ethnic classification adopted for reporting purposes in federal government publications (Office of Federal Statistical Policy and Standards, 1978).[1] Many of the large data sets analyzed in the chapters that follow used these categories, and vital rates and population figures with which the smaller studies are compared tend to use them. But within these categories there is much diversity (cultural, socioeconomic, behavioral, genetic) that is relevant to health outcomes. Several of the chapters address some of the challenges associated with identifying membership in particular groups.

It is common for researchers concerned with health outcomes (including mortality) to control for race and ethnicity in their analyses. Such procedures statistically adjust for a range of factors that are known to be related to health and that vary across racial and ethnic groups. Of late, however, there has been renewed interest in understanding these racial and ethnic differences and their potential implications for the mix and distribution of health states within the population. Socioeconomic arguments cite the consequences of lifelong poverty. Relevant factors include both early-life differences, such as birth weight and childhood nutrition, and midlife variables, such as access to employer-provided health insurance, the strain of physically demanding work, and exposure to a broad range of toxins, both behavioral (e.g., smoking) and environmental (e.g., workplace exposures). Over the life cycle, these factors combine to increase the demand for health care, while potentially limiting consumption of necessary health services. In late life, these factors may affect the age of onset of both morbidity and disability, the severity of symptoms, and ultimately the age at, and cause of, death. Recent research also highlights the enduring effects of education. Increased education appears to lower the risks for some chronic diseases—most notably, coronary heart disease and, perhaps most intriguingly, organic dementias—while retarding the pace of disease progression for other conditions (Snowdon et al., 1996; Feinstein, 1993).

---

[1]The Office of Management and Budget has issued a proposed statistical directive allowing multiple racial and ethnic classification, to replace the system set up in 1979. For a discussion of the history of the current system and issues affecting proposed revisions, see Edmonston et al., 1996.

In contrast to these socioeconomic explanations, cultural theories emphasize differences in norms regarding lifestyle and self-care behaviors, contacts with health care providers, and treatment compliance. Moreover, the experience of racial and ethnic discrimination may have adverse psychological and physiological effects, in addition to limiting the quantity and quality of health care received. Still other research suggests that there are race-related genetic factors both for predisposing conditions, such as hypertension and diabetes mellitus, and for life-threatening conditions, such as aplastic anemia.

Most commonly, competing causal explanations are examined independently of one another, although it is unlikely that any one approach can solely account for differences observed by race or ethnicity. The Committee on Population believed that it would be worthwhile to bring together experts from a variety of disciplines to examine and evaluate alternative models. The overarching goal of the committee's 1994 workshop, which was sponsored by the National Institute on Aging, was to make progress in understanding the extent to which racial and ethnic differences reflect differences in socioeconomic status, health-promoting behaviors, access to health care, genetics, and other factors.

Ideally, we would have had papers that addressed all aspects of health—both total and cause-specific mortality, morbidity, and disability—for each of the major ethnic and racial groups in the United States, as well as providing systematic consideration of the potential causal factors mentioned above. Data limitations, funds, and the current status of the field did not allow us to fill each cell of the multidimensional matrix. Rather, we chose to focus on critical cells in which either research is most advanced or the need for information is greatest—something we hope will itself be a substantial contribution. Accordingly, the nine papers in this volume range from overviews of racial and ethnic differences in the measures of health outcomes to in-depth looks at particular causal factors to investigations of specific diseases or specific ethnic groups.[2] The result of our pragmatic approach has been a primary focus on black-white differentials, given that the bulk of available data and analysis have highlighted these. Nevertheless, several of the papers provide insight into the health of the growing proportion of the elderly who are Hispanic or Asian/Pacific Islanders.

The academic disciplines represented include the social and behavioral sciences, demography, epidemiology, genetics, and medicine. The data sources used were even more diverse, including censuses, death registries, administrative records from Social Security and Medicare, national surveys (e.g., the National Longitudinal Mortality Survey, the National Long Term Care Survey, the Health

---

[2]At the workshop, we also benefited from two additional presentations on specific diseases—one on hypertension by Norman Anderson and another on cancer by Harold Freeman. We refer you to their published work (e.g., Anderson and McManus, 1996; Freeman, 1991). Also, Burton Singer made a presentation of work in progress, jointly authored with Carol Ryff, entitled "Social Ordering/ Health Linkages: Pathways and Allostasis," which delved into psychosocial, physiological, and chemical aspects of stress and their implications for health.

and Retirement Survey, the Asset and Health Dynamics of the Oldest Old [AHEAD] survey, the National Medical Expenditures Survey), and small area studies (e.g., the New Haven Established Populations for the Epidemiologic Study of the Elderly, the Ni-Hon-San Studies of Japanese and Japanese Americans, the North Manhattan Aging Project).

The volume begins with papers by Irma Elo and Samuel Preston and by Kenneth Manton and Eric Stallard that assess overall differences in mortality among racial and ethnic groups of older Americans and, in particular, investigate the often-observed crossover of mortality rates of blacks and whites in late life. Both papers recognize problems associated with age reporting that may contribute to the apparent black-white crossover in mortality. Elo and Preston (Chapter 2) bring the keen perspective and tools of demography to the issue. They review and evaluate several studies using different data sets and estimation techniques to address the crossover question. Only one study, which is based on a relatively small sample, fails to detect a crossover, but this study is noteworthy because the data set on which it is based has been so painstakingly constructed. The authors and M. Hill matched death certificates of blacks ages 60 and older in 1980 and 1985 with records from the U.S. census and records from the Social Security Administration. Their findings of age misreporting from these matched data are used to correct the age distribution of deaths among blacks. When the corrected distribution is compared with the distribution for whites, no crossover in mortality at older ages is evident.

Manton and Stallard (Chapter 3) link racial and ethnic patterns of age-specific mortality to age patterns of specific disease processes, namely, osteoporosis and hip fracture, heart diseases and stroke, and cancers. They argue that these processes, in combination with the mortality selection of frail persons, provide evidence of a crossover at later ages. Their analysis of death certificates in particular reveals a crossover, even when allowing for a plausible degree of age misreporting. Manton and Stallard conclude their paper with an analysis of disability and active life expectancy and find that older blacks, despite their survival advantage, experience more disability than whites, who they suggest are more subject to acute disease.

Although these first two papers come to conflicting conclusions on the mortality-crossover issue, we believe that both make important contributions to the debate and that together they highlight the value of different approaches and the need for further work on the question. The two papers agree that there is Hispanic advantage in survival at older ages relative to whites and blacks. Elo and Preston's analysis also highlights the possible contribution of immigrant status to the mortality advantage both for Hispanics and for Asians and Pacific Islanders. They argue that this advantage may be due in part to the selectivity of migration. (Immigrants may be among the healthiest and hardiest individuals in their countries of origin.) But the apparent mortality advantage for immigrants may also be partly an artifact of measurement: some immigrants return to their countries of origin in old age, and thus their deaths are not reported in the United States. Moreover, as noted in other papers in the volume, older Hispanics, despite their apparent mortality advantage, report more physical and functional health problems than do non-Hispanic whites.

The next set of four papers focuses on possible causal pathways to racial and ethnic differentials in health. James Smith and Raynard Kington (Chapter 4) focus on the complex interactions linking race, socioeconomic status, and health. Their review of the literature indicates that taking socioeconomic differences into account eliminates a significant proportion of observed racial differences in health status. Moreover, most of the difference in mortality is eliminated. Smith and Kington use data from the new Health and Retirement Survey (HRS) and the AHEAD survey, which provide the best information to date on the income and wealth of older Americans. They estimate models that allow for nonlinear effects of economic variables and that include risk factors, such as smoking, drinking, and exercise. They find that the effects on health status of being black or Hispanic relative to being non-Hispanic white are substantially reduced by the inclusion of measures of income and wealth. The risk factors, though in some cases statistically significant, have only modest collective effects on racial and ethnic differences in health status in these models. Finally, Smith and Kington present a preliminary investigation of reverse causation that indicates that the feedbacks from health to current socioeconomic status are probably more important than the effects of socioeconomic status on health in the short run.

Taking a step back from health outcomes, Lisa Berkman and Jewel Mullen (Chapter 5) focus on black-white differences in health-damaging and health-promoting behaviors, controlling where possible for socioeconomic status. They base their observations on a general review of the literature, as well as their own analyses of data from the New Haven Established Populations for the Epidemiologic Study of the Elderly. Despite greater apparent concern on the part of blacks than whites about their health, blacks do not consistently adopt more beneficial behaviors than whites. Older blacks engage in less physical activity and are more likely to be obese (especially women), but they are less likely to consume alcohol than whites. Racial differences in smoking patterns are complex, with older blacks less likely to have ever smoked but, if they have, less likely to have quit. Lack of exercise and obesity are associated with hypertension and diabetes, both of which have been reported to be twice as common among blacks than among whites. Berkman and Mullen also explore the role of social networks and social support in influencing health, but find few racial differences in summary measures of social support.

José Escarce and Frank Puffer (Chapter 6) examine the use of medical care of older blacks and whites, yet another possible factor underlying differences in health outcomes. Using data from the 1987 National Medical Expenditure Survey, they analyze racial differences in total medical care expenditures (irrespective of source of payment), physician visits, and inpatient hospital nights. They estimate two types of models: one that adjusts for variables that primarily describe need for medical care and one that includes additional demographic and socioeconomic characteristics and represents more of what they call a demand perspective. In the latter, although blacks were slightly less likely than whites to have some medical expenses, there were no significant differences in the level of expenditure, conditional on having at least some. In the former, which included only age, sex, race, health status, and measures of attitudes and beliefs about health care, race had a larger effect: whites were significantly more likely than blacks to have at least some medical expenditures and some physician visits. Moreover, conditional on some utilization, blacks had lower levels of use. Escarce and Puffer conclude that racial differences in the quantity of medical care received by elderly people in the United States have largely disappeared, but that the care that blacks receive may not fully reflect their differential health needs. Thus, older blacks may still be underserved by health care services.

James Neel (Chapter 7) also focuses on black-white differences in health, but examines possible genetic bases for these differences. Despite the "avalanche" in the discovery of genetic variation since World War II, Neel argues that most variation has no effect on survival. Among the polymorphisms that have been related to health are those in the code for human leukocyte antigens, which are associated with autoimmune disorders in middle or late life. Although these polymorphisms are present in both blacks and whites, the establishment of an association between an allele and a disease in one group does not necessarily imply that it exists in another, and in this case, the association has been established only in white populations. Another association currently receiving great attention is that of Alzheimer's disease and the type ε4 allele of the apolipoprotein E system, but once again research on the link among whites is more advanced.

Next Neel highlights two diseases—hypertension and diabetes—that, depending on the definitions of disease used, are relatively more prevalent among blacks than whites. He notes the familial nature of both, but reminds us that familial patterns do not necessarily reflect genetic differences per se. Both diseases are heterogeneous and are caused by multiple factors, but a number of rare subtypes with strong genetic linkages have been identified.

In sum, knowledge about the genetic basis of racial differentials in adult and late-life diseases is meager. Neel concludes by noting that blacks and whites are generally very similar genetically and that differences in environment play a strong role in determining how inherited susceptibilities are expressed. Until researchers become more adept at measuring and controlling for these factors, it will be difficult to reach conclusions regarding racial differences in susceptibility to complex diseases.

The final three papers of the volume focus on either specific diseases or specific ethnic groups. Barry Gurland and his associates (Chapter 8) highlight a disease not discussed at length in the earlier papers, but one with important implications for the quality of life and the need for long-term care. They report on a study in North Manhattan of dementia among Hispanics, blacks, and non-Hispanic whites, in which particular care is taken to minimize ethnic and racial biases in diagnosis, some of which may be based in differences in educational attainment. They find that Hispanics and blacks have a higher age-adjusted prevalence of dementia than non-Hispanic whites. However, in a multivariate analysis that controls for education and sex, ethnic and racial differences are not statistically significant. They propose three hypotheses for the relation of education to dementia: (1) that education is curtailed relatively early owing to precursors of dementia, and thus there is reverse causation; (2) that low educational attainment is associated with other deprivations that are related to dementia; and (3) that education builds and maintains a robust neurobiological structure.

To understand the implications of dementia for quality of life and to further test the possibility of ethnic or racial bias in diagnosis, the Gurland team examines the prevalence of memory complaints, functional impairments, and depression among those with advanced dementia and those with border-zone dementia in the three racial/ethnic groups, and they find similar patterns. There are, however, striking differences in service utilization by dementias, with non-Hispanic whites much more likely to be in nursing homes than the other two groups and with blacks likely to be relatively greater users of home care and hospitals. Hispanics and blacks are also more likely to use emergency clinics than whites.

The penultimate paper provides insight into the role of culture by studying coronary heart disease among Japanese Americans and Japanese in Japan. Dwayne Reed and Katsukiko Yano (Chapter 9) compare three groups of men, all of whose grandparents were native Japanese and all of whom were born between 1900 and 1919, but who were distinguished by their residence in the mid- to late-1960s in three different locations: California, Hawaii, and Japan. At baseline examination, age-adjusted prevalence rates indicated generally greatest risk factors for coronary heart disease among the Californians and lowest among those in Japan. The only exception was for smoking, which was highest in Japan. A similar pattern, with Hawaiians intermediate, is found for myocardial infarction and coronary heart disease over various follow-up periods.

Further analysis by birthplace of the group residing in Hawaii found that birth in Japan or extended residence there when younger was generally associated with lower risk factors for coronary heart disease. Various measures of retention of Japanese culture were also predictive of lower risk factors, but in multivariate models of coronary heart disease that included these risk factors, the cultural measures did not have significant effects. Nor were measures of psychosocial stresses statistically significant. The study suggests the important role that modifying high-risk behavior can play in reducing coronary heart disease, highlights cultural influences on those risk factors, and suggests the potential for alterations in risk through community-level interventions.

The final paper, by Kyriakos Markides and colleagues (Chapter 10), reviews the health of older Hispanics, who currently make up only a very small proportion of older Americans but whose numbers are likely to increase rapidly in the future. The authors note the overall advantage of Hispanics in comparison with non-Hispanic whites and blacks in mortality, but caution that there is significant intragroup heterogeneity, with Cuban Americans most advantaged, Puerto Ricans least, and Mexican Americans intermediate. They also note that the Hispanic mortality advantage holds for most major causes of death; only diabetes and liver disease/cirrhosis are exceptions. Given Hispanics' generally lower socioeconomic status as well as their relatively more vulnerable risk profiles, this advantage is difficult to explain. Speculation has focused on protective cultural effects, as well as selective immigration, but the authors cite conflicting evidence of effects of immigrant status on broader indicators of health and reinforce the fact noted earlier that the Hispanic advantage in mortality is not accompanied by a Hispanic advantage in disability.

As a group, these nine papers increase our sophistication in thinking about racial and ethnic differences among older Americans. Besides providing the best estimates to date of differences in mortality and other aspects of health, they underscore the critical interactions of socioeconomic status and environment with race and ethnicity and provide perspective on the roles of culture and immigration experience.

Many of the issues that motivated this volume remain unresolved. Gaps in nationally representative data sets are partially at fault. Several studies provide detailed measures of adult health transitions and late-life socioeconomic status, but no study provides a full range of comparable life-history measures for the individual, no less the family. We lack, of course, survey data linked with genetic markers, and the ethical and legal obstacles to building such an integrated data set are formidable. Finally, there is a continuing need to clarify analytically what it is we mean by racial and ethnic differences. Such research moves us into more refined discussions of unobserved heterogeneity. It also requires that we generate testable hypotheses of how culturally distinct differences emerge and the extent to which such differences are diluted through intermarriage or socioeconomic integration. These are topics that have not commanded much thoughtful reflection in the demography of aging but that are clearly an important part of any emerging research agenda in the field.

REFERENCES

Anderson, N.B., and C. McManus
     1996   *Hypertension in Blacks Across the Life Course: A Biopsychosocial Analysis.* New York: Springer.
Edmonston, B., J. Goldstein, and J.T. Lott, eds.
     1996   *Spotlight on Heterogeneity: The Federal Standards for Racial and Ethnic Classification.* Washington, DC: National Academy Press.

Feinstein, J.S.
  1993   The relationship between socioeconomic status and health: A review of the literature. *Milbank Quarterly* 71(2):279-322.
Freeman, H.P.
  1991   Race, poverty, and cancer. *Journal of the National Cancer Institute* 83(8):526-527.
Hobbs, F.B., with B.L. Damon
  1996   Sixty-five plus in the United States. Current Population Reports, Special Studies, P23-190. Washington, DC: Bureau of the Census.
Office of Federal Statistical Policy and Standards
  1978   *Federal Statistical Policy Directive No. 15: Race and Ethnic Standards for Federal Statistics and Administrative Reporting.* Washington, DC: U.S. Department of Commerce.
Snowdon, D.A., S.J. Kemper, J.A. Mortimer, L.H. Greiner, D. Wekstein, and W.R. Merkesbery
  1996   Linguistic ability in early life and cognitive function and Alzheimer's disease in late life: Findings from the Nun Study. *Journal of the American Medical Association* 275(7):528-532.

2

Racial and Ethnic Differences in Mortality at Older Ages

Irma T. Elo and Samuel H. Preston

INTRODUCTION

This paper evaluates evidence regarding racial and ethnic differences in mortality in the United States. In keeping with the theme, we emphasize mortality at older ages; specifically, we deal with ages 45 and above and attempt to extend the analyses to ages 100 and older. We focus on recent estimates rather than attempting a broader historical overview. We give our main attention to mortality rates from all causes combined, although we refer to studies of racial and ethnic differences in mortality by cause of death in a later section.

We deal with four major groups: African Americans, Hispanics, Asian Americans and Pacific Islanders, and whites (or, on occasion, non-Hispanic groups). The analyses are organized by type of data sources available: vital statistics/census-derived rates, linked data files, and extinct generation methods.

VITAL STATISTICS AND CENSUS DATA

African Americans and Whites

Mortality estimates for whites and African Americans based on vital statistics and census data have consistently shown black death rates to exceed white rates until some age above the mid-seventies; at that point, black death rates have historically "crossed over" white rates and have declined relative to white rates thereafter. In Table 2-1 and Figures 2-1 and 2-2, we show estimates of age-specific death rates by 5-year age groups above age 45 for African Americans and whites (as well as for Asian/Pacific Islanders and Hispanics) in 1989. The rates

TABLE 2-1   Death Rates Based on Vital Statistics and Census Data: Whites, African Americans, Asian/Pacific Islanders, and Hispanics, 1989

| Age Group | Death Rates (per 1,000) | | | | Ratios | | |
	Whites	African Americans	Asian/ Pacific Islanders	Hispanics	African-Americans to White Rates	Asian/Pacific Islanders to White Rates	Hispanic to White Rates
Males							
45-49	4.41	10.82	2.35	4.89	2.45	0.53	1.11
50-54	6.96	15.92	3.69	6.56	2.29	0.53	0.94
55-59	11.63	22.63	6.10	9.23	1.95	0.52	0.79
60-64	18.46	31.86	10.55	14.30	1.73	0.57	0.77
65-69	27.97	44.94	15.33	20.54	1.61	0.55	0.73
70-74	43.27	60.40	25.28	32.01	1.40	0.58	0.74
75-79	65.97	81.83	42.29	47.91	1.24	0.64	0.73
80-84	102.57	109.82	70.47	71.95	1.07	0.69	0.70
85-89	152.97	148.70	121.50	108.20	0.97	0.67	0.71
90-94	240.73	201.59	—	160.76	0.84	—	0.63
95+	310.51	233.67	—	—	0.75	—	—
Females							
45-49	2.36	5.19	1.37	1.92	2.20	0.58	0.81
50-54	3.99	7.85	2.55	3.12	1.97	0.64	0.78
55-59	6.50	11.75	3.99	4.92	1.81	0.61	0.76
60-64	10.15	17.98	5.45	7.75	1.77	0.54	0.76
65-69	15.48	25.21	8.64	12.12	1.63	0.56	0.78
70-74	24.28	34.83	13.33	18.32	1.43	0.55	0.75
75-79	38.46	50.72	22.90	28.03	1.32	0.60	0.73
80-84	64.56	73.33	42.90	47.67	1.14	0.66	0.74
85-89	108.88	110.05	101.44	79.53	1.01	0.70	0.73
90-94	189.08	159.18	—	153.25	0.84	—	0.72
95+	288.03	231.88	—	—	0.80	—	—

Note: For Asians and Pacific Islanders, the final, open-ended age interval begins at age 85+; for Hispanics at age 90+. The ratios to white rates for the open-ended interval are based on comparable rates for whites.
SOURCE: Based on data from National Center for Health Statistics, 1993; Hollman, 1993; 1989 NCHS Mortality Detailed Data Tape.

are obtained in a conventional manner, using 1989 deaths from vital statistics in the numerator (National Center for Health Statistics [NCHS], 1993) and the Census Bureau's estimates of population on July 1, 1989, in the denominator (Hollman, 1993).[1] The crossover to lower African-American mortality occurs in the age interval 85 to 89 for males and 90 to 94 for females. At younger ages,

---

[1]Census estimates are based on a reconciliation of cohort counts in the 1980 and 1990 censuses, with the addition of information from Medicare at older ages. Typical patterns of census undercounts by age, sex, and race are preserved in the estimates. Because population estimates are presented in thousands, we choose the final open-ended interval for African Americans and whites to be age 95 and older and to be lower for other groups.

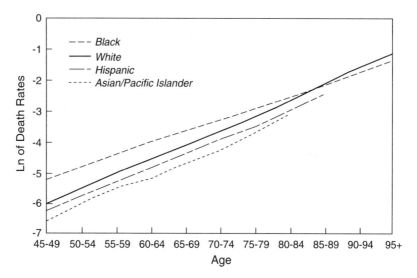

FIGURE 2-1 Death rates, white, African-American, Asian/Pacific Islander, and Hispanic females, 1989. SOURCES: Based on data from National Center for Health Statistics, 1993; Hollman, 1993; 1989 NCHS Mortality Detailed Data Tape.

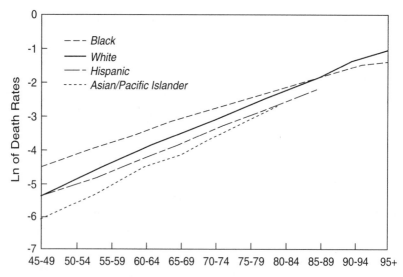

FIGURE 2-2 Death rates, white, African-American, Asian/Pacific Islander and Hispanic males, 1989. SOURCES: Based on data from National Center for Health Statistics, 1993; Hollman, 1993; 1989 NCHS Mortality Detailed Data Tape.

age-specific death rates for African Americans exceed white rates by as much as two to one, and there is a gradual, but steady, narrowing of the differential as age advances (Table 2-1 and Figures 2-1 and 2-2). Throughout the 20th century, black-white mortality differentials have been characterized by the occurrence of the greatest relative disadvantage for blacks in middle age, followed by a slower rate of increase in black death rates relative to white rates.

Many observers have attributed the crossover to the "survival of the fittest," suggesting that adverse conditions faced by African Americans at younger ages subject the weakest members of a cohort to high mortality with only the most robust reaching old age (e.g., Jackson, 1980; Markides and Mindel, 1987; Otten et al., 1990; Manton et al., 1991; Zopf, 1992). Manton and others have further formalized this notion into arguments involving unobserved heterogeneity (Manton and Stallard, 1981; Manton et al., 1981, 1987). These views have dominated much of the literature on mortality of elderly African Americans. Yet evidence from other populations suggests that cohorts who have experienced unfavorable conditions in early life also tend to experience elevated mortality at older ages (Elo and Preston, 1992; Mosley and Gray, 1993).

An alternative explanation for the crossover phenomenon is the poor quality of vital statistics and census data used to estimate African-American mortality, on which much of the evidence for the crossover has been based (Zelnik, 1969; Coale and Kisker, 1986, 1990). Zelnik and Coale and Kisker cite the likelihood that misreporting of age and other forms of error have seriously biased African-American death rates at older ages. The unreliability of age data for older African Americans undoubtedly reflects the fact that many of their births were never registered. Most were born in the South, where few states were members of the birth-registration area before 1920 (Shapiro, 1950).

Substantial evidence exists to support the notion that the misreporting of age is a serious source of bias in estimates of mortality at older ages, particularly among African Americans. The first study to reveal serious inconsistencies in age reporting in vital statistics and census data was the 1960 Matched Records Study, which linked death certificates registered in May to August 1960 to the 1960 Census of Population (NCHS, 1968; Kitagawa and Hauser, 1973). In only 44.7 percent of nonwhite male and 36.9 percent of nonwhite female matched cases was the same age reported in the two sources. Ages reported on the death certificate were systematically younger than those reported on the census record, and discrepancies increased sharply with age and were pronounced even in 5-year age groups. Such inconsistencies were less pronounced for whites than nonwhites; 74.5 percent of the ages agreed in the two sources for white males and 67.9 percent for white females.[2] Corrections for age discrepancies in the two

---

[2]Because African Americans made up 92 percent of the total nonwhite population in the 1960 Census of Population, these results mostly reflect age reporting among African Americans (tabulated from the Bureau of the Census, 1983:Table 45).

sources led to only relatively small changes in the white rates at older ages but substantially increased estimated death rates for nonwhites. The racial crossover in mortality moved from the age interval 75 to 79, based on uncorrected rates, to the last open-ended age interval, 85 and older, after corrections were made for age inconsistencies (Kitagawa and Hauser, 1973:Table 6.1).

More recent evidence of inconsistencies in vital statistics and census data come from evaluations of intercensal changes in cohort size and intercensal deaths. These results for each of the intercensal decades from 1930-1940 to 1980-1990 show increasing amounts of inconsistency between vital statistics and census data for African Americans as age advances (Elo and Preston, 1994). Mortality rates based on these data are likely to be highly unreliable. Similar analyses for whites, on the other hand, have concluded that vital statistics and census data for the most recent decade, 1980-1990, are highly consistent up to age 94, with consistency levels similar to those found in Sweden and the Nether-lands, countries with population registers (Shrestha and Preston, 1995).

Coale and Kisker (1990) have suggested that African-American vital statis-tics deaths from age 65 to age 70 are more numerous than Medicare deaths, but that at ages above 80 they are 7 percent to 10 percent incomplete. They base their conclusion on a comparison of census populations with reconstructed popula-tions inferred from registered deaths. The authors interpreted this finding as a suggestion of possible underregistration of African-American deaths at advanced ages, but the finding is also consistent with greater overstatement of age in the census than in death statistics, a pattern revealed by the 1960 matching study discussed above. Although we have uncovered no studies of possible under-registration of deaths, Shryock and Siegel (1973) assert death underregistration to be less than 1 percent in 1967.

Another potential problem with the use of vital statistics and census data is inconsistency of the reporting of race on death certificates and on the census records. Available evidence suggests that this is not an important issue for African Americans or whites.[3] The 1960 Matched Records Study found, for example, that 98.2 percent of African Americans (all ages combined) had the same race reported on the death certificate as on the census record; if we ignore whether the same individual was represented in the two totals, the net difference was only 0.3 percent (NCHS, 1969).[4] A more recent study linking records from 12 Current Population Surveys (CPS) with the National Death Index for 1979 to 1985 found a similarly high correspondence in the reporting of race among

---

[3]We should note that an increase in interracial marriages in recent years has raised the potential for inconsistent race reporting for the offspring of such marriages on death certificates and on birth and census records (see, e.g., Hahn et al., 1992; Robinson and Gist, 1992). Such inconsistencies do not, however, affect the results discussed in this paper.

[4]In this linkage study, the total number of African Americans in the census was 34,994, whereas the total number reported as African American on the death certificate was 35,085, a net difference of $1 - (34,994/35,085) = 0.003$ (tabulated from NCHS, 1969:Table 2).

African Americans; for 98.2 percent the same race was reported on the death certificate as in the CPS record, with a net difference of 0.4 percent (Sorlie et al., 1992). The consistency in the reporting of race is even higher for whites; in the 1960 study, 99.8 percent of the whites had the same race recorded on the death certificate and the census record (NCHS, 1969), and in the 1979-1985 CPS/death certificate link the agreement for whites was 99.2 percent (Sorlie et al., 1992).

Hispanics

The recent addition of a Hispanic-origin item to death certificates on a state-by-state basis starting in 1978 permits a (nearly) national level calculation of death rates from vital statistics and censuses for Hispanics. Estimated death rates for the self-identified Hispanic population in 1989 are presented in Table 2-1 and Figures 2-1 and 2-2. Because published numbers of deaths for Hispanics are available only in 10-year age categories, we have derived the numerators from a tabulation of the NCHS death files for 1989. Death certificates in which the Hispanic-origin field is classified as Mexican, Puerto Rican, Cuban, Central or South American, or other Hispanic origin are included. Population denominators are based on the Census Bureau's estimates of the Hispanic population on July 1, 1989; Hispanic identification is based on responses to the 1980 and 1990 Hispanic origin questions included in the two censuses (Hollman, 1993). Because Louisiana, New Hampshire, and Oklahoma did not tabulate data on deaths by Hispanic origin (NCHS, 1993:Table 7-7), these states, representing about 1 percent of the older Hispanic population, are excluded from the numerator and the denominator. Hispanic residents of other states who died in Louisiana, New Hampshire, or Oklahoma are also necessarily excluded from the numerator in the calculation of death rates. The number of Hispanic deaths may thus be slightly underestimated and may lead to a small downward bias in the death rates shown in Table 2-1.

Except for males aged 45 to 49, death rates for the Hispanic population are below those of the white population for both sexes at all ages. The proportionate gap between Hispanics and whites tends to increase with age, so that Hispanic death rates are 26 percent to 30 percent below those of whites at ages 80 to 84 and 85 to 89. Similar differences in Hispanic and white death rates at ages 45 and above are revealed by the mortality estimates, also based on vital statistics and census data, incorporated into the Census Bureau's population projections (Day, 1993). The difference between Hispanic and white rates increases as age advances, with the ratios of Hispanic to white rates declining from 1.02 at ages 45 to 49 to 0.71 at ages 80 to 84 for males and from 0.88 at ages 45 to 49 to 0.72 at ages 80 to 84 for females (Bureau of the Census, unpublished tabulations).[5] The

---

[5]The Census Bureau's mortality estimates are based on NCHS death data for age, sex, race and Hispanic origin. The denominator data in the calculation of the death rates are based on 1990 census data adjusted for net census coverage error with the use of demographic analysis (for further detail, see Day, 1993:xxxvii).

results of Table 2-1 are consistent with Hispanic/non-Hispanic differences in 1979 to 1981 in 15 reporting states; at all ages above 44, Hispanic males and females had death rates below the national average in these 15 states (NCHS, 1990).

The pattern revealed in Table 2-1 is also consistent with earlier analyses of Hispanic mortality at a subnational level. Most of these studies focused on Texas and California, where persons of Mexican origin dominate among the Hispanic group, or on New York, where Puerto Ricans dominate. Rather than using self-identification, the studies identify the Hispanic-origin population either by applying a Spanish surname classification system to deaths and population or by using the identification of place of birth to classify those born outside the United States. Studies using place of birth to identify the Hispanic-origin population sometimes focus separately on Mexican, Puerto Rican, or Cuban-born persons.

One of the most detailed studies compares age-specific death rates of various Hispanic subgroups with those of whites during 1979-1981 (Rosenwaike, 1987). The study uses 10-year age groups up to age 75 and above, and deals separately with persons born in Mexico, Puerto Rico, and Cuba. Of the 24 age, sex, and origin groups for which comparisons with whites are made at ages 45 and older, only 4 show higher death rates for Hispanics (Puerto Rican males at ages 45 to 54 and 55 to 64; Puerto Rican and Mexican females at 65 to 74). Cubans, a relatively high-status immigrant group, show exceptionally low mortality in all comparisons. All three Hispanic-origin groups have lower age-standardized death rates than whites for diseases of the heart, cerebrovascular diseases, and malignant neoplasms, with the exception of heart disease among Puerto Rican women.

Bradshaw and Liese (1991) provide a useful chronological review of studies of Hispanic mortality in the Southwest and California. Most of the studies are based on Spanish surname classifications. In general, studies of relative mortality among older Hispanics since 1950 show older Hispanic males to have lower mortality than older non-Hispanic males. The picture for females is more complex. Early studies usually found older Hispanic females to be at a disadvantage, but this disadvantage has typically been reduced or reversed in more recent years (e.g., Rosenwaike and Bradshaw, 1989). Female Hispanics appear to have made faster progress relative to non-Hispanics than have male Hispanics. This tendency was observed (for all ages combined) in the Hispanic study with the longest historical sweep, an analysis of mortality among people with Spanish surnames from 1940 to 1980 in Bexar County, Texas (San Antonio) (Frisbie, 1991:Table 3:3). If the results in Table 2-1 are correct, Hispanic females have achieved mortality conditions every bit as favorable as Hispanic males.

The question, of course, is whether Table 2-1 is credible. There are several potential sources of error. First, misreporting of age may be a serious problem for Hispanics, as it is for blacks. The only study that we know of that provides direct evidence about age reporting patterns among Hispanics in the United States is a study by Kestenbaum (1992) that linked 1987 death certificates from Texas and

Massachusetts to the Social Security Administration's Master Beneficiary Record File. This study shows that for Hispanics, age reporting in the two sources was more consistent than for African Americans but less consistent than for non-Hispanic whites. At death certificate ages 65 and above, ages agreed for 88.4 percent of Hispanic, 72.6 percent of African-American, and 94.6 percent of non-Hispanic white decedents. At death certificate ages 85 and above, the respective percentages were 81.7 percent, 63.2 percent, and 91.7 percent. Only 21 percent of the Hispanic population aged 65 and older resided in these two states in 1990, and thus the above results may not accurately reflect age reporting patterns among the Hispanic population nationwide (Bureau of the Census, 1992a, 1992b, 1992c). Nevertheless, the results suggest that age reporting problems are more prevalent among Hispanic Americans than non-Hispanic white Americans.

Indirect evidence further suggests that inconsistencies in age reporting between death certificates and census records could lead to biased estimates of Hispanic mortality at older ages. Rosenwaike and Preston (1984) use intercensal methods to compare the consistency of recorded deaths and population counts by cohort in the censuses of 1960 and 1970. Using data on the Puerto Rican-born population from the censuses and vital statistics systems of both the United States and Puerto Rico, they find large inconsistencies at older ages. For example, there were 25 percent too many persons reported at ages 75 and above in the 1970 census relative to the number expected from the 1960 census and intercensal deaths. This inconsistency is much larger than that found using the same basic method on data for African Americans for the same or later periods (Elo and Preston, 1994). Dechter and Preston (1991) demonstrate that these inconsistencies are large and pervasive in Latin America.

An additional problem, not serious for blacks or whites, is a potential disparity between ethnic identification systems used for deaths and for population counts. Rosenwaike and Bradshaw (1988) examine death certificates and coding instructions for vital statistics offices in five states that were using the Hispanic-origin question. They find that the ethnic systems are "demonstrably incomparable" with census systems, especially for subcategories of the Hispanic population.

Fortunately, the Sorlie et al. (1992) study investigates the comparability of Hispanic identification in the CPS and on death certificates for states using the Hispanic-origin question on death certificates. They find net underreporting of Hispanic-origin question on death certificates, but the discrepancy was not large: in a linked file, 600 decedents were identified as Hispanic on the CPS, and 563 death certificates identified an Hispanic origin. Sixty-two people were listed as Hispanic on the CPS but not on the death certificate, and 25 on the death certificate but not on the CPS. The numbers pertain to all ages; no age breakdown is available. The net error of 6.6 percent in the Sorlie et al. study suggests that Hispanic death rates in Table 2-1 should be raised by this amount as a first approximation.

Results are reported only for the matched sample in which Hispanic-origin field is filled out on the death certificate. A failure to report on this field on death certificates may bias estimates of Hispanic mortality computed in the conventional manner. In 1989, for example, information on Hispanic origin was missing on about 3 percent of the death certificates at ages 45 and above.[6] In contrast, when the Hispanic-origin field is not filled out on a census form, the Census Bureau uses various imputation procedures to assign a value to the missing data.

The only other linked data set that permits an investigation of the comparability of classifications is the Kitagawa-Hauser (1973) study of U.S. death certificates and 1960 census records. Their only result pertaining to the Hispanic population relates to persons born in Mexico. Correction for inconsistencies in reporting left the death rate unchanged for Mexican-born males and reduced the uncorrected death rate by 2 percent for Mexican-born females. Consistent with results reported earlier, corrected age-standardized death rates for Mexican-born males were 16 percent below those of white natives aged 35 and older in 1960, whereas corrected female rates were 1 percent higher (Kitagawa and Hauser, 1973:104, 106).

Asian Americans and Pacific Islanders

Death rates for Asian Americans and Pacific Islanders as a group in 1989 are shown in Table 2-1 and Figures 2-1 and 2-2. Because published figures for this group are also available only in 10-year age intervals, we have obtained data for the numerators from the NCHS Mortality Detail Files for 1989. The numerator data consist of all deaths that were classified as Chinese, Japanese, Hawaiian (including part-Hawaiian), Filipino, and other Asian or Pacific Islander. Population estimates used in the denominator include persons who reported themselves in one of the Asian and Pacific Islander groups listed on the census form, who wrote in responses specifying one of the Asian countries not listed, or who identified themselves as belonging to one of the Pacific Islander cultural groups. The denominator data are again based on Census Bureau's population estimates for July 1, 1989 (Hollman, 1993).

Mortality among Asian Americans and Pacific Islanders appears to be lower than for any other group shown in Table 2-1. The greatest advantage relative to whites is indicated for males in the age range 45 to 49 to 55 to 59, where the rates for Asian/Pacific Islanders are only about half of the rates for white males. At ages above 75, male rates are still 33 percent to 36 percent below those of white males. The advantage of Asian/Pacific Islander females relative to white females is also substantial; death rates for Asian/Pacific Islander females are 34 percent to

---

[6]The tabulation is based on deaths that occurred in the District of Columbia and 47 states, excluding Louisiana, New Hampshire, and Oklahoma.

46 percent below white female rates at ages 45 to 49 through 80 to 84, and 30 percent below the white rates at ages 85 and older.

Previous studies based on vital statistics and census data have similarly documented low mortality among Asian Americans. Yu et al. (1985) estimated mortality in 1979-1981 among Chinese, Japanese, and Filipinos, the three largest Asian groups in the United States. No sex-specific tabulations were shown. All estimated rates above age 45, shown for 10-year age intervals, were well below the rates for whites. Filipinos showed strikingly low mortality; death rates for Filipinos were 41 percent to 69 percent below white rates. Except in the final, open-ended age interval, 85 and above, Japanese had lower mortality rates than the Chinese, although both were well below those of whites. Among the Japanese, at ages 45 to 54 to 75 to 84, estimated death rates were 40 percent to 59 percent below white rates; among the Chinese, death rates fell below the white rates by 21 percent to 49 percent. Similar results have been shown for Asian-American males and females in 1979-1981 at ages 45 to 64 (U.S. Department of Health and Human Services, 1985:Figures 6 and 7). In addition, state-level studies from California and Hawaii have shown mortality to be lower for Japanese and Chinese than for white Americans (for a review, see Barringer et al., 1993).

A more recent set of mortality estimates for Asian/Pacific Islanders has been prepared by the Bureau of the Census in conjunction with its population projections (Day, 1993). These estimates pertain to fiscal year 1992. The Bureau's estimates are also based on vital statistics and census data, although the definition of Asian/ Pacific Islanders differs from that used in Table 2-1. For the calculation of age-specific death rates, the estimated number of deaths was obtained by subtracting deaths of American Indians, provided by the Indian Health Service, from the deaths of "other races." This procedure was employed because NCHS death data by race were available only for whites, blacks, and other races for the time period of interest. Thus, deaths of the Asian/Pacific Islander population are a residual category once deaths for whites, African Americans, and American Indians are excluded (Day, 1993:xxxvii). The denominator data come from the 1990 census with adjustment for net census coverage error by the use of demographic analyses. The Bureau's estimates also place Asian/Pacific Islander death rates well below those of whites for both men and women. In the age range from 45 to 49 to 80 to 84, the death rates for Asian/Pacific Islander males are 34 percent to 45 percent below white male rates; for females, the relative advantage ranges from 20 percent to 44 percent (Bureau of the Census, unpublished tabulations).

The estimates discussed above, however, must be viewed with extreme caution. The main difficulty in estimating accurate levels of mortality from vital statistics and census data for Asian Americans and Pacific Islanders stems from problems in comparability of race reporting in the two sources. Although most studies that have examined the bias resulting from the lack of agreement in the denominator and numerator data for Asian Americans have focused on estimates of infant mortality (e.g., Frost and Shy, 1980; Yu, 1984; Wang et al., 1992),

Sorlie et al.'s (1992) study, discussed above, covers the entire age range. The discrepancies between the baseline race identification taken from the CPS and the matching death certificate were much larger for Asian/Pacific Islanders than for whites, African Americans, or Hispanics. The agreement for Asian/Pacific Islanders was only 82.4 percent, and the race of the decedent was more often classified as white on the death certificate than on the CPS. No detail by age or sex was available, although the authors noted that "the rates of agreement did not vary much by sex or age group of the decedent" (Sorlie et al., 1992:182). The total number of deaths classified as Asian/Pacific Islander in the CPS surveys was 272 versus 242 on the matching death records, leading the authors to conclude that death rates for Asian/Pacific Islanders calculated from vital statistics and census data are likely to be underestimated by 12 percent (272/242 = 1.12). Even if the Asian/Pacific Islander death rates in Table 2-1 were multiplied by 1.12, they would still be well below those of white Americans.

The only other national-level study that has examined the comparability of race classifications on death certificates and census records for Asian Americans over the entire age range is the 1960 Matched Records Study, discussed previously. In 1960, percentage agreement was high for Japanese (97.0%), somewhat lower for Chinese (90.3%), and very low for Filipinos (72.6%) (NCHS, 1969). Comparable estimates for the same subgroups are not possible from the National Longitudinal Mortality Survey (NLMS). We know of no studies that have examined consistency of age reporting in vital statistics and census data for Asian Americans and Pacific Islanders. However, a strong emphasis on age in East Asian cultures appears to be associated with unusually accurate age reporting (Coale and Bannister, 1994).

The large influx of Asian immigrants since the mid-1960s and the increasing diversity of the Asian/Pacific Islander population as a whole undoubtedly contribute to the uncertainties in the comparability of vital statistics and census data used in the estimates of mortality. Mortality levels are also likely to vary among the Asian/Pacific Islander subgroups and raise questions of the relevance of mortality estimates for the Asian/Pacific Islander group as a whole (Barringer et al., 1993).

LINKED STUDIES

Estimates of mortality based on data sources where information for deaths and population at risk comes from a single file avoid the racial and ethnic classification problems created by dual data sources discussed above. Data sources of this type available for estimating mortality among older Americans are Social Security and Medicare files, the NLMS, and subnational studies.[7]

---

[7]Recently data from the National Health Interview Survey (NHIS) linkage with the National Death Index have also become available and provide another source of linked data for analyses of mortality. These data are based on a linkage of records for individuals aged 18 and above from the 1986-1990 NHIS with the National Death Index for years 1986 through 1991.

Social Security and Medicare Data

We first focus on two studies that have explicitly examined black-white mortality differentials based on Social Security and Medicare data. We then briefly discuss studies of Hispanic mortality. We know of no studies that have used Social Security and Medicare data to estimate mortality among Asian Americans and Pacific Islanders.

Comparisons of death rates based on vital statistics and census data with those obtained from Social Security and Medicare data suggest that conventionally constructed death rates underestimate African-American mortality at older ages. Coale and Kisker (1990) have shown, for example, that in 1980, nonwhite rates calculated from registered deaths and census counts are substantially lower than Medicare rates from about age 82 to age 95 for both males and females. Most ratios of death rates calculated from death registration and census data divided by Medicare death rates for nonwhites fell well below 0.95, while white mortality schedules from the two data sources showed close correspondence up to age 95. Above age 95, however, the mortality schedules for both whites and nonwhites from both sources appeared flawed. The authors' final estimates of mortality showed nonwhite death rates to be above white rates up to age 90, with the estimated rates above age 90 being slightly lower for nonwhites than for whites.

These results undoubtedly reflect inconsistencies between age reporting in Social Security data and on death certificates. Linked studies of death certificates with Social Security Administration (SSA) records have shown particularly large inconsistencies in age reporting for African Americans. The previously cited study by Kestenbaum (1992) based on death data from Massachusetts and Texas found, for example, that only 72.6 percent of African Americans whose age at death on the death certificate was 65 and over had the same age reported in the two sources; for the 85 and older age group, the percentage was even lower, 63.2 percent. Consistent with findings from previous studies, age reporting among non-Hispanic whites was much more compatible; ages agreed for 94.6 percent and 91.7 percent of non-Hispanic white decedents aged 65 and above and 85 and above, respectively.

Similarly, findings based on a national sample of African-American decedents aged 65 and older in 1985 show large discrepancies in age reporting on the death certificate and a matching SSA record (Elo et al., 1996). Only 63 percent of decedents aged 65 and older had the same exact age reported in the two sources; discrepancies were pronounced even in 5-year age groups, with only 82 percent of the decedents falling within the same 5-year age group on death certificates and the matching SSA records. Comparability of age reporting for whites was not examined. In both studies, when ages disagreed, the death certificate age was much more likely to be younger than the age at death based on SSA records, except among the oldest old.

Perhaps the most careful analyses of old age mortality based on Social Security and Medicare data was conducted by Kestenbaum (1992). The author compared white and black mortality differentials at ages 85 and older based on Social Security and Medicare data from which records for certain subpopulations thought to have most unreliable information had been excluded. Black mortality exceeded or was the same as white mortality up to age 87 for males and up to age 88 for females, at which ages the rates crossed over. The author concluded that "allowing some margin for error, we can assert confidently that white mortality exceeds black mortality after age 90" (Kestenbaum, 1992:572).

Because age data on SSA records are reported by the decedents several years or decades prior to death, whereas the death certificate age is reported by relatives or others, it is generally believed that an individual's age at death based on Social Security records is more accurate than the age recorded on the death certificate. Furthermore, SSA now requires verification of alleged age as a condition for entitlement to program benefits and enrollment in Medicare. The superiority of age reporting in Social Security is supported by results from a three-way matching study linking a sample of death certificates for African Americans aged 65 and older in 1985 to records for those same individuals in U.S. censuses of 1900-1920 and to Social Security records (Preston et al., 1996).

Among the oldest cohorts, however, there are reasons to suspect the accuracy of age reporting even in the SSA files. Problems with SSA data among the oldest old stem from the relatively lax procedures used in the past to verify an individual's age. Prior to November 1965, an individual filing for Social Security benefits was not usually required to provide proof of age as long as the alleged age was the same as on a request for a Social Security card filed at least 5 years earlier (Deutch, 1973); this was the practice even though SSA made no systematic attempt to verify the date of birth reported on the initial application forms (Aziz and Buckler, 1992). Thus, SSA information on date of birth has not been strictly verified for many persons born near or before the turn of the century. Even after stricter verification procedures were instituted in 1965, many elderly persons who could not obtain a birth certificate were allowed to submit various documents of lesser quality as proof of age (Social Security Administration, 1988).

We are not aware of any analysis of Hispanic mortality that uses data from the Social Security Administration. However, when the Census Bureau undertook projections of the Hispanic population in 1986, it investigated mortality among Spanish surnamed persons aged 65 and older in Medicare files during the period 1968-1979. The unpublished analysis is summarized in Spencer (1986). Death rates for elderly Hispanics computed from Medicare files were lower than those of elderly whites or blacks. These rates were the principal basis for the life-table values at baseline used in projections. At age 65, female life expectancy estimated for 1983 was 19.36 years and male life expectancy was 15.84 years (Spencer, 1986:Table B-2). These are 0.5 and 1.3 years higher than the respective life expectancies for whites in 1982 (NCHS, 1985:11).

National Longitudinal Mortality Survey

An alternative source of data for estimating mortality for various racial and ethnic groups is the NLMS. Below, we show mortality estimates obtained from the NLMS Public Use Sample, which is based on five CPS surveys conducted between March 1979 and March 1981. The NLMS contains 637,324 individual records that have been linked to the National Death Index (NDI) for the years 1979-1985.[8] This record linkage identified 22,649 deaths that had occurred within the 5-year period following the date of the CPS interview to members of the five CPS cohorts (for details on the linkage procedures, see Rogot et al., 1986).[9] Because no other follow-up of individuals included in the five CPS cohorts was attempted, all individuals who were not linked to the NDI were considered to be alive at the end of the 5-year follow-up period.[10] These procedures are likely to result in some deaths being missed because of a lack of perfect detection of deaths in the NDI. Rogot et al. (1992:2) have noted that "there is some ascertainment loss, of perhaps 5%, occurring in the matching process because of recording errors in the files being matched."

There are reasons to suspect that the success in matching to the NDI differs by characteristics of the decedent, including race. Curb et al. (1985), for example, found significant variation by race and sex in the identification of known deaths in the NDI in 1979-1981. Deaths of African Americans and women were less likely to be located in the NDI than those of whites and men. The main explanation given for this finding was Social Security number discrepancies in the NDI and in the identifying information of the decedent used in the match. Boyle and Decouflé (1990) also found that in a match to the NDI, nonwhite deaths were missed more often than white deaths in a follow-up study of randomly selected Vietnam veterans. We have no way of knowing whether the

---

[8]The NLMS Public Use Data File is a subset of the larger NLMS database consisting of 12 census samples numbering about 1.3 million persons in the United States. Eleven of the twelve cohorts were taken from CPS surveys conducted from March 1973 through March 1985, with one sample drawn from the 1980 Census of Population. Sample individuals were then matched to the NDI beginning in 1979, when the NDI was established, with plans to continue mortality follow-up through 1993 (Rogot et al., 1992).

[9]The five CPS surveys were conducted in March 1979, April, August, and December 1980, and March 1981.

[10]We should note, however, that the March 1981 CPS cohort was followed only through the end of 1985, or approximately 4 years and 9 1/2 months. We cannot distinguish which sample individuals belong to this cohort, and we must accept a 5-year follow-up period for them as well (National Institutes of Health, 1992).

linkage rates varied by race or ethnicity in the NLMS, but it is possible that they were more complete for whites than for African Americans and perhaps Hispanics.[11] We have elsewhere shown that estimates of white male and female death rates by educational attainment at ages 55 to 64 through 75 to 84 based on the NLMS are comparable to those estimated from the National Health and Nutrition Survey Epidemiologic Follow-up Study (NHEFS) for a roughly similar time period (Preston and Elo, 1995).

The NLMS data on socioeconomic and demographic characteristics come from the interview data from the CPS surveys, in which the interviewer contacts, by personal interview or through the telephone, the most knowledgeable adult member of the household, who provides information on all household members. Our samples for these analyses consist of 86,802 males and 104,372 females aged 45 to 89, of whom 11,165 and 8,584 respectively, had died during the 5-year follow-up period.[12] Because of the small number of deaths for Asian/Pacific Islanders and Hispanics, direct calculation of death rates is not feasible. Therefore, to assess racial and ethnic differences in mortality, we estimate a logit regression model where the dependent variable is the log odds of the probability of dying during the 5-year follow-up period.[13] The estimated coefficients are then translated into age-specific death rates by 5-year age groups. Race/ethnicity is a combined categorical variable. Categories are non-Hispanic white, non-Hispanic African American, non-Hispanic Asian/Pacific Islander, and Hispanic. Note that Hispanic individuals can be of any race; the other groups exclude all individuals who identified themselves as Hispanic.

Tables 2-2 and 2-3 present the estimated coefficients from the logit models. Model 1 presents the main effects for the various racial/ethnic groups; Model 1a further distinguishes between native- and foreign-born Hispanics and Asian/Pa-

---

[11]Because one of the key fields in establishing a successful link to the NDI is the individual's Social Security number, if the reporting of this information either in the CPS or on death certificates varies by race or ethnicity, linkage rates are likely to vary by the same characteristic. In a national sample of 1985 African-American death certificates at ages 65 and above, the Social Security number was missing for 9 percent of female and 5 percent of male decedents (tabulations by the authors); the sample did not include whites. In Kestenbaum's (1992) study of death certificate linkage with the SSA's Master Beneficiary Record File, only 2.3 percent of death certificates of persons aged 65 and older were missing a Social Security number or had an invalid number recorded. The Kestenbaum sample, however, was heavily weighted towards non-Hispanic whites. Of the 121,127 linked cases, 104,288, or 86.1 percent, were non-Hispanic whites (Kestenbaum, 1992:Table 3). These results suggest that reporting of Social Security numbers on death certificates may be more complete for whites than for other racial or ethnic groups.

[12]We exclude from the sample individuals whose race on the CPS was coded as either American Indian or "other" nonwhite, other than African American or Asian/Pacific Islander, and for whom race was missing (total = 1,244).

[13]Age is treated as a linear variable. That the logit of death rates or death probabilities is highly linear in age was first demonstrated by actuaries in the 1930s (e.g., Perks, 1932) and has been repeatedly reaffirmed (e.g., Himes et al., 1994). Addition of an age-squared term to Model 3 did not significantly improve the fit of the model.

TABLE 2-2   Coefficients of Equations Predicting the Log Odds of Dying in a
5-Year Period: Males Aged 45 to 89, 1979-1985, National Longitudinal
Mortality Survey[a]

Characteristic	Model 1	Model 1a	Model 2	Model 3[b]
Age	0.0926	0.0927	0.0956	0.0826
	(0.001)	(0.001)	(0.001)	(0.001)
Race/ethnicity[c]				
Black	0.2934	0.2935	2.1379	0.0610
	(0.039)	(0.039)	(0.228)	(0.042)
Asian/Pacific Islander	–0.4393		–0.4376	–0.4461
	(0.105)		(0.106)	(0.107)
Asian/Pacific Islander Native born		–0.3589		
		(0.171)		
Asian/Pacific Islander Foreign born		–0.5526		
		(0.154)		
Asian/Pacific Islander Birthplace unknown		–0.3028		
		(0.251)		
Hispanic	–0.4041		0.3542	–0.5462
	(0.071)		(0.413)	(0.072)
Hispanic Native born		–0.1020		
		(0.107)		
Hispanic Foreign born		–0.6246		
		(0.124)		
Hispanic Birthplace unknown		–0.4838		
		(0.175)		
Age-race/ethnicity interactions				
Age/black			–0.0282	
			(0.003)	
Age/Hispanic			–0.0115	
			(0.006)	
Constant	–7.8178	–7.8245	–8.0209	–7.5322
	(0.071)	(0.072)	(0.077)	(0.081)
Log likelihood	–28,897.9	–28,890.9	–28,866.0	–28,553.2
Sample size	86,802	86,802	86,802	86,802

[a]White is used as the reference category; standard errors are in parentheses.

[b]Model 3 includes controls for education, income, current residence, and marital status.

[c]White, black, and Asian/Pacific Islander categories exclude all Hispanics. Hispanics can be of
any race.

TABLE 2-3   Coefficients of Equations Predicting the Log Odds of Dying in a 5-Year Period: Females Aged 45 to 89, 1979-1985, National Longitudinal Mortality Survey[a]

Characteristic	Model 1	Model 1a	Model 2	Model 3[b]
Age	0.0921	0.0922	0.0941	0.0862
	(0.001)	(0.001)	(0.001)	(0.001)
Race/ethnicity[c]				
Black	0.3402	0.3403	1.6733	0.1806
	(0.041)	(0.041)	(0.251)	(0.043)
Asian/Pacific Islander	−0.5081		−0.5014	−0.5480
	(0.144)		(0.144)	(0.146)
Asian/Pacific Islander Native born		−0.3309		
		(0.228)		
Asian/Pacific Islander Foreign born		−0.6754		
		(0.219)		
Asian/Pacific Islander Birthplace unknown		−0.4559		
		(0.356)		
Hispanic	−0.2495		−0.2431	−0.3970
	(0.080)		(0.080)	(0.081)
Hispanic Native born		−0.0174		
		(0.125)		
Hispanic Foreign born		−0.4128		
		(0.138)		
Hispanic Birthplace unknown		−0.3225		
		(0.196)		
Age-race/ethnicity interactions				
Age/black			−0.0197	
			(0.004)	
Constant	−8.5145	−8.5187	−8.6590	−8.3985
	(0.081)	(0.081)	(0.086)	(0.094)
Log likelihood	−25,790.9	−25,787.8	−25,776.7	−25,673.7
Sample size	104,372	104,372	104,372	104,372

[a]White is used as the reference category; standard errors are in parentheses.

[b]Model 3 includes controls for education, income, current residence, and marital status.

[c]White, black, and Asian/Pacific Islander categories exclude all Hispanics. Hispanics can be of any race.

cific Islanders. Because place of birth was missing for a sizable fraction of the sample, we have further distinguished this group from the foreign- and native-born Hispanics and Asian/Pacific Islanders. The purpose of Model 1a is to investigate the hypothesis that the relatively low mortality of Asian/Pacific Islanders and Hispanics reflects the fact that many of these individuals are recent migrants to the United States. Previous studies have noted the unusually low mortality of Hispanic, Asian, and other foreign-born adults in the United States (e.g., Elo and Preston, 1996; Kestenbaum, 1986; Rosenwaike, 1987). In Model 2 we introduce interactions between age and race/ethnicity; only interactions significant at least at the 10 percent level are included. Model 3 repeats the same analysis as Model 1 with controls for education, income, marital status, and current residence (central city, metropolitan area outside central city, and nonmetropolitan area).

Table 2-4 and Figures 2-3 and 2-4 present the age-specific death rates by 5-

TABLE 2-4   Predicted Death Rates: Whites, African Americans, Asian/Pacific Islanders, and Hispanics, National Longitudinal Mortality Survey, 1979-1985

Age Group	Death Rates (per 1,000)				Ratios		
	Whites	African Americans	Asian/ Pacific Islanders	Hispanics	African-American to White Rates	Asian/Pacific Islander to White Rates	Hispanic to White Rates
Males							
45-49	4.58	10.88	2.97	3.92	2.38	0.65	0.86
50-54	7.33	15.08	4.77	5.94	2.06	0.65	0.81
55-59	11.70	20.82	7.63	8.98	1.78	0.65	0.77
60-64	18.55	28.59	12.17	13.52	1.54	0.66	0.73
65-69	29.12	38.99	19.28	20.25	1.34	0.66	0.70
70-74	45.09	52.71	30.24	30.07	1.17	0.67	0.67
75-79	68.42	70.46	46.75	44.17	1.03	0.68	0.65
80-84	101.11	92.95	70.80	63.89	0.92	0.70	0.63
85-89	144.66	120.72	104.37	90.63	0.83	0.72	0.63
Females							
45-49	2.28	5.03	1.38	1.79	2.21	0.61	0.79
50-54	3.64	7.26	2.21	2.86	1.99	0.61	0.79
55-59	5.80	10.45	3.53	4.56	1.80	0.61	0.79
60-64	9.20	14.99	5.63	7.25	1.63	0.61	0.79
65-69	14.54	21.41	8.93	11.49	1.47	0.61	0.79
70-74	22.80	30.37	14.12	18.10	1.33	0.62	0.79
75-79	35.36	42.71	22.16	28.24	1.21	0.63	0.80
80-84	53.96	59.35	34.39	43.49	1.10	0.64	0.81
85-89	80.56	81.28	52.54	65.71	1.01	0.65	0.82

SOURCE: Calculations by the authors from the National Longitudinal Mortality Survey public use file, based on coefficients presented in Tables 2-2 and 2-3, Model 2.

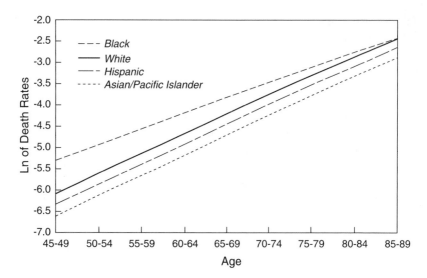

FIGURE 2-3 Death rates, white, African-American, Asian/Pacific Islander, and Hispanic females, ages 45 to 69, 1979-1985. SOURCE: Based on data from the National Longitudinal Mortality Survey.

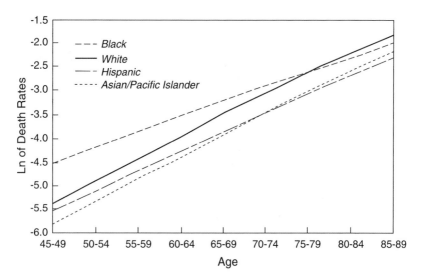

FIGURE 2-4 Death rates, white, African-American, Asian/Pacific Islander, and Hispanic males, ages 45 to 89, 1979-1985. SOURCE: Based on data from the National Longitudinal Mortality Survey.

year age groups up to age 85 to 89 that are predicted from the coefficients shown in Tables 2-2 and 2-3, Model 2.[14] Because the NLMS excluded persons who were in institutions at the beginning of the follow-up period, death rates based on the NLMS are below the national level recorded in vital statistics, particularly at older ages. The predicted death rates for white and African-American males and females at the youngest age interval shown in Table 2-4 (45 to 49) are similar to the rates based on U.S. life tables in 1983 (near the midpoint of the follow-up period), but they begin to diverge thereafter, with the largest differences recorded at the oldest ages (cf. NCHS, 1986).

African Americans

As shown in Tables 2-2 and 2-3, African Americans have higher mortality than whites, Asian/Pacific Islanders, or Hispanics. The coefficients for African Americans in Model 1 for both sexes in NLMS are large and highly significant. As age advances, however, the racial gap in white and black death rates begins to narrow as is indicated by the significant and negative interaction terms between age and being African American (Tables 2-2 and 2-3, Model 2). This convergence is clearly evident in Table 2-4 and Figures 2-3 and 2-4, which present the predicted death rates by 5-year age groups. At ages 45 to 49 and 50 to 54, African-American death rates are twice as high as white rates, but the differentials narrow substantially thereafter, as was the case with similar comparisons presented in Table 2-1. For males, the predicted death rates cross over in the age interval 80 to 84; for females the rates have become nearly identical by age 85 to 89, the last age interval shown. In the 1983 U.S. life tables, the black-white mortality crossover for both males and females occurred in the age interval 85 and older, the final, open-ended, age interval shown (NCHS, 1986).

Hispanics

The results from the NLMS also place mortality of older Hispanic Americans below that of non-Hispanic whites. The ratios of Hispanic to white rates in Table 2-4 are not very different from those derived from dual data sources in Table 2-1. The ratios are actually somewhat lower for males in Table 2-4. Female ratios, on average, are slightly higher in Table 2-4 than in Table 2-1. Consistently with many earlier studies, Sorlie et al. (1993), also based on the NLMS, have further demonstrated lower mortality at ages 45 and above for all

---

[14]The coefficients were translated into age-specific death rates as follows: $[\ln(e^k + 1)]/5 = \mu$ (x to $x+n$); where k represents the sum of the appropriate coefficients from Model 2 in Tables 2-2 and 2-3. For example, the death rate among white males in the age interval 45-49 is obtained as follows: $[\ln(e^{(-8.0209 + 44.5*0.0956)} +1]/5 = 0.00458$. The calculations shown in Table 2-4 use more precision than the coefficients shown in Tables 2-2 and 2-3.

Hispanic subgroups (Mexican, Puerto Rican, Cuban, and other Hispanic) relative to non-Hispanics.

An examination of Model 1a suggests that much of the Hispanic advantage is due to exceptionally low mortality among Hispanics born outside the United States (Tables 2-2 and 2-3). The results from the NLMS in fact suggest that the mortality of U.S.-born Hispanics is not significantly different from that of non-Hispanic whites for either males or females. The mortality of those for whom a birthplace was not reported appears closer to that of the foreign born. The low mortality of the foreign born is often interpreted as reflecting the positive selection of migrants on such attributes as healthiness. But it is also possible that the advantage of nonnatives reflects in part the difficulties of following them up in the U.S. death records, since it is likely that some may have died abroad. It is also, of course, possible that the linkage of the CPS cohorts to the NDI was more successful for native- than for foreign-born Hispanics, an outcome that would lead to an underestimate of mortality among the foreign born. We have no way of knowing whether this was in fact the case.

We should also exercise some caution in drawing firm conclusions from the above results because of the relatively small number of deaths in the NLMS, which also prevents us from conducting more detailed analyses of mortality by cause of death that could shed further light on the observed patterns. Nevertheless, the above results underscore the importance of distinguishing between the native born and the foreign born in studies of health and mortality among the U.S. Hispanic population. There is clearly a need for further studies in this area. Data collection efforts that provide large enough sample sizes and that institute stringent follow-up procedures are needed if we hope to obtain accurate estimates of mortality for the Hispanic population in the United States.

Asian Americans and Pacific Islanders

The results based on the NLMS also confirm the low mortality of Asian Americans and Pacific Islanders relative to whites and other racial and ethnic groups. The relative advantage appears somewhat greater for females than for males (Tables 2-2 and 2-3). As was the case with Hispanics, results from Model 1a suggest that a portion of the lower mortality of Asian/Pacific Islanders is attributable to the low mortality among the foreign born. The findings for the native-born Asian Americans and Pacific Islanders further imply that their mortality is also lower than that of non-Hispanic whites, although the small number of deaths makes the results unstable and reaches significance only for males.

The results from the NLMS indicate that mortality estimates based on vital statistics and census data seem to exaggerate the relative mortality advantages of Asian/Pacific Islander males and females in comparison with white Americans. Ratios of Asian/Pacific Islander death rates to those of whites range from 0.52 to 0.69 for males in Table 2-1, compared with a range of 0.65 to 0.72 in Table 2-4.

The respective numbers for females are 0.54 to 0.70 and 0.61 to 0.65. This exaggeration is most likely the result of underestimation of mortality for this ethnic group based on data obtained from dual sources. As noted above, the consistency of race reporting for this subpopulation in death statistics and census records is low, much lower than for other racial and ethnic groups. Even so, the NLMS results continue to suggest that Asian/Pacific Islanders in the United States have extremely low mortality in comparison with whites and African Americans.

Subnational Studies

A number of studies have used data from small-scale, subnational data collection efforts, in addition to national data, to examine black-white mortality differentials at older ages. Wing et al. (1985), for example, analyzed data collected in the community-based Evans County (Georgia) Study to examine the black-white mortality crossover. These data, together with data from the Charleston Heart Study (Charleston County, South Carolina), were reanalyzed by Manton et al. (1991). The Evans County data consist of a 20-year follow-up of 3,102 persons aged 15 to 75 in 1960-1962, and the Charleston Heart Study data are based on a 25-year follow-up of 2,181 individuals aged 35 to 97 in 1960-1961. In both studies, the age of the participants was obtained by a personal interview at the start of the study.

Manton et al. (1991) examined the age pattern of black and white mortality and tested the sensitivity of the mortality crossover to different specifications of the hazard function and the use of different ages at the start of the follow-up. The age at the start of the follow-up had little effect on the results, and the same was true for the hazard functions specified. The authors found strong evidence for a racial crossover in mortality for females (at age 92). The results for males were more ambiguous. According to the authors (1991:1057):

> The relatively small differences in black/white male mortality rates in middle age caused the crossover to be less significant for males. . . . Nonetheless, the difference is in the hypothesized direction and the hazard function yields a crossover at an age [80-84] consistent with other studies. This, coupled with the strong evidence for a crossover in female mortality, indicates that the crossover is a real phenomenon.

The convergence of black and white death rates at older ages has also been documented in the Alameda County (California) study by Kaplan et al. (1987). The authors examined the association between behavioral and demographic risk factors during a 17-year follow-up among subjects who were at least 38 years of age at the baseline interview in 1965. Age-stratified proportional hazard analyses were conducted to compare risk factor associations and mortality at ages 60 to 69 and 70 and older with two younger age groups (38 to 49 and 50 to 59). As noted above, a convergence of black and white death rates at older ages was observed; at ages 70 and older, black mortality was insignificantly lower than white mortality; the relative hazard for blacks relative to whites was 0.76 with a 95 percent confidence interval of 0.52 to 1.12, when other risk factors were controlled for (Kaplan et al., 1987:Table 4).

The results from all studies discussed thus far, whether based on vital statistics and census data or on a single source, show a similar age pattern of differentials between white and black mortality. African-American death rates exceed white rates at younger ages, with the two rates slowly converging as age advances until, at the oldest ages, African-American death rates fall below those of whites. We have suggested that inconsistencies in age reporting in vital statistics and census data could account for this pattern when dual data sources are used for mortality estimates. But even when a single data source is used, a racial crossover is observed. It is possible that differences between African Americans and whites in the accuracy of age reporting at the baseline could lead to the observed mortality patterns. If, for example, net overstatement of age is more common among African Americans than whites, this could produce a racial crossover in death rates at older ages because the reported black death rates at a given age would actually pertain to what is, on average, a younger age group. None of the studies has made an attempt to verify the accuracy of baseline age reporting or of differences in the accuracy of age reporting by race. Even estimates based on Social Security and Medicare data are affected by a lack of stringent age verification procedures for the oldest old at the time when they applied for Social Security benefits. Studies that have examined age reporting patterns among whites and African Americans suggest that age reporting appears more accurate for whites than blacks. We address the implications of age misreporting bias for the observed racial crossover in mortality in the next section.

EXTINCT GENERATION ESTIMATES

An alternative method of estimating mortality at older ages is to track deaths by age in a birth cohort until the last member of the cohort has died. One can then reconstitute the size of the cohort and death rates at all previous ages. The extinct generation method is the principal procedure being used in a major international analysis of mortality trends at older ages (Kannisto, 1994).

Elo and Preston (1994) have used the extinct generation method to reconstruct African-American mortality back to 1930 for cohorts born before 1890. When reassembled into age-specific death rates for various periods of time, the extinct generation estimates show lower death rates above age 80 or 90 than do conventional vital statistics/census methods in 1930, 1940, and 1970, the only years investigated. Many of the extinct generation death rate series do not increase with age. The authors argue that net overstatement of age on death certificates is the likely source of these anomalies.

To investigate the effect of age misstatement on African-American mortality at older ages, the authors have matched a sample of 5,262 death certificates of African Americans dying at ages 60 and above in 1985 or 1980 to records from U.S. censuses of 1900, 1910, and 1920 and to records of the SSA: 56.8 percent of the death certificates were matched to an early census and 88.1 percent to Social Security records; for 50.5 percent of death certificates, a three-way match was attained (Preston et al., 1996).

This study shows that ages on death certificates are subject to serious error. In only about 70 percent of death certificates did the age at death agree with that available from *either* of the other two sources. With respect to both alternative sources, the pattern of age misstatement on death certificates was one of net understatement. Nevertheless, too many deaths are registered at ages 95 and above as well as at ages 60 to 69.

In order to convert the corrected distribution of age at death into age-specific death rates, the authors used a variant of the extinct generation method. In particular, they used an intercensal growth correction to transform the age distribution of deaths in 1985 into what the distribution would be in a cohort subject to 1985 death rates for the rest of its life. The resulting life table death rates are presented in Table 2-5. Corrected death rates are somewhat higher than uncorrected death rates at 85 to 89 and much higher than uncorrected rates at ages over 90. The racial crossover in mortality when compared to the uncorrected white death rates for 1985 has disappeared.

TABLE 2-5   Estimated Age-Specific Death Rates by Race: United States, 1985 (Death Rates per 1,000)

	Females			Males		
	African Americans			African Americans		
Age Group	Death Certificate Age[b]	Final Age[c]	Whites[a]	Death Certificate Age[b]	Final Age[c]	Whites[a]
65-69	26.3	22.7	16.1	46.0	44.0	30.3
70-74	38.7	35.4	25.2	65.0	62.4	47.5
75-79	54.9	52.9	40.1	87.6	91.1	71.5
80-84	83.8	70.2	67.8	123.4	114.4	109.2
85-89	118.5	128.9	115.1	160.5	168.8	162.5
90-94	153.4	198.7	188.6	199.2	272.3	238.2
95+	214.3	290.8	271.2	232.8	323.2	317.7

[a]White rates are based on registered deaths in 1985 and the Census Bureau's estimates of population on July 1, 1985.

[b]Death rates based on age as reported on the death certificate.

[c]Death rates based on deaths corrected for age misstatement. The final, open-ended, age group for males and females is 95+.

SOURCE: Preston et al., 1996.

The Preston et al. (1996) study is the most painstaking attempt to establish corrected ages at death for older African Americans, and it is the only study that fails to reveal a crossover between white and black death rates. These two features are likely to be related to one another. Nevertheless, the results are based on a relatively small number of linked cases and an unconventional methodology. If the authors are correct, their conclusions should be validated within the next 10 to 15 years through Social Security data for cohorts whose ages have been subject to improved verification.

CAUSES OF DEATH

The major causes of death for people aged 45 and above are diseases of the heart, malignant neoplasms, and cerebrovascular disease. It would be surprising if racial and ethnic differences in death rates from all causes combined were not principally attributable to differences in death rates from these causes. Table 2-6 presents age-standardized death rates at ages 45 and older from these causes in 1989-1991 for the major racial and ethnic groups that we are dealing with. The rates use preliminary death rates supplied by NCHS and census-based population estimates; they are calculated by the U.S. Department of Health and Human Services (NCHS, 1994). As noted earlier, differences in racial and ethnic classification systems between deaths and population estimates have probably biased downward death rates for Hispanics (perhaps by 7% or so) and Asian/Pacific Islanders (12%).

For every comparison of all-cause death rates between whites and another group that can be made in Table 2-6, the three identified causes account for a majority of the all-cause discrepancy. Nearly always, they operate in concert. Hispanics and Asian/Pacific Islanders have lower age-standardized death rates than whites from all causes and from each of the three causes (although differences for cerebrovascular disease are minor and in one case negligible); blacks have higher mortality than whites from all three causes.

In addition to the excess mortality of blacks from the three causes shown in Table 2-6, mortality from diabetes is an important source of black-white mortality differentials at ages 45 and older. Death rates from diabetes are two to three times higher for blacks than for whites at these ages, although the racial differentials narrow at older ages (Manton et al., 1987; NCHS, 1993). Diabetes is also an important factor contributing to the excess mortality from heart disease and stroke among African Americans. Relative to whites, African Americans have been shown to have a twofold excess risk of diabetes at ages 45 and above, with females having higher prevalence than males. Data on multiple-cause mortality, an important source of information for describing mortality at older ages, further show that diabetes is frequently identified as a contributing cause of death at older ages (Manton et al., 1987).

TABLE 2-6   Age-Standardized Death Rates at Ages 45 and Older by Race/
Ethnicity for Certain Major Causes of Death: United States, 1989-1991 (Deaths
per 100,000)

Cause of Death	Whites	Blacks	Asian/Pacific Islanders	Hispanics
Males				
All causes	2,030	3,039	1,158	1,484
Diseases of the heart	726	969	373	485
Cerebrovascular diseases	99	194	99	84
Malignant neoplasms	565	870	335	352
Females				
All causes	1,223	1,776	714	892
Diseases of the heart	376	597	205	271
Cerebrovascular diseases	84	148	81	63
Malignant neoplasms	380	457	215	238

SOURCE: Compiled from NCHS, 1994: Tables 32-35.

The excess mortality of African Americans from heart disease and stroke also reflects differences in the distribution of other risk factors between blacks and whites. The increased prevalence and severity of hypertension among blacks than whites are well established and are considered important factors contributing to their poorer health outcomes (e.g., Johnson et al., 1986; Manton et al., 1987; Svetkey et al., 1993; NCHS, 1994:Table 78). A much higher prevalence of obesity among black women than other race/sex groups also places them at an increased risk of mortality (NCHS, 1994:Table 80).

The higher prevalence of cigarette smoking among black than among white males has also contributed to the higher African-American male mortality from heart disease, stroke, and lung cancer. The male differentials in lung cancer mortality are similar to those for all cancers combined, shown in Table 2-6. In contrast, age-adjusted death rates from lung cancer at ages 45 and older were higher for white than for African-American women in 1989 (NCHS, 1993). These distinct patterns undoubtedly reflect past cohort differentials in smoking habits.

The black disadvantage in cancer mortality and morbidity is also evident when we examine cancer incidence and survival. For many of the most important cancers, age-adjusted cancer incidence rates in 1991 were higher for black than for white males, including cancers of the oral cavity and pharynx, esophagus, stomach, colon, pancreas, lung, and prostate. For females, incidence rates were also higher for cancers of the colon, pancreas, lung and bronchus, and cervix uteri (NCHS, 1994:Table 67). In contrast, the age-adjusted incidence rate for breast cancer was lower for black than for white women. Five-year relative cancer survival rates are also generally lower for blacks than for whites. In the period 1983-1990, for example, the 5-year relative survival rates from cancers of all sites was 35.7 percent for black males versus 50.8 percent for white males; the respective rates for females were 45.5 percent and 59.8 percent. Of the specific cancer sites for which data were shown—11 for males and 10 for females— survival rates were lower for blacks than for whites in all but two cases for males and one for females (NCHS, 1994:Table 68).[15]

Some of the poorer cancer survival rates among blacks seem to be attributable to differences in the stage of the disease at the time of the diagnosis (Brawn et al., 1993; Eley et al., 1994). A study (Ragland et al., 1991) that examined stage-specific survival rates for cancers for which mortality is considered avoidable by early diagnosis (colon, rectum, bladder, breast, cervix, uterine corpus, and prostate), for example, found no significant stage-specific differentials in survival by race for colon, male rectal, and prostate cancer. Stage-specific survival differences did, however, persist for male bladder, female rectal, and breast cancer. It has been suggested that racial differentials in survival from breast cancer may be linked to nutritional status and lower levels of serum albumin and hemoglobin (Coates et al., 1990).

Stroke mortality has declined rapidly in recent years, a decline that has been attributed to favorable trends in risk factors (Higgins and Thom, 1993). Black-white differentials in stroke mortality, however, remain substantial (Table 2-6). Among factors contributing to cerebrovascular mortality on which blacks are adversely distributed are socioeconomic status, prevalence of hypertension and diabetes, and prevalence of cigarette smoking among males.

The extent to which well-established risk factors (smoking, systolic blood pressure, total serum cholesterol level, body mass index, alcohol intake, and diabetes) account for black-white mortality differentials was recently investigated by Otten et al. (1990) in a national sample of adults based on data drawn from the National Health and Nutrition Survey Epidemiological Follow-up Study (1971-1984). At ages 35-77, major cardiovascular diseases accounted for 56.1 percent of the racial differences in mortality (both sexes combined), with cerebrovascular diseases alone accounting for 28.0 percent. Cancer accounted for an additional 18 percent (Otten et al., 1990:Table 2). In an analysis of all-cause mortality, the above six risk factors accounted for 31 percent of the excess mortality of African Americans at ages 35 to 54 and all of the much smaller black excess at ages 55 to 77.

Using a more detailed list of causes of death than shown in Table 2-6 for Hispanics, Markides and Coreil (1986) identify a "Mexican-American" pattern of mortality, which has extended to the Hispanic population as a whole in more recent years (Sorlie et al., 1993). The pattern includes unusually high death rates

---

[15]Data on cancer incidence and survival rates come from the Surveillance, Epidemiology, and End Results Program of the National Cancer Institute and are based on 11 population-based registries throughout the United States and Puerto Rico. These data are not limited to ages 45 and above (NCHS, 1994:270).

from diabetes, cirrhosis of the liver, and homicide and unusually low death rates from cardiovascular diseases and cancer. Sorlie et al. (1993) show that Hispanic death rates are low for cancer at all major sites, including the lung. As noted earlier, Rosenwaike (1987) examines 1979-1981 age-adjusted death rates by cause for persons born in Cuba, Mexico, and Puerto Rico. Mexicans and Puerto Ricans have much higher death rates than whites from diabetes, cirrhosis, and homicide; Cubans show a significant excess mortality only for homicide.

CONCLUSIONS

In this paper, we examine recent evidence on racial and ethnic differences in mortality in the United States at ages 45 and above. The four racial and ethnic groups included are African Americans, Hispanics, Asians and Pacific Islanders, and whites. We review evidence based on various types of data sources, including vital statistics and census data, linked data files, and extinct generation methods. The data for estimating adult and old age mortality in the United States appear most reliable for whites. Various sources of data error, including age misreporting, inconsistencies in the coding of race and ethnicity, and difficulties of following the foreign born in vital statistics data, create uncertainties in mortality estimates for other racial and ethnic groups.

A comparison of mortality estimates among whites and African Americans shows a convergence in white and black death rates at oldest ages. At younger ages, age-specific death rates for African Americans exceed white rates by as much as two to one, with a gradual narrowing of the differentials as age advances, until at the oldest ages, African-American death rates fall below those of whites. This pattern of differentials has been documented in vital statistics and census data, linked data files, and Social Security/Medicare data. Substantial evidence exists, however, to support the view that age misreporting has biased mortality estimates at older ages for African Americans. Age reporting inconsistencies in vital statistics and census data and age misreporting in death statistics, both of which are more pronounced for African Americans than whites, seriously bias comparisons of age-specific death rates based on dual data sources and on extinct generation estimates. Differences in age reporting accuracy at the baseline interview in linked data files could also produce the observed mortality patterns. None of the studies based on linked data sets have attempted to verify the accuracy of age reporting at the baseline interview. At the oldest ages, age reporting in Social Security/Medicare data also has not been strictly verified.

The only study that has systematically investigated the effects of age misreporting on mortality estimates among African Americans has demonstrated that age-specific death rates for African Americans at the oldest ages are biased downward. Mortality estimates based on corrected age distribution of deaths are substantially higher than estimates based on uncorrected data at ages 85 and above. When compared to mortality estimates for whites at these ages, no evidence for a racial crossover in mortality is found. Uncertainty about white rates at ages 95+, however, prevents firm conclusions about racial differences in mortality at the highest ages. This is the only study reviewed here which does not show a racial crossover in mortality. It is also the only one that has attempted to establish corrected ages at death for African Americans.

Mortality estimates for Hispanics and for Asian/Pacific Islanders place their mortality below that of white Americans. The proportionate gap between Hispanics and whites increases with age, while the Asian/Pacific Islander advantage is larger at younger than at older ages. In both cases, a portion of the lower mortality is attributable to the low mortality among the foreign born, particularly among Hispanics. It is often assumed that the low mortality of the foreign born is related to the healthy migrant effect, but it is also possible that deaths of the foreign born are missed in U.S. death records because some of these individuals may have died abroad. Inconsistencies in the reporting of race in vital statistics and census data also bias mortality estimates downward for both Hispanics and Asian/Pacific Islanders. Age misreporting at older ages introduces an additional source of bias in estimates of mortality among Hispanics, although this bias appears to be less severe than for African Americans. Nevertheless, mortality estimates based on linked data sources suggest that mortality among both Hispanics and Asian/Pacific Islanders is below that of white Americans.

REFERENCES

Aziz, F., and W. Buckler
    1992   The status of death information in Social Security Administration files. Pp. 262-267 in
            Proceedings of the Social Statistics Section, American Statistical Association. Washington, DC: American Statistical Association.
Barringer, H.R., R.W. Gardner, and M.J. Levin
    1993   *Asian and Pacific Islanders in the United States.* The Population in the United States in
            the 1980s. Census Monograph Series. New York: Russell Sage Foundation.
Boyle, C.A., and P. Decouflé
    1990   National sources of vital status information: Extent of coverage and possible selectivity in
            reporting. *American Journal of Epidemiology* 131(1):160-168.
Bradshaw, B.S., and K.A. Liese
    1991   Mortality of Mexican-origin persons in the southwestern United States. Pp. 81-94 in
            Mortality of Hispanic Populations, Ira Rosenwaike, ed. New York: Greenwood Press.
Brawn, P.N., E.H. Johnson, D.L. Kuhl, M.W. Riggs, V.O. Speights, C.F. Johnson, P.P. Pandya, M.L.
        Lind, and N.F. Bell
    1993   Stage at presentation and survival of white and black patients with prostate carcinoma.
            Cancer 71(8):2569-2573.
Bureau of the Census
    1983   *Census of Population: 1980. General Population Characteristics. United States Summary.* Final report PC80-1-B1. Washington, DC: U.S. Department of Commerce.
    1992a   *1990 Census of Population: General Population Characteristics, Massachusetts.* Washington, DC: U.S. Department of Commerce.
    1992b   *1990 Census of Population: General Population Characteristics, Texas.* Washington, DC: U.S. Department of Commerce.

1992c   *1990 Census of Population: General Population Characteristics, United States.* Washington, DC: U.S. Department of Commerce.

Coale, A.J., and J. Bannister
1994   Five decades of missing females in China. *Demography* 3(3):459-479.

Coale, A.J., and E.E. Kisker
1986   Mortality crossover: Reality or bad data? *Population Studies* 40:389-401.
1990   Defects in data on old-age mortality in the United States: New procedures for calculating mortality schedules and life tables at the highest ages. *Asian and Pacific Population Forum* 4(1):1-31.

Coates, R.J., W.S. Clark, J.W. Eley, R.S. Greenberg, C.M. Huguley Jr., and R.L. Brown
1990   Race, nutritional status, and survival from breast cancer. *Journal of the National Cancer Institute* 82(21):1684-1692.

Curb, J.D., C.E. Ford, S. Pressel, M. Palmer, C. Babcock, and C.M. Hawkins
1985   Ascertainment of vital status through the National Death Index and the Social Security Administration. *American Journal of Epidemiology* 121(5):754-766.

Day, J.C.
1993   *Population Projections of the United States, by Age, Sex, Race, and Hispanic Origin: 1993 to 2050.* Current Population Reports, Bureau of the Census, Series P-25, No. 1104. Washington, DC: U.S. Department of Commerce.

Dechter, A., and S.H. Preston
1991   Age misreporting and its effects on adult mortality estimates in Latin America. *Population Bulletin of the United Nations* 31/32:1-17.

Deutch, J.
1973   Proof of age policies—Past, present, and future. Unpublished internal memorandum by the Evaluation and Measurement System Staff, to the Assistant Bureau Director, Program Policy. U.S. Department of Health, Education, and Welfare. Washington, DC.

Eley, J.W., H.A. Hill, V.W. Chen, D.F. Austin, M.N. Wesley, H.B. Muss, R.S. Greenberg, R.J. Coates, P. Correa, C.K. Redmond, C.P. Hunter, A.A. Herman, R. Kurman, R. Blacklow, S. Shapiro, B.K. Edwards
1994   Racial differences in survival from breast cancer: Results of the National Cancer Institute black/white cancer survival study. *Journal of the American Medical Association* 272(12):947-954.

Elo, I.T., and S.H. Preston
1992   Effects of early-life conditions on adult mortality: A review. *Population Index* 58(2):186-212.
1994   Estimating African-American mortality from inaccurate data. *Demography* 31(3):427-458.
1996   Educational differentials in mortality: United States, 1979-85. *Social Science and Medicine* 42(1):47-57.

Elo, I.T., S.H. Preston, I. Rosenwaike, M. Hill, and T.P. Cheney
1996   Consistency of age reporting on death certificates and Social Security records among elderly African Americans. *Social Science Research* 25:292-307.

Frisbie, W.P.
1991   Mortality Among Mexican Americans and Mexican Immigrants. Final report to the National Institute of Child Health and Human Development. Austin: Department of Sociology, University of Texas. Unpublished.

Frost, F., and K.K. Shy
1980   Racial differences between linked birth and infant death records in Washington state. *American Journal of Public Health* 79:974-976.

Hahn, R.A., J. Mulinare, and S.M. Teutsch
1992   Inconsistencies in coding of race and ethnicity between birth and death in U.S. infants. *Journal of the American Medical Association* 267(2):259-263.

Higgins, M., and T. Thom
    1993   Trends in stroke risk factors in the United States. *Annals of Epidemiology* 3(5):550-554.
Himes, C.L., S.H. Preston, and G.A. Condran
    1994   A relational model of mortality at older ages in low mortality countries. *Population Studies* 48(2):269-291.
Hollman, F.
    1993   *U.S. Population Estimates by Age, Sex, Race, and Hispanic Origin: 1980 to 1991.* Current Population Reports, Series P-25, No. 1095. Bureau of the Census. Washington, DC: U.S. Department of Commerce.
Jackson, J.J.
    1980   *Minorities and Aging.* Belmont, CA: Wadsworth.
Johnson, J.L., E.F. Heineman, G. Heiss, C.G. Hames, and H.A. Tyroler
    1986   Cardiovascular disease risk factors and mortality among black women and white women aged 40-64 years in Evans County, Georgia. *American Journal of Epidemiology* 123(2):209-220.
Kannisto, V.
    1994   *Development of Oldest Old Mortality, 1950-1990.* Odense, Denmark: Odense University Press.
Kaplan, G.A., T.E. Seeman, R.D. Cohen, L.P. Knudsen, and J. Guralnik
    1987   Mortality among the elderly in the Alameda County study: Behavioral and demographic risk factors. *American Journal of Public Health* 77(3):307-312.
Kestenbaum, B.
    1986   Mortality by nativity. *Demography* 23(1):87-90.
    1992   A description of the extreme aged population based on improved Medicare enrollment data. *Demography* 29:565-580.
Kitagawa, E.M., and P.M. Hauser
    1973   *Differential Mortality in the United States: A Study of Socioeconomic Epidemiology.* Cambridge, MA: Harvard University Press.
Manton, K.G., C.H. Patrick, and K.W. Johnson
    1987   Health differentials between blacks and whites: Recent trends in mortality and morbidity. *Milbank Quarterly* 65 (Suppl. 1):129-199.
Manton, K.G., and E. Stallard
    1981   Methods for evaluating heterogeneity of aging processes in human populations using vital statistics data: Explaining the black/white mortality crossover by a model of mortality selection. *Human Biology* 53:47-67.
Manton, K.G., E. Stallard, and J.W. Vaupel
    1981   Methods for comparing the mortality experience of heterogeneous populations. *Demography* 18:389-410.
Manton, K.G., E. Stallard, and S. Wing
    1991   Analyses of black and white differentials in the age trajectory of mortality in two closed cohort studies. *Statistics in Medicine* 10:1043-1059.
Markides, K.S., and J. Coreil
    1986   The health of Hispanics in the southwestern United States: An epidemiologic paradox. *Public Health Reports* 101:253-265.
Markides, K.S., and C.H. Mindel
    1987   *Aging and Ethnicity.* Newbury Park, CA: Sage Publications.
Mosley, W.H., and R. Gray
    1993   Childhood precursors of adult morbidity and mortality in developing countries: Implications for health programs. Pp. 69-100 in *The Epidemiological Transition: Policy and Planning Implications for Developing Countries*, James Gribble and Samuel H. Preston, eds. Washington, DC: National Academy Press.

National Center for Health Statistics

1968   Comparability of age on the death certificate and matching census record, United States, May-August 1960. *Vital and Health Statistics* 2(29).

1969   Comparability of marital status, race, nativity, and country of origin on the death certificate and matching census record, United States, May-August 1960. *Vital and Health Statistics* 2(34).

1985   *Vital Statistics of the United States, 1982. Life Tables.* Volume II, Section 6. Hyattsville, MD: Public Health Service.

1986   *Vital Statistics of the United States, 1983. Life Tables.* Volume II, Section 6. Hyattsville, MD: Public Health Service.

1990   Deaths of Hispanic origin, 15 reporting states, 1979-81. *Vital and Health Statistics* 20(18).

1993   *Vital Statistics of the United States 1989.* Volume II, Mortality, Part A. Hyattsville, MD: Public Health Service.

1994   *Health, United States, 1993.* Hyattsville, MD: Public Health Service.

National Institutes of Health

1992   National Longitudinal Mortality Study. Public use file documentation. Bethesda, MD: National Institutes of Health.

Otten, M.W., S.M. Teutsch, D.F. Williamson, and J.S. Marks

1990   The effect of known risk factors on the excess mortality of black adults in the United States. *Journal of the American Medical Association* 263:845-850.

Perks, W.

1932   On some experiments in the graduation of mortality statistics. *Journal of the Institute of Actuaries* 63:12.

Preston, S.H., and I.T. Elo

1995   Are educational differentials in adult mortality increasing in the United States? *Journal of Aging and Health* 7(4):476-496.

Preston, S.H., I.T. Elo, I. Rosenwaike, and M. Hill

1996   African-American mortality at older ages: Results from a matching study. *Demography* 33(2):193-209.

Ragland, K.E., S. Selvin, and D.W. Merrill

1991   Black-white differences in stage-specific cancer survival: Analysis of seven selected sites. *American Journal of Epidemiology* 133(7):672-682.

Robinson, J.G., and Y.J. Gist

1992   The effect of alternative race classification rules on the annual number of births by race: 1968-1989. Presented at the annual meeting of the Population Association of America, Denver, CO.

Rogot, E., P. Sorlie, and N.J. Johnson

1986   Probabilistic methods in matching census samples to the National Death Index. *Journal of Chronic Diseases* 39(9):719-734.

Rogot, E., P.D. Sorlie, N.J. Johnson, and C. Schmitt

1992   *Mortality Study of 1.3 Million Persons by Demographic, Social, and Economic Factors: 1979-1985 Follow-up.* NIH publication 92-3297. Bethesda, MD: National Institutes of Health.

Rosenwaike, I.

1987   Mortality differentials among persons born in Cuba, Mexico, and Puerto Rico residing in the United States, 1979-81. *American Journal of Public Health* 77(5):603-606.

Rosenwaike, I., and B. Bradshaw

1988   The status of death certificates for Hispanic population of the Southwest. *Social Science Quarterly* 69:722-736.

1989   Mortality of the Spanish surname population of the Southwest: 1980. *Social Science Quarterly* 70:631-641.

Rosenwaike, I., and S.H. Preston
    1984   Age overstatement and Puerto Rican longevity. *Human Biology* 56(3):503-525.
Shapiro, S.
    1950   Development of birth registration and birth statistics in the United States. *Population Studies* 4:86-111.
Shrestha, L., and S.H. Preston
    1995   Consistency of census and vital registration data on older Americans: 1970-1990. *Survey Methodology 21(2):167-177.*
Shryock, H.S., and J.S. Siegel
    1973   *The Methods and Materials of Demography.* Rev. ed. Volume 2. Washington, DC: Bureau of the Census.
Social Security Administration
    1988   *Social Security Handbook: 1988.* 10th ed. Baltimore, MD: Social Security Administration.
Sorlie, P.D., E. Backlund, N.J. Johnson, and E. Rogot
    1993   Mortality by Hispanic status in the United States. *Journal of the American Medical Association* 270(20):2464-2468.
Sorlie, P.D., E. Rogot, and N.J. Johnson
    1992   Validity of demographic characteristics on the death certificate. *Epidemiology* 3(2):181-184.
Spencer, G.
    1986   *Projections of the Hispanic Population: 1983 to 2080.* Current Population Reports, Series P-25, No. 995. Bureau of the Census. Washington, DC: U.S. Department of Commerce.
Svetkey, L.P., L.K. George, B.M. Burchett, P.A. Morgan, and D.G. Blazer
    1993   Black/white differences in hypertension in the elderly: An epidemiologic analysis in central North Carolina. *American Journal of Epidemiology* 137(1):64-73.
U.S. Department of Health and Human Services
    1985   *Report of the Secretary's Task Force on Black and Minority Health.* Volume II: Crosscutting Issues in Minority Health. Washington, DC: U.S. Department of Health and Human Services.
Wang, X., D.M. Strobino, and B. Guyer
    1992   Differences in cause-specific infant mortality among Chinese, Japanese and White Americans. *American Journal of Epidemiology* 135(12):1382-1393.
Wing, S., K.G. Manton, E. Stallard, C.G. Hames, and H.A. Tryoler
    1985   The black/white mortality crossover: Investigation in a community-based study. *Journal of Gerontology* 40(1):78-84.
Yu, E.
    1984   The low mortality rates of Chinese infants: Some plausible explanatory factors. *Social Science and Medicine* 16:253-262.
Yu, E.S., C-F. Chang, W.T. Liu, and S.H. Kan
    1985   Asian-white mortality differences: Are there excess deaths? Pp. 209-251 in *Report of the Secretary's Task Force on Black and Minority Health.* Volume II: Crosscutting Issues in Minority Health. Washington, DC: U.S. Department of Health and Human Services.
Zelnik, M.
    1969   Age patterns of mortality of American Negroes 1900-02 to 1959-61. *Journal of the American Statistical Association* 64(326):433-451.
Zopf, P.E., Jr.
    1992   *Mortality Patterns and Trends in the United States.* Studies in Population and Urban Demography, no. 7. Westport, CT: Greenwood Press.

3

Health and Disability Differences Among Racial and Ethnic Groups

Kenneth G. Manton and Eric Stallard

INTRODUCTION

Racial and ethnic differences in the age patterns of incidence and prevalence of chronic morbidity and disability are important because they provide data on (1) biological mechanisms, endogenous and exogenous, of age-related morbidity, (2) how the quality of life for groups changes over age and time, and (3) lead indicators of future mortality and disability trends that aid in the development of health policy by improving mortality, health service, and population forecasts.

We have previously examined epidemiological, demographic, and other data on racial and ethnic health differences (Manton et al., 1987). Here we examine more recent biomedical and epidemiological research on African-American, white, and Hispanic differences in health and disability. Though data on racial and ethnic health differences have improved and have generated many new hypotheses, there are many areas in which no definitive studies have been done for different racial and ethnic groups. Consequently, there is often little consensus on the magnitude or age dependence of racial and ethnic differences in health or on the biological mechanisms underlying many differences.

Since the scientific record on racial and ethnic health differences, especially at late ages, is incomplete, we must assemble available data into a coherent description to compare age-related health differences across racial and ethnic groups. For this purpose, a life-table model of the age relation of three health processes—disability, morbidity, and mortality—is useful. Figure 3-1 portrays changes in two hypothetical cohorts, one with high mortality and one with low mortality, as linked life-table functions.

High Mortality

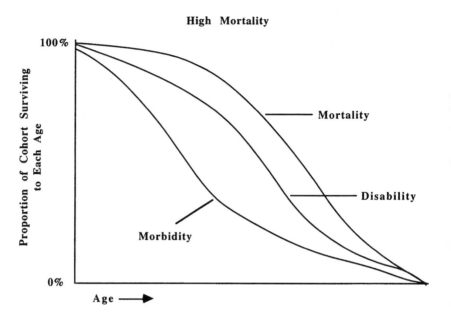

Low Mortality

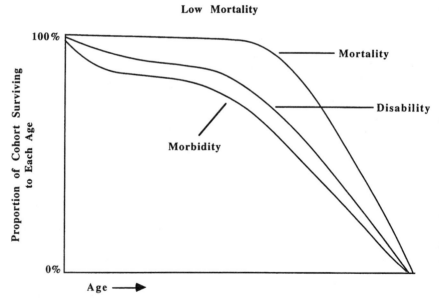

FIGURE 3-1 Interrelations of morbidity, disability, and mortality in two hypothetical populations. SOURCE: Duke University Center for Demographic Studies.

The area between curves for each cohort represents the person-years lived free of morbidity and disability, with morbidity but free of disability, or with both morbidity and disability. The high-mortality cohort reflects a population with more time spent in morbid states but less time spent with disability (e.g., in developing countries, where acute and long-term medical care for disabled elderly persons is scarce, or in socioeconomically disadvantaged groups). The low-mortality cohort spends less time in morbid states, but more time with disability.

The first scenario suggests that in populations with low life expectancy, people spend time in clinically latent morbid states and that once disability occurs, the lack of social and long-term care infrastructure causes rapid terminal declines due to a loss of physical homeostasis (e.g., Colantonio et al., 1992). It is uncertain whether this scenario holds for U.S. African Americans and Hispanics who, often socioeconomically disadvantaged over much of the life course, may have greater social resources and relatively equitable access to medical and postacute services at age 65 through Medicare—and to long-term care services through Medicaid. In populations with high life expectancy, health care may defer chronic morbidity to later ages, with disabled people able to live a long time with adequate long-term care. This scenario, however, may not occur even in economically advanced countries. In Japan, one of the world's richest economies, only 6 percent of gross national product was spent on health services in 1990 even though, because of high life expectancy and declining fertility, the population is aging. Consequently, the health services provided to the elderly are limited, with many elderly enduring stays of 6 months or more in acute care hospitals because of a lack of long-term care and rehabilitation facilities (Okamoto, 1992).

The two hypothetical models represent scenarios against which the health experience of U.S. racial and ethnic groups can be compared. Race-related physiological differences (e.g., hypertension; Cooper and Rotimi, 1994) may produce more complex scenarios than the ones shown in Figure 3-1, as may differences in access to health care.

Ideally, longitudinal data on levels and types of disability, on flows into and out of morbidity and disability states, and on age- and gender-specific effects of diseases on mortality are used to construct such models. For example, a disabling event prevalent in U.S. postmenopausal women is hip fracture. The natural history of hip fractures, like that of other events and conditions, has evolved. The mean age for hip fractures in Britain increased from 67 years in 1944 to 79 years in 1990 (Keene, 1993). This 12-year shift marked a change in hip fracture's natural history. At age 67, hip fractures often do not involve the hip socket and are due to exogenous forces. Hip fractures at later ages often involve the hip socket, are due to osteoporosis, and require more health care. Such age changes in disease presentation could affect U.S. racial and ethnic differences in disability and mortality because African-American and Hispanic females have lower risks of hip fracture than white females.

Unfortunately, longitudinal data are not equally available for the groups reviewed. Consequently, we need to assess the quality and scope of the literature on racial and ethnic differences on specific diseases and conditions and then integrate these various findings. This is a multistep process.

First, we review data on the racial and ethnic differences in the risks of specific diseases and in the rates at which the diseases progress. When possible, we make gender-specific comparisons because racial and ethnic health differences often vary in degree, and sometimes in direction, by gender. Since many studies of racial and ethnic groups were done for individual diseases, studies of racial and ethnic differences have to be reviewed for a number of areas. Thus, the first stage of the review provides insight into racial and ethnic differences in disease-specific mechanisms and their age and gender dependence.

Since most disease-specific studies are of select populations, as a second stage we review the age relation of racial and ethnic differences in health, disability, and mortality in two sets of national data. First, we examine age patterns of total and cause-specific mortality by race to determine if they are consistent with the epidemiological data on racial and ethnic differences in the age dependence of disease processes. This is logical since racial and ethnic differences in disease in large part cause racial and ethnic differences in mortality age patterns. Second, we examine the National Long Term Care Surveys, where race-specific disability and mortality trajectories can be linked.

Thus, an assemblage of data is used to identify (1) the age dependence of disease mechanisms, (2) mortality and morbidity linkages, and (3) disability and mortality linkages. These relations, from different data sets, provide information to construct models like Figure 3-1.

MAJOR MORBIDITY PROCESSES AND THEIR AGE DEPENDENCE ACROSS RACIAL AND ETHNIC GROUPS

There are few studies that describe a number of diseases in a longitudinally followed elderly population. One such study (Guccione et al., 1994), though representing only whites, provides a context in which to discuss racial and ethnic differences in disease. In the study, 2,731 people were followed for 38 years to determine which of 10 conditions caused one or more of seven disabilities in people aged 64 to 98. The proportion of disability due to each condition, adjusted for age, sex, and comorbidity, is presented in Table 3-1. Stroke and heart disease caused disability on all seven functions. Diabetes, osteoarthritis, and hip fracture were also responsible for significant disability.

These results suggest that as a minimum, we should examine studies on hip fractures (osteoporosis), stroke, and heart disease in African Americans and Hispanics, and that it would be good to examine atherosclerosis, hypertension, diabetes, and anemia as well. In the review we look for differences between racial and ethnic groups (e.g., hip fractures are more prevalent among white females).

TABLE 3-1 Percentage of Disability Attributable to Specific Conditions After Adjustment for Age, Sex, and Comorbidity, by Condition and Activity for 2,731 Whites Followed for 38 Years in the Framingham Heart Study

Activity	Knee Osteo-arthritis	Hip Fracture	Diabetes	Stroke	Heart Disease	Congestive Heart Failure	Claudication	Chronic Obstructive Pulmonary Disease	Depressive Sympto-matology	Cognitive Impairment
Stair climbing	16.7	9.1	9.8	12.8	5.2	7.6	3.1	7.4	15.4	—a
Walking a mile	15.4	4.9	4.3	9.3	9.3	2.4	6.8	5.2	10.4	—a
Heavy home chores	—a	2.8	2.2	6.7	15.3	3.9	1.2	3.8	4.0	—a
Housekeeping	16.7	7.8	2.6	12.6	13.4	6.5	0.0	6.5	15.9	3.4
Cooking	0.5	7.1	6.8	14.7	8.9	3.3	3.1	—a	4.3	7.3
Grocery shopping	1.2	7.5	3.5	16.7	13.0	1.6	—a	4.5	15.4	7.8
Carrying bundles	16.6	7.3	4.6	12.6	2.3	6.6	3.0	4.0	16.6	8.6

aAdjusted odds ratio < 1; attributable fraction not computable.
SOURCE: Guccione et al., 1994:Table 5. Copyright 1994 by the American Public Health Assocation. Reprinted by permission.

We examine age differences in disease as well as risk factors and disease mechanisms. We examine other prevalent diseases (notably cancer) that are not listed in Table 3-1. Also, to describe possible physiological mechanisms, we occasionally refer to cross-national data to distinguish social from physiological factors in racial and ethnic differences in disease. A complication in reviewing disease mechanisms is that there are racial and ethnic differences in disease interactions (e.g., atherosclerosis and osteoporosis, diabetes and stroke), especially at later ages.

Osteoporosis and Hip Fracture

Osteoporosis is usually viewed as a disease of postmenopausal women that accelerates with age. Two separate mechanisms have been proposed for osteoporosis. One, prevalent from age 55 to 74, is related to bone density and the rapidity of postmenopausal declines in estrogens. A second, dominating after age 75, is due to age differences in vitamin D metabolism (e.g., in the kidney and liver) and intestinal absorption of calcium (Eastell et al., 1991).

The morbidity of both types of osteoporosis is manifest in two ways. The first is increased risk of hip, spinal, and wrist fractures. Hip fracture is often studied because its consequences are severe—hip fracture mortality is estimated to be between 5 percent and 20 percent with long-term nursing home care necessary for 15 percent to 33 percent of patients (Boult et al., 1991). Spinal fractures have a slower course. A second effect of osteoporosis is its interaction with atherosclerosis. Here we discuss racial and ethnic differences in the effect of osteoporosis on hip fracture. Interaction with atherosclerosis is deferred to the discussion of heart disease and stroke.

Early onset osteoporosis is a disease of postmenopausal women that accelerates with age and is often associated with hip fracture. Hip fracture is more prevalent in white than in African-American or Hispanic women. Hip fracture rates begin to increase exponentially at age 70 for white women. They start to increase exponentially for white men and black women at age 75 and for black men past age 85. Since the incidence rates of hip fracture double every 5 years, this means that white men and black women have half the incidence of white women. Hispanic female rates are similar to black female rates (Kellie and Brody, 1990; Riggs and Melton, 1992). Possible explanations for racial differences in the incidence of hip fracture (and the rate of osteoporotic changes) are differences in bone density at menopause (possibly due to early differences in nutrition, physical activity, and body mass) and in the postmenopausal production of sex and parathyroid hormones.

One way to understand physiological differences in osteoporosis in racial and ethnic groups is to examine differences between males and females. The risk of hip fracture is lower, and occurs at later ages, in males than in females. Edelstein and Barrett-Connor (1993) found that body mass relative to height was associated with bone mineral density for both genders. However, whereas lean body mass predicted bone density in *both* genders, fat mass predicted a larger proportion of bone mineral density in women than men, possibly because of the conversion of androgens to estrogens in adipose tissue. Thus, both mechanical (i.e., weight-bearing physical activity) and hormonal factors likely affect bone density.

To analyze the effect of hormones on bone mineral density in elderly African-American, Hispanic, and white females, researchers often study serum estrone, the dominant type of estrogen produced postmenopausally. In postmenopausal women it is produced by aromatization of androstenedione in adipose (fat) tissue. Cauley et al. (1994) examined serum estrone levels to see if they explained differences in bone mass in black and white females. Serum estrone levels were higher in African-American than in white women, and bone mass was 23 percent to 27 percent greater in black women. Levels of serum estrone were related to bone mass differences among white, postmenopausal women. Bone mass decreased linearly with age for white, but not black, females. This could be due to several factors. Black-white differences in body mass explained most differences in serum estrone. However, nonobese black females had greater bone mass than nonobese white females. Race still significantly predicted bone mass differences after serum estrone was controlled for. Edelstein and Barrett-Connor's (1993) study of gender differences in bone density suggests that female racial differences in bone mass that are not explained by serum estrone might be due to the greater lean body mass of African-American females in comparison with white females and to the mechanical effects of greater muscle mass on physical activity and bone metabolism. The greater bone density of African-American females may be due to higher body mass and to greater postmenopausal production of estrone due to a higher proportion of body fat, factors that could increase the risk of hypertension and adult onset diabetes. If, instead, greater bone density is due to greater lean body mass and physical activity in African-American females, then the metabolic and circulatory effects of a higher body mass would be less likely to cause stroke and heart disease. Other risk factors for African-American women, including thinness, prior stroke, using walking aids, and alcohol consumption, were also risk factors for white women. Lower hip fracture risks for Hispanic females are also associated with greater body mass. Racial and ethnic differences in the risk of osteoporosis and hip fracture among females may involve several additional factors.

First, late onset osteoporosis (age 75 and older) is linked to age changes in vitamin D metabolism (in the kidney and liver) and intestinal absorption of calcium (Eastell et al., 1991). Vitamin D increases osteoclastic activity (i.e., a breaking down of the bone matrix by cells in the constant remodeling of bone tissue) *and* bone resorption (decreases in bone mass). Thus, both too little and too much vitamin D causes osteoporosis (Moon et al., 1992). This effect, however, differs by race. Blacks are less sensitive than whites to both vitamin D toxicity and deficiency (Taussig, 1966; Seelig, 1969). Studies of blacks aged 68 to 93 and whites 70 to 89 showed that hypovitaminosis D with secondary hyperparathyroidism occurred often in blacks (Perry et al., 1993). However, even with lower vitamin D levels, there was less bone resorption (and less turnover of skeletal mass) in U.S. blacks. In native Africans the incidence of hip fracture is even lower—only half that of U.S. blacks. A lower rate of bone formation was also indicated by lower serum osteocalcin in U.S. blacks. Blacks had higher ionized calcium levels than whites with similar parathyroid hormone levels; this suggests that bone metabolism is less sensitive to parathyroid hormone in blacks. The reduced sensitivity may be an adaptation in blacks to (1) a higher melanin content of the skin, which therefore produces less vitamin D, and (2) a lower intake of dairy products because of a high prevalence of intestinal lactase deficiency (Pollitzer and Anderson, 1989). A decreased sensitivity to parathyroid hormone and greater stability of skeletal mass in African-American females thus appear as important in their lower risk of osteoporosis as body mass differences and their effects on the postmenopausal production of sex hormones. Consistent with findings on the two types of osteoporosis, vitamin D and calcium supplementation, at least in white women, decreased hip fracture to advanced ages (e.g., in a group with a mean age of 84; Chapuy et al., 1994). Supplemental estrogens reduced the risk of fracture in black women, as it did for white women, up to age 75 (Grisso et al., 1994).

Heart Diseases and Stroke

U.S. heart disease and stroke mortality has changed markedly (DeStefano et al., 1993; Ghali et al., 1990; Pathological Determinants of Atherosclerosis in Youth Research Group, 1993). Although U.S. mortality for most types of heart disease and stroke has declined, racial differences in mortality are still marked: the age-adjusted mortality rates from major cardiovascular diseases for blacks is 1.5 times the rate for whites (Singh et al., 1996:Table 12).

Congestive heart failure is an exception to the general trend toward lower mortality from cardiovascular disease. Congestive heart failure occurs at late ages and reflects the cumulative effect of prior ischemic heart disease, hypertension, and atherosclerosis. Mortality from congestive heart failure increased until at least 1988 (Centers for Disease Control and Prevention, 1994). Mortality increases were paralleled by increased morbidity and service use and affected all race and gender groups. Age-standardized congestive heart failure hospitalization rates increased 60 percent for both whites and blacks from 1973 to 1986 (Ghali et al., 1990). This is consistent with declines from 1980 to 1989 in nonfatal coronary heart disease at ages 45 to 54—with increases at ages 75 to 84 (DeStefano et al., 1993).

Changes in other circulatory diseases differ by race and gender. To better differentiate African-American, Hispanic, and white trends in circulatory disease (Sempos et al., 1988), we identified factors affecting race and age trends of several processes related to circulatory events: atherosclerosis, diabetes, body iron stores, and hypertension.

Atherosclerosis

Atherosclerosis is a degenerative process that increases the risk of many circulatory diseases. It affects coronary heart disease, stroke, and, at late ages, peripheral vascular disease. Thus, in some senses the relation of atherosclerosis (the age-dependent process) to heart disease and stroke (the morbid events) parallels the relation of osteoporosis (the age-dependent process) to hip and other fractures (the morbid events). An evaluation of African-American and Hispanic differences in the progression of atherosclerosis is handicapped by a lack of longitudinal studies; the Framingham Heart Study, for example, studied only whites. The two best known longitudinal studies of circulatory disease containing significant numbers of African Americans and whites are the Charleston Heart Study and the Evans County study. There are, however, cross-sectional studies of risk factors for circulatory disease that represent African Americans and whites; a few represent Hispanics. Other studies examine differences in pathologies of the circulatory system in African Americans and whites at death.

One widely studied risk factor for atherosclerosis is cholesterol. Some data suggest that atherosclerosis in whites is more susceptible to cholesterol than in blacks (Eggen et al., 1965; Strong, 1972). In the 28-year follow-up of the Charleston Heart Study, the dependence of coronary heart disease mortality on cholesterol differed in African Americans and whites. White female cholesterol values had a J-shaped relation to mortality (i.e., mortality was higher at both very low and very high values of cholesterol). At intermediate values, mortality risk was lowest. The cholesterol-mortality relation was linear for African-American females. The increase in the risk of coronary heart disease with an increase of 1 standard deviation in cholesterol was 60 percent for white, compared with 40 percent for black, females (Knapp et al., 1992). For males, both the Charleston Heart Study and the Evans County Study suggest higher risk of coronary heart disease for whites than for blacks. In Charleston, black men and women had lower total cholesterol at baseline. Cholesterol was not a significant predictor of risk for black males (Keil et al., 1993).

To examine African-American, Hispanic, and white differences in the national distribution of, and changes in, total cholesterol, the National Health and Nutrition Examination Surveys for 1976 to 1980 (NHANES II) and for 1988 to 1991 (NHANES III; Sempos et al., 1993) can be used. Declines in cholesterol were similar for whites, African Americans, and Hispanics—though the proportion in a high-risk group was 8 percentage points lower for both African Americans and Hispanics than for whites. Lower cholesterol levels in African Americans and Hispanics may be due to differences in activity and nutrition. Studies showed that black Seventh Day Adventists with vegetarian (or partly vegetarian) diets had lower cholesterol than blacks eating an omnivorous diet; that is, a dose-response effect between cholesterol and nutritional factors (e.g., fats) was evident for African Americans as it is for whites (Melby et al., 1994).

Total cholesterol is a general indicator of the risk of coronary heart disease. There is growing interest in cholesterol subtypes and other lipoproteins. High-density lipoprotein (HDL) cholesterol protects against atherosclerosis by transporting lipids away from atheromas (irregularly distributed lipid deposits in the large- and medium-sized arteries). Low-density lipoprotein (LDL) cholesterol accelerates atherosclerosis, as may very low density lipoproteins (VLDL) or triglycerides, because LDL is trapped in atheromas after being oxidized. Other lipoproteins—for example, lipoprotein (a) [Lp(a)] or apolipoprotein E (Apo E)—also predict racial differences in atherosclerosis.

Lp(a) is associated with heart disease, stroke, and peripheral vascular disease. It appears to prevent blood clots from being dissolved by blocking plasminogen—an enzyme responsible for thrombolysis. It may also increase the uptake of LDLs by atheromas (Valentine et al., 1994).

The Atherosclerosis Risk in Communities (ARIC) study (1986 to 1989) of 14,254 persons measured HDL, LDL, and Lp(a) for blacks and whites of both genders. Lp(a) strongly discriminated black and white risks of coronary heart disease. Lp(a) levels were twice as high among blacks of both genders as among whites. Few environmental factors affected Lp(a). Selby et al. (1994) showed that Lp(a) levels had genetic determinants and that levels were higher in African-American than in white women. A genetic determination of Lp(a) levels for U.S. blacks is consistent with findings that blacks from the Sudan (Sandholzer et al., 1991), Ghana (Helmhold et al., 1991), and the People's Republic of the Congo (Parra et al., 1987) had Lp(a) levels similar to U.S. blacks. Also consistent with a genetic determination is the fact that racial differences in Lp(a) levels exist at early ages. The Coronary Artery Risk Development in Young Adults (CARDIA) study of 5,115 persons aged 18 to 30 found mean Lp(a) values twice as high for blacks as for whites—with black medians three times as high—results consistent with the Houston, Texas (Gayton et al., 1985), Bogalusa Heart (Srinivasan et al., 1991), and ARIC studies.

HDL and LDL in ARIC, in contrast, were similar for women of both races. Black men had more HDL than white men. White men had 16 percent to 26 percent higher triglyceride levels and the lowest HDL levels. Thus, HDL and triglyceride levels suggest lower risks of coronary heart disease for black men. The per-unit risk of elevated Lp(a) is less in blacks than whites, suggesting that Lp(a) interacts with other metabolic factors in blacks (Marcovina et al., 1993). If Lp(a) inhibits plasminogen, it might elevate black risks of stroke (Shintani et al., 1993). If Lp(a) increases cholesterol uptake in atheromas, this suggests interactions with cholesterol—an effect that could be dampened because black males have lower LDL and higher HDL levels.

Thus, Lp(a) and hypertension may explain the higher mortality from strokes for blacks than whites in middle and late-middle ages. Since Lp(a) has genetic determinants, and mortality selection has been shown in a number of twin studies to eliminate elevated genetic risks of mortality from coronary heart disease by age 85 (e.g., Marenberg et al., 1994; Carmelli et al., 1994; Reed et al., 1991; Heller et al., 1993), these age patterns of disease risk (and mortality selection) could contribute to a convergence of mortality patterns in blacks and whites owing to a different age dependence of circulatory diseases related to atherosclerosis at late ages.

Apo E is important in circulatory disease and dementia. One study suggested that the effects of Apo E differ in men and women (Ferrières et al., 1994). In some studies, Apo E2 and E4 subtypes lowered Lp(a), a fact significant for black circulatory disease risks. E2 was associated with reduced, and E4 with elevated, risks of heart disease (Tiret et al., 1994). E2 was associated with higher stroke risks—possibly interacting with diabetes (Couderc et al., 1993). The effects of E2 were stronger in postmenopausal females (Schaefer et al., 1994), lowering LDL twice as much as for premenopausal females.

Racial differences in atherosclerosis are also evaluated by studying circulatory pathologies in African Americans and whites. The Pathobiological Determinants of Atherosclerosis in Youth (PDAY, 1993) study collected material on thoracic and abdominal aortas and right coronary arteries in 1,532 autopsied black and white, male and female, subjects aged 15 to 34 for 1987 to 1990. PDAY did not show more coronary artery raised lesions in white, than black, males. This differed from the International Atherosclerosis Project (Guzmán et al., 1968) and other earlier studies (Strong and McGill, 1963; Eggen and Solberg, 1968). In autopsies of 1,243 blacks and whites aged 30 to 69 in New Orleans (Eggen et al., 1965) and in the International Atherosclerosis Project, where 23,000 autopsies from 15 geographic locations and four race-sex groups were assessed (Strong, 1972), there was less calcification of atheromas in blacks than in whites. Strong concluded that race differences were due to such factors as diet, activity, smoking, and stress. One dietary factor could be vitamin D consumption and age differences in its metabolism and its effects on calcium. The New Orleans study of autopsies from the 1950s to the 1960s suggested that atherosclerosis was 10 years of age more advanced in whites than in blacks. Differences between the findings of PDAY and the International Atherosclerosis Project may be due to recent decreases in the prevalence of atheromas in white males and a stable prevalence in black males.

Diabetes Mellitus (Adult Onset)

There are two types of diabetes mellitus. One, juvenile onset, is due to the autoimmunological destruction of pancreatic cells that produce insulin. Here we examine adult onset diabetes mellitus, which is not insulin dependent but is associated with degenerative changes in glucose and fat metabolism. Further references to diabetes are to the adult type.

Diabetes is more prevalent in U.S. blacks than whites (Cowie et al., 1993). In the 16-year follow-up of NHANES I the age-adjusted incidence was 15 percent for black women and 10.9 percent for black men. White women had an incidence of 7.0 percent; white men, 6.9 percent. Risk factors for diabetes include body mass index (body weight in kilograms divided by height in meters squared, i.e., kg/m^2), although age-adjusted diabetes risks were higher for both lean (body mass index < 20) and overweight (body mass index > 26) blacks. Low education and low activity were also associated with the incidence of diabetes (Lipton et al., 1993). However, known risk factors do not fully explain the higher prevalence of diabetes among blacks. Thus, genetic differences in metabolic adaptation to obesity by race may be involved (Cowie et al., 1993). The relative risk of diabetes for those with one diabetic parent was 2.3; with two diabetic parents, 3.9. Efforts to find a genetic factor have focused on maternal mitochondrial DNA (Lin et al., 1994). Changes in mitochondrial DNA have been suggested as a general marker of aging and degenerative disease (Wallace, 1992).

In NHANES, diabetes was found to be higher in most Hispanic groups (Flegal et al., 1991). Though body mass index and socioeconomic status (which affect early nutrition) are important determinants of diabetes in Hispanics, so may be genetic determinants of body fat distribution and tissue resistance to insulin. As was true for blacks, adjustment for standard risk factors left a diabetes risk of 1.9 for Hispanics relative to whites (Marshall et al., 1993).

The excess risk of diabetes in blacks may be recent (in the last 30 years). Among male draftees aged 18 to 45 in 1924, black diabetes rates were one-third those of whites. They were two-thirds of white rates by 1944. In the 1960s in Chicago, blacks had low diabetes rates despite high rates of obesity. Though U.S. data show that black women had relatively high, but stable, obesity over the past 30 years, black females did not have higher diabetes rates in the 1960s. Diabetes rates for blacks and whites apparently crossed over in the 1970s. Because these increases (e.g., a 105% increase for black men from 1973 to 1983) were inconsistent with moderate increases in black obesity, other risk factors are likely to be involved (Lipton et al., 1993).

One hypothesis is that the incidence of diabetes reflects poor nutrition in mothers of low socioeconomic status. Poor maternal nutrition may affect the fetal development of such organs as the pancreas and liver, and this may show up later in life as chronic diseases (e.g., Barker and Meade et al., 1992; Barker and Godfrey et al., 1992). This hypothesis suggests that pancreatic beta-cell failure ᵈ the lessened ability to produce insulin are due to poor fetal and early postna- ᵗⁱtion. Evidence of this is also suggested by analyses of Civil War veterans ᶜ1994). In groups with genetically high risks of diabetes, such as the the problem may relate more strongly to insulin resistance (the "thrifty phenotype" hypothesis) than to insulin production (McCance et al., 1994). In Pima Indians, selective mortality of infants of low birthweight may play a significant role in the incidence of diabetes at later ages. Other models of diabetes incidence emphasize the role of insulin resistance or the genetics of the production of glucokinase, which is linked to diabetes in U.S. blacks—but not whites (Yki-Järvinen, 1994).

So far we have examined the incidence of diabetes. We are also interested in the racial and ethnic differences in age progression of diabetes—as we were for atherosclerosis. Important in diabetes progression is the degree of glycemic (blood sugar) control as measured by glycosylated hemoglobin (GHb). Small differences in GHb are related to the risk of diabetic complications (e.g., retinal degeneration). In one study there was a significant difference in GHb means (10.5% vs. 8.4%) for blacks and whites reporting diabetes. Race and GHb were also associated in those not reporting diabetes. Insulin use significantly reduced this association. Some consequences of GHb elevation occurred 4 to 7 years before diabetes was diagnosed (Harris et al., 1992). Thus, one factor affecting diabetes progression, and its morbid consequence, may be differences between blacks and whites in access to health care and the identification and control of elevated GHb. In Hispanics, no relation of socioeconomic status to blood glucose was found (Haffner et al., 1989).

Although the effect of diabetes on stroke and other circulatory disease risks is well known, the process may differ in whites, blacks and Hispanics (Sempos et al., 1988). Comparisons of racial and ethnic groups in similar environments have elucidated some of these differences. Diabetes prevalence among South Asians in England (19.6%) was 4.3 times that among British white males (4.8%), as indicated by mean serum insulin fasting and 2-hour glucose loading levels. Among African-Caribbean men in England, diabetes prevalence (14.6%) was almost as high as among South Asians, but insulin and triglycerides were lower and HDL was higher (McKeigue et al., 1991). For South Asians, high resistance to insulin produced increased central obesity and elevated triglyceride levels (Sheu et al., 1993). The natural history of diabetes in South African blacks is characterized by an accelerated (relative to whites) decline in beta-cell function, which produces insulinopenia (i.e., low levels of insulin). Insulinopenia may be the reason diabetes has fewer macrovascular complications for blacks than for whites (Joffe et al., 1992). The risks of coronary heart disease in diabetics could be due to central obesity associated with the failure of insulin to suppress release of nonesterified fatty acids from intra-abdominal fat cells. This increases triglycerides, reduces production of HDL cholesterol, and increases atherogenesis (the formation of lipid deposits in the arteries). Thus, elevated triglyceride levels, with insulin resistance, glucose intolerance, and hyperinsulinemia (high levels of insulin), can occur independently of high total cholesterol levels. Hyperinsulinemia in central obesity (e.g., high levels of IGF-1, insulin growth factor) may stimulate smooth muscle growth, adversely affecting vasculature and microvasculature in white males (McKeigue et al., 1991, 1993). In white males, higher insulin levels were associated with circulatory disease. Indeed, all excess circulatory disease risk in white males could be related to hyperinsulinemia. White female risks were elevated in those whose fat distribution resembles that of typical males (Modan et al., 1991; Fontbonne, 1991). Plasma insulin was a better marker than hypertension of abnormal glucose tolerance in obese males in the Paris Prospective Study (Fontbonne et al., 1988). The different metabolic mechanisms of diabetes in black males, and their higher levels of HDL, may explain the lower risk of coronary heart disease in blacks (as in Hispanics).

As for coronary heart disease, there was evidence of selective survival, with people age 80 and older having less variability in insulin and blood pressure levels, body mass index, and waist-hip ratios. Thus, people with better physiological control of insulin, blood glucose, and body mass index have better survival to late ages (Campbell et al., 1993; Bild et al., 1993).

Body Iron Stores

The role of physiological iron in disease is complex. Both elevated and depressed levels produce morbidity. For blacks, the risk is often due to nutritional deficiencies that produce anemia. Salive et al. (1992) found elderly black males and females (36.4% and 30.3%, respectively) over twice as likely to be anemic as white males and females (14.3% and 11.6%, respectively). Hemoglobin means converged for males and females above age 90 (i.e., 136 g/L vs. 132 g/L), though twice as many males (40.0% < 130 g/L) had anemia as females (20.7% < 120 g/L). Male iron levels can be reduced by physical activity (Lakka et al., 1994). Thus, physical activity could affect the risk of cardiovascular disease by reducing iron levels—along with having other positive metabolic effects.

The higher prevalence of anemia among blacks may lower the late-age risk of circulatory disease by slowing the oxidation of LDL in atheromas. Among white males, elevated iron levels may accelerate atherosclerosis because free iron oxidizes LDL cholesterol; that is, hypercholesterolemia (high total cholesterol levels) and body iron levels interact (Kiechl et al., 1994). In 847 men and women aged 40 to 79, serum ferritin (a measure of iron in the body) predicted carotid artery disease in both sexes and was synergistic with hypercholesterolemia (Salonen et al., 1992). In men, ferritin levels varied moderately with age. For women, ferritin increases were marked for those age 50 to 59 (i.e., postmenopausally). Hematocrit, another measure of iron in the blood, was related to high blood pressure (Smith et al., 1994) possibly owing to higher blood viscosity (Löwick et al., 1992). The ability of ferritin levels to predict coronary heart disease declined for the elderly owing to nutritional deficits, differential survival, and the lower variance of ferritin. Differences in gender risk also moderated with age (dropping from 2.4 to 1 to 1.4 to 1 by age 80; Matthews et al., 1994). Thus, excess risk of coronary heart disease in white males may be partly explainable by higher iron stores in males than in females up to, and past, the age of menopause. After the age of menopause, white female iron stores are stable while iron stores of white males start to decrease. Atherosclerosis risks increase with age more rapidly for postmenopausal white females than for white males of similar ages (Matthews et al., 1994; Sullivan, 1989); this may be due to the interaction of iron stores with the release of calcium into the blood (and its uptake by smooth muscle cells) because of menopausal changes in bone metabolism. This explanation is suggested by the association of increased stroke risks in women with osteoporosis. Low bone density was one of the strongest risk factors for stroke in women; that is, there is a 74 percent increase in mortality per 1 standard deviation decrease in the bone density of the heel (Browner et al., 1991). One hypothesis is that in addition to calcium release, production of parathyroid hormone is increased, which causes both smooth muscle cell absorption of calcium and hypertension (Browner et al., 1993). Thus, the age acceleration of the risk of circulatory disease should be greater for white than for black or Hispanic females because of the more rapid progression of osteoporosis (and skeletal calcium release) in white females (Moon et al., 1992).

Hypertension

Hypertension is an important cause of certain types of heart disease and stroke in blacks, Hispanics, and whites. The prevalence of hypertension peaks at younger ages for blacks than for whites (Svetkey et al., 1993). In whites, older age was associated with hypertension. This pattern appears due to mortality selection; that is, the early elevation of blood pressure in blacks caused early mortality from stroke, coronary heart disease, and renal disease to be higher than for whites. In elderly whites, diabetes was the best predictor of hypertension. It was not significant for blacks.

Hypertension has many causes. Recently, interest has focused on the genetic determinants of renin (an enzyme affecting kidney function) and angiotensinogen (a protein affecting vasodilation, dilation of the blood vessels) as factors in hypertension (Dzau and Re, 1994). A single gene codes for angiotensinogen. Its mutation may predispose a person to hypertension (Jeunemaitre et al., 1992; Griendling et al., 1993). This mutation was found in 36 percent of whites with normal blood pressure (normotensives) and 47 percent of white hypertensives. The frequency of this mutation among blacks is 80 percent to 90 percent (Rotimi et al., 1994). Though predisposing to hypertension, the mutation is not sufficient in that West Africans (as opposed to U.S. blacks) have little hypertension (Cooper and Rotimi, 1994). Psychosocial stress and behavioral or environmental factors (e.g., sodium intake) also play important roles.

Hypertension can affect health by causing left ventricular hypertrophy, a risk factor for congestive heart failure. Angiotensin-converting enzyme (ACE) inhibitors are beneficial, not only in reducing blood pressure but also in reversing left ventricular hypertrophy (Lindpaintner, 1994). The effects of ACE on growth factors for smooth muscle and left ventricular hypertrophy are significant findings about the mutation in the angiotensinogen gene (Caulfield et al., 1994; Schunkert et al., 1994). That is, renin (an enzyme) and angiotensinogen (a protein) can also affect hypertension by stimulating the proliferation of smooth muscle cells in blood vessels (Dzau and Re, 1994; Dzau, 1994).

At late ages, systolic hypertension elevates stroke, total mortality, and mortality from coronary heart disease (Rutan et al., 1988). Diastolic hypertension is less of a risk at late ages; its decline may indicate progression of aortic atherosclerosis (Witteman et al., 1994). Thus, interventions in hypertension in the elderly have to be carefully targeted. Antihypertensive drugs have different efficacy in different age and racial groups, which suggests different, age-evolving race-specific (and ethnic-specific) etiologies for hypertension. Calcium channel blockers were most effective in young (under 60 years) and old (over 60 years) black males. Captopril worked best in young white males. Beta blockers worked best for older white males. The lesser effect of captopril in black males is consistent with the lesser prognostic significance of left ventricular hypertrophy in black males (Sutherland et al., 1993). Calcium channel blockers and diuretics may be effective in black males because black males tend to have hypertension due to low renin levels—possibly associated with hyperaldosteronism (excessive production of a steroid hormone produced by the adrenal cortex) and electrolyte imbalances (Materson et al., 1993).

Complex hormonal feedback systems affect hypertension, with different systems having greater effects in some racial and ethnic groups. Both the kidneys and the adrenal glands help control blood pressure. Hyperaldosteronism is associated with higher levels of production of androgen (a male hormone) and with higher levels of kidney dysfunction (White, 1994). Kidney failure rates, and the need for dialysis, are six times higher for blacks than whites, partly because of hypertension (Mathiesen et al., 1991) though the black risks of kidney failure are not fully explained by differences in the prevalence or severity of hypertension (Perneger et al., 1993). Kidneys produce both renin and erythropoietin (a protein that enhances the formation of red blood cells). Thus, kidney damage may cause hypertension but, owing to declines in erythropoietin, may moderate atherosclerosis by reducing the availability of iron (i.e., an antagonism of two risk factors). The adrenals produce aldosterone, which affects electrolyte and mineral-corticoid equilibrium. Thus, dysfunction of aldosterone production affects both sodium and potassium retention and androgen production.

Cancers

Table 3-1 did not include cancers, possibly because disability is associated with cancer's terminal phases, which may be relatively short. Nonetheless, there are significant differences in the incidence, diagnosis, and treatment of cancer among whites, African Americans, and Hispanics, and these affect the age pattern of cancer morbidity and mortality. For example, the age-adjusted mortality rate from malignant neoplasms for blacks is 1.35 times the rate for whites (Singh et al., 1996:Table 12).

One difficulty in studying cancer is that it represents over 35 diseases. Some cancers are so lethal (e.g., pancreatic and liver) that there are no major racial or ethnic differences in survival. We selected to review cancers that reflect well-identified racial and ethnic differences. In some, early detection affects survival, with few racial and ethnic differences after adjustment has been made for stage at diagnosis. In others, after stage at diagnosis has been controlled for, survival differences existed (e.g., bladder, female rectal, breast, cervical, and uterine cancer; Ragland et al., 1991). We examined breast and cervical cancer because there are different risk factors and types of disease present in blacks, Hispanics, and whites. Indeed there may be a negative correlation between cervical and breast cancer risk owing to their joint dependence on reproductive behavior. We examined racial and ethnic differences in prostate cancer because of large racial and ethnic differences in incidence and because its risk rises at late ages. We examined multiple myeloma, a cancer prevalent at late ages, because there are large racial differences in its incidence.

Prostate Cancer

The incidence and mortality of prostate cancer from 1986 to 1990 were higher for black than for white males. For both there are increases to very old ages. Prostate cancer, diagnosed early, has a good prognosis. Consequently, prostate cancer often occurs on death certificates as a contributing cause of death at late ages (Manton et al., 1991). This is due to the relatively long survival of males diagnosed at earlier ages with prostate cancer. In addition, prostate cancer is frequently diagnosed at a nonlethal stage in males dying at late ages of other causes. However, even latent tumors were more prevalent in U.S. blacks and whites than in Japanese (Yantani et al., 1982).

There is some evidence that prostate cancer risk is related to low levels of the active form of vitamin D (Corder et al., 1993). Indeed, vitamin D isomers may be involved in regulating cell differentiation and growth in a number of tissues because vitamin D interacts with the receptor sites of other hormones. Another hypothesis suggests that higher prostate cancer risks for black males are due, in part, to 10 percent higher testosterone levels in black than in white males. Higher testosterone levels in black women (than in white women) in the first trimester of pregnancy may affect the male offspring's hypothalamic-pituitary-testicular feedback system (Ross and Henderson, 1994), raising the offspring's testosterone production. Production of the 5-alpha reductase enzyme, which converts testosterone into its active forms, may have genetic determinants. For example, the activity of 5-alpha reductase is lower in Japanese and Chinese males. Their prostate cancer risks are lower than for U.S. whites and only a 30th of risks for black males. Additionally, there is a twofold to threefold increase in the risk of prostate cancer from a polyunsaturated fatty acid that can only be obtained from dietary sources—alpha-linoleic acid. The level of alpha-linoleic acid is positively related to the consumption of red meat and butter. It is negatively related to the consumption of dark fish. Hence, alpha-linoleic acid may aid the progression of a tumor (rather than function as a tumor initiator) since the incidence of microscopic prostate cancer at autopsy is the same in the United States and Japan—despite much higher clinically significant prostate cancer rates in the United States (Yantani et al., 1982). Also implicated in the risk of prostate cancer is the lower intake of linoleic acid (which comes from vegetable sources such as corn oil). A low linoleic acid intake was found in African-American males (Kaul et al., 1987). Thus, the pattern of high red meat intake (increasing alpha-linoleic acid) and low vegetable intake (decreasing linoleic acid) could explain the high prostate cancer risks of U.S. blacks and whites, as opposed to Japanese and Chinese (who eat more fish and vegetables); such a pattern would operate by affecting synthesis of eicosanoids (which affect inflammatory response in tissue) or blocking the products of 5-alpha reductase activity (and altering testosterone metabolism; Gann et al., 1994).

Such factors may also affect the risk of prostate cancer in Hispanic males. White Hispanic and non-Hispanic males had incidence rates of prostate cancer (age standardized) nearly identical to black Hispanic males. Black non-Hispanic males had nearly double the prostate cancer risk of black Hispanic males. The lower risk of prostate cancer for black Hispanic males may be due to the heavy reliance on various vegetable staples (e.g., black beans) in the diet despite the use of considerable fat in cooking (Trapido et al., 1990, 1994a).

Breast Cancer

Breast cancer is prevalent among females but, if diagnosed early, has good cure rates. Four risk factors for breast cancer were the same for blacks and whites (age at first birth, parity, surgical menopause, benign breast disease), and two (family history and breast feeding) were different in magnitude. Early age at menarche, contraceptive use, and smoking had more complex black-white differences (Mayberry and Stoddard-Wright, 1992). This complexity may be because breast cancer, like many other diseases reviewed, changes in nature with age of onset. Early onset breast cancer is generally histologically more aggressive, grows rapidly, has genetically determined risks, and is not estrogen-receptor positive. This form of breast cancer is frequently manifested premenopausally. Late onset breast cancer is histologically less aggressive, slower growing, dependent on reproductive history, and often estrogen-receptor positive.

There are racial and ethnic differences in overall breast cancer behavior. Breast cancer has a high lifetime prevalence (about 12%) and is treatable in the early stages. Data from the National Cancer Institute's Surveillance of Epidemiology and End Results program show that 5-year relative survival rates increased from 63 percent to 76 percent in whites in the last 25 years. In black women, survival improved from 46 percent to 64 percent. Poorer survival for black women is, in part, due to their greater chance of receiving a diagnosis at a late stage. Limited access to health care, usual source of care (e.g., white women have more frequent access to private clinics or physicians as indicated by the higher availability of private health insurance for whites [92.7%] versus blacks [58.9%]), higher body mass index, and lower mammography rates were associated with a diagnosis at a late stage for blacks (Hunter et al., 1993). Three factors—histological tumor grade, patient delay, and a physician breast exam—explained half of the black excess mortality for stage III and IV (vs. stage I and II) disease.

Overall survival is significantly worse for both black and Hispanic women. However, adjustment for tumor stage eliminated white-Hispanic differences, but not white-black differences. The interval before diagnosis does not explain the differences because black women were diagnosed at younger ages than whites. There were some racial differences in treatment. Blacks and whites received similar systemic therapy for node-positive breast cancer. For node-negative disease, however, blacks received less systemic therapy. There were identifiable racial differences in tumor biology. Black women, relative to whites, (1) were younger at diagnosis, (2) were estrogen-receptor negative and progesterone-receptor negative, (3) had larger tumors (27.7% > 5 cm), and (4) had tumors with a higher proliferation factor, all suggestive of blacks' having a higher risk of the early onset, aggressive form of the disease (Elledge et al., 1994). Hispanics had biologically more aggressive tumors than whites. However, blacks had significantly more aggressive tumors than Hispanics.

Both blacks and Hispanics have a lower incidence of breast cancer (Trapido et al., 1994b). This may be because there are two types of breast cancer. The early, aggressive disease is not affected by age at pregnancy or by fertility behavior and is related to genetic factors. It is more prevalent in black females (and apparently Hispanics). However, although more aggressive, it is less prevalent than late onset breast cancer. Late onset breast cancer is less aggressive and less influenced by genetic factors and more dependent on reproductive history (Manton and Stallard, 1992). In populations with low fertility and later age at first pregnancy (MacMahon et al., 1973), postmenopausal disease is more prevalent. Thus, in whites there is a higher overall prevalence of breast cancer owing to the greater risk of postmenopausal disease. In blacks, overall prevalence is lower, but there is a greater proportion of the aggressive early onset form of the disease. The early form of the disease, with its genetic determinants, tends to be removed from the black population at early ages due to mortality selection.

Cervical Cancer

Cervical cancer is of interest because when detected early (by Pap smear), it is treatable. Cervical cancer risks, which are related to early onset of sexual activity (and infection with human papilloma virus; risk ratio = 23.5; Becker et al., 1994), are higher in both blacks and Hispanics than in whites. However, the incidence of cervical cancer is much lower for both white and nonwhite Hispanics than for non-Hispanic blacks. Cervical and breast cancer risks are negatively correlated because of their different relation to sexual and reproductive behavior. Black non-Hispanics have the lowest breast cancer risks, whites and nonwhite Hispanics are intermediate (and similar), and non-Hispanic whites have by far the highest risks. Although Hispanics and blacks are in high-risk groups for cervical cancer, they are significantly less likely to undergo a Pap test. However, if cancer screening is available in prepaid health plans, Hispanics use it as often as whites (Perez-Stable et al., 1994).

Multiple Myeloma

Multiple myeloma is a cancer of plasma cells producing proteins for the immune system. It has a poor prognosis: a 5-year survival rate of 27 percent. Incidence and mortality for blacks (measured from 1986 to 1990) are twice the rates of whites. In contrast to many cancers, it continues to increase in incidence to advanced ages. Because myeloma is related to the aging of the immune system, it may be more an indicator of generalized aging processes than are many specific chronic diseases that have well-characterized risk factors. Thus, racial differences in multiple myeloma may reflect racial differences in generalized aging rates better than other diseases. This is suggested by data on a precursor condition to multiple myeloma called monoclonal gammopathy of unknown significance (MGUS). At current levels of life expectancy, multiple myeloma occurs in one-third of MGUS cases. As life expectancy increases and mortality from other diseases is deferred, higher proportions of the cases of MGUS may convert to multiple myeloma.

MGUS is defined by the detection of an abnormal immunological protein on electrophoresis. In whites it is 6 percent prevalent below age 80, 14 percent prevalent over age 90, and 19 percent over age 95 (Radl et al., 1975). MGUS has significant racial differences. It is rare (as is multiple myeloma) in Japanese, while blacks, consistent with their higher myeloma risk, have higher rates of MGUS than whites (Bowden et al., 1993; Singh et al., 1990). In contrast, Japanese have higher levels of normal immunoglobulins (i.e., IgG and IgA); this suggests that the Japanese have had long-term exposures to antigens that elevated these immunoglobulins but lack the genetic susceptibility that blacks have to produce monoclonal gammopathies. These data suggest racial differences both in the functioning of the immune system at late ages and in environmental exposures to immunological challenges.

White Hispanics and non-Hispanics have similar age-standardized incidence rates for multiple myeloma for both genders. In contrast, for black Hispanics and non-Hispanics (both genders), there is about a threefold elevation of multiple myeloma risks (Trapido et al., 1994a, 1994b). Thus, Hispanic status does not affect multiple myeloma risk but being black rather than white does.

Other data suggest that mortality selection will eventually operate on dysfunction of the immunological system—but at extreme ages. The risks of autoantibodies to the thyroid, pancreas, and other organs are not selected out of populations until almost age 100 (Takata et al., 1987; Mariotti et al., 1992).

Disease Interactions

To fully explain racial and ethnic differences in disease risks and progression, we must consider interactions of multiple diseases and multifactorial syndromes. For example, the "X syndrome" in circulatory disease—the clustering of insulin resistance, hyperinsulinemia, hyperglycemia, high triglycerides, and low HDL (Feskens and Kromhout, 1994)—involves aspects of both lipoprotein and glucose metabolism, which differ in blacks and whites. There appear to be metabolic differences in diabetes between black and white males (e.g., low insulin production in black male diabetes; insulin resistance in white male diabetics) that lower circulatory diseases for blacks.

Osteoporosis and atherosclerosis in postmenopausal females may be related to each other owing to changes in the production of estrogen and racial differences in the metabolism of vitamin D. Vitamin D is metabolized in the kidney and liver. As osteoporosis progresses and parathyroid hormone increases (especially in whites), the cells in artery walls absorb more calcium, and hypertension increases. White females are more susceptible to this process than black females. Another factor in this process may be body iron levels, which depend on kidney function (and the production of erythropoietin). A decline in kidney function may decrease body iron stores but increase hypertension. Blacks are more susceptible to kidney dysfunction than whites owing to the combined effects of hypertension and diabetes. Anemia may moderate atherosclerosis in blacks by reducing the potential for LDL to be oxidized and trapped in atheromas. The rise in iron levels in females postmenopausally, along with the progression of osteoporosis, may be responsible for the more rapid acceleration of atherosclerosis and mortality postmenopausally among white than among black women. If hemoglobin drops too low, the blood's oxygen-carrying capacity is impaired, and this aggravates cardiac ischemia. Differences in diabetes associated with hormonal factors and hyperinsulinemia may affect black-white differences in the age dependence of mortality risks at late ages, as may differences in Lp(a). If much of late onset dementia (85 and older) is due to circulatory disease (Skoog et al., 1993), there may be racial differences in dementia onset (Aronson et al., 1990), which is also suggested by the role of Apo E in atherosclerosis and the interactions of Apo E with Lp(a) that affect blood clotting. Racial and ethnic differences in dementia have been underresearched and require specialized longitudinal studies of risk factors in black, white, and Hispanic populations. Thus, there is a complex set of feedbacks that differ in Hispanics, blacks, and whites. We will need longitudinal data and specialized models to identify and describe these multiple disease interactions.

Health Care

There are differences in the type and quality of care delivered to racial and ethnic groups (Ayanian, 1994). Examples have been discussed for coronary heart disease, breast cancer, and diabetes. Medical innovations can have race- and ethnic-specific effects on both disease progression and mortality.

Two studies examined general differences in the quality of care by race and socioeconomic status. Kahn et al. (1994) examined the quality of care received by black or indigent Medicare beneficiaries. Similar results were found for both groups vis-à-vis whites and the affluent. In studying measures of quality of care (e.g., history taking, physical exam, chest X rays, common diagnostic tests, standard therapies) for 9,932 patients in hospitals in five states, they found that in urban teaching and nonteaching hospitals and in rural hospitals, blacks and the indigent received poorer care on average. An "apparent" advantage for blacks and the poor was that *in aggregate* they received more care in urban teaching hospitals. Since urban teaching hospitals had better care on average, estimates of racial quality of care differentials were downwardly biased. Peterson et al. (1994) examined racial differences in rates of coronary angiography, angioplasty, and bypass graft surgery in 33,641 men in Veterans Administration hospitals. Black veterans were less likely than white veterans to receive these procedures. Thus, there were racial differences in the quality of care in a common health-care system, although it was difficult to demonstrate mortality consequences.

In addition, medical innovations affect blacks, whites, and Hispanics differently owing to differences in disease risks and mechanisms. Initially, little could be done medically to control coronary heart disease, which was more prevalent in white males. Bypass surgery and thrombolytic agents can now reduce myocardial damage done by infarcts and allow heart attack survivors to live longer, even at ages 80 and older (Ko et al., 1992). In the second phase of the Thrombolysis in Myocardial Infarction (TIMI-II) trials, thrombolysis produced equally favorable outcomes (1-year mortality) in blacks and whites (Taylor et al., 1993). In Hispanics, outcomes were better than in the other two groups even though Hispanic (and black) profiles of risk factors appeared to be worse. Thus, while outcomes for all three groups were equally favorable, the higher incidence of coronary heart disease among whites means that successful treatment for coronary heart disease produces more total benefits for whites.

ACE-II inhibitors reduce the hospital use, disability, and mortality risks of congestive heart failure (SOLVD Investigators, 1991). Reductions in hospital use are considerable; about 350 stays were avoided per 1,000 persons in 3 years of follow-up. ACE-II inhibitors may also reverse left ventricular hypertrophy, a morbid condition related to hypertension that is prevalent among blacks. ACE-II inhibitors may also have beneficial effects in diabetes, again a condition more prevalent in blacks. By 1991, physicians increasingly prescribed ACE-II inhibitors and calcium channel blockers whereas newly treated hypertensives were half as likely to use diuretics, which have adverse effects in diabetics (Psaty et al., 1993). Thus, given the higher risks of hypertension, left ventricular hypertrophy, and diabetes for blacks, the use of ACE-II inhibitors may have greater per capita benefits for them.

Tighter control of insulin and blood glucose reduces the consequences of diabetes (Williams, 1994). This, however, requires intensive access to medical care and a high degree of patient involvement. With whites having greater access to health care, this may benefit white more than black diabetics. Strict dietary control and exercise can affect cholesterol (Ornish et al., 1990) and may be responsible for the secular changes in black-white differences in the rate of atherosclerotic progression noted between the PDAY and earlier studies. A recent anticholesterol drug trial shows significant reductions in total mortality as well as mortality from coronary heart disease. In this trial, 4,444 people with a prior heart attack had a total mortality rate 30 percent lower than that expected over 5 years. This drug could be of most benefit to white males, who have the lowest HDL levels and the greatest heart disease and atherosclerosis risks from hypercholesterolemia.

Effective treatment of hypertension has increased the age of chronic renal failure from the fourth to the fifth decade of life, a shift most evident for blacks (Qualheim et al., 1991). This shift may be extended because of the beneficial effects of ACE inhibitors on renal failure in diabetics (Chan et al., 1992). People aged 65 and older have become the fastest growing group in the end-stage renal disease program (59,000, or 40% of the end-stage renal disease population in 1990), and blacks are a large proportion (34.9%) of all persons on dialysis. Blacks, however, are a smaller proportion (17.9%) of those receiving kidney transplants. The growth of the dialysis population is highest at ages 75 and above, possibly owing to the use of erythropoietin (starting in 1988 in end-stage renal disease) to combat the anemia caused by dialysis. Thus, Medicare's end-stage renal disease program has benefits for both blacks and whites, but provides different services for blacks (more dialysis) than whites (more transplantation).

BLACK, HISPANIC, AND WHITE TOTAL AND CAUSE-SPECIFIC
MORTALITY DIFFERENCES

There are two reasons for analyzing black, white, and Hispanic age differences in disease mechanisms. One is to study the age-specific effects of the risks, incidence, and management of diseases in different racial and ethnic groups. The second is to discover whether it is plausible that racial and ethnic differences in the age trajectory of mortality are due to the different age risks of specific diseases in the three groups and to the effects of mortality selection on the age prevalence of specific conditions. The morbidity data suggest that black, white, and Hispanic morbidity risks are multifactorial and complex and are unlikely to be proportional across age. For example, hypertension and diabetes, two risk factors for stroke, may raise the mortality of blacks relative to whites in middle age. At older ages, whites (especially males) are at greater risk for atherosclerosis than blacks; this suggests that whereas blacks susceptible to stroke die at earlier ages, white circulatory mortality risks may accelerate more rapidly at later ages. A similar pattern may occur for white females; their greater osteoporosis risk relative to black females may cause their risks of atherosclerotic heart disease to increase more rapidly postmenopausally.

The need to examine the mechanisms of specific diseases and subsequently their contribution to cause-specific (and total) mortality at specific ages is amplified by the greater uncertainty about the accuracy of age reporting at later ages in population data for U.S. blacks than for whites. Uncertainty about data quality also exists for Hispanics because their mortality is advantaged relative to whites and because Hispanics are a racially mixed group that is hard to define in population data. Thus, the morbidity review provides independent information that can be used to assess the plausibility of the race- or ethnic-specific age trajectory of mortality rates calculated from cause-specific and total mortality data. This is especially important for studies in the United States, which does not have long-standing population registries (like Sweden) or vital statistics programs (like Great Britain) to provide high-quality population and mortality data at late ages. In the United States the problem is compounded because the level and structure of age-reporting errors in census and mortality data may differ; error structures may also differ across censuses. To avoid the problem of using data sources with different error structures in life-table calculations, we calculated extinct cohort tables for U.S. whites and nonwhites using only the age at death reported on death certificates. To see if this is a reasonable strategy, we first examined the quality of age reporting on death certificates relative to other sources in matched record studies.

Table 3-2 compares ages at death reported on death certificates (grouped into 5-year age categories) for three racial groups and ethnic groups with ages at death reported on Medicare data from the Master Beneficiary Record (MBR) for 124,507 matched cases in 1987 for Massachusetts and Texas. This allows us to

TABLE 3-2 A Comparison of the Mean Age at Death and Ratio of the Number of Deaths Calculated from Death Certificates for Persons Assigned to a Given Medicare Master Beneficiary Record Age Group

MBR Age Group	MBR Mean Age	Whites (Non-Hispanic)			Hispanics			Blacks				
		DC Mean Age	Difference (2) – (1)	Ratio of DC to MBR Counts (%)	DC Mean Age	Difference (5) – (1)	Ratio of DC to MBR Counts (%)	DC Mean Age	Difference (8) – (1)	Ratio of DC to MBR Counts (%)	Ratio of DC to SSA Counts (%)	Ratio of DC to Census Counts (%)
	(1)	(2)	(3)	(4)	(5)	(6)	(7)	(8)	(9)	(10)	(11)	(12)
65-69	67.5	67.53	0.03	100.73	67.64	0.14	101.64	67.68	0.18	106.93	105	104
70-74	72.5	72.50	0.00	100.22	72.54	0.04	100.37	72.34	-0.16	104.44	102	99
75-79	77.5	77.50	0.00	100.21	77.47	-0.03	101.01	77.22	-0.28	104.37	95	97
80-84	82.5	82.47	-0.03	100.27	82.40	-0.10	101.02	81.96	-0.54	99.89	103	100
85-89	87.5	87.45	-0.05	99.93	87.35	-0.15	97.97	86.63	-0.87	93.88	82	82
90-94	92.5	82.44	-0.06	98.64	92.31	-0.19	96.16	91.20	-1.30	85.28	83	79
95-99	97.5	97.32	-0.18	99.81	97.03	-0.47	100.58	95.58	-1.92	88.22	108	102
100+	102.5	101.99	-0.51	103.32	100.60	0.90	116.67	99.40	-3.10	101.10	131	165

Note: DC = death certificate; SSA = Social Security Administration.
SOURCE: Columns 1 to 10 are derived from Kestenbaum, 1992:Table 3; data for 1987 in Massachusetts and Texas; columns 11 and 12, from Preston et al., 1996:Figure 1 data for 1985 in the United States.

quantify the size and direction of errors in age reporting on death certificates for blacks, whites, and Hispanics for ages 65 to 100 and above (Kestenbaum, 1992). The rows in Table 3-2 refer to age groups in the MBR files. In column 1, the mean age within each MBR age group is assumed to be the midpoint of the 5-year age interval. Columns 2, 5, and 8 present the mean ages in the death certificate files for the same people. The death certificate files may classify some of these people in younger or older age groups, leading to discrepancies in the estimated mean ages. Columns 3, 6, and 9 display the discrepancies. For whites, the differences are small, except for the last two age groups (–0.18 and –0.51). For Hispanics, the differences are also small, with only the last two age groups exceeding ±0.2 year. For blacks, all but the first two of the differences exceed ±0.2 year with what appears to be a substantial downward bias at older ages.

Misclassification of age in the death certificate files may lead to underestimates and overestimates of the actual number of deaths in the various age groups. Columns 4, 7, and 10 display the ratios of (1) the number of deaths for matched cases in each age category for ages at death reported on the death certificate to (2) the number of deaths in the age categories generated from the MBR. For whites, all but two of the age groups are within 1 percent. For Hispanics, all but three are within 2 percent. For blacks, only one is within 1 percent, and two are within 2 percent. For blacks there were substantially more deaths reported on death certificates up to age 79 and fewer from ages 80 to 99. Deficits in the three older age categories from 85 to 99 were large for the death certificate data (i.e., –6.1%, –14.7%, –11.8%). These cases apparently were in the three lower age categories due to the underreporting of age at death on death certificates for blacks. The number of blacks (92) reported as age 100 and above on death certificates was similar to that in the MBR (91).

Also in Table 3-2 are two sets of ratios for blacks from Preston et al. (1996:Figure 1). Columns 11 and 12 refer to a sample of 2,657 deaths among African Americans in 1985 that were linked both to Social Security Administration (SSA) records and to the 1900-1920 U.S. censuses. The similarity of the census and SSA age distributions was used to argue for their accuracy relative to that of death certificate ages. SSA age was assumed to be most reliable because it was one of two sources where age agreed in 91 percent of 1,087 two-way agreements in the sample.

Preston's results differ from Kestenbaum's (1992). Both showed that the number of deaths reported at ages 65 to 69 was overstated on death certificates. For ages 70 to 84, the number of deaths recorded from death certificates may be overstated or understated. The number of deaths recorded from death certificates at ages 85-94 is understated, but the two studies disagreed on magnitude. For ages 95-99 the number of deaths recorded from death certificates may be overstated or understated. For ages 100 and above, the number of deaths from the death certificates is overstated, but the two studies disagreed on magnitude.

A difficulty in assessing mortality rates above age 100 is that the number of cases is small. Thus, it is important to assess the statistical precision of the results of match studies above age 100 to see if real differences are being identified. In the data in Preston et al. (1996), there appeared to be 26 death certificate, 20 SSA, and 16 census deaths above age 100 (calculated from the ratios in Table 3-2 and the 52 deaths reported at age 100 and older on death certificates, and with a three-way match rate of 50.5% assumed). If the number of deaths above 100 recorded by the SSA is assumed to be the most accurate and we assume that the 20 deaths are Poisson distributed, then the standard error of the estimate is 4.5, and a 2-standard error confidence interval ranges from 11 to 29 deaths. This confidence interval includes both the death certificate (26) and the census estimates (16) of deaths. Thus, the numbers of deaths reported above age 100 in the three sources are not significantly different.

In Kestenbaum (1992), 92 blacks had ages at death greater than 100 on death certificates, compared with 91 blacks in the MBR. The standard error for the 91 persons with ages at death over 100 in the MBR is 9.5, with a 2-standard error confidence interval of 72 to 110 deaths. This clearly includes the 92 deaths above age 100 recorded on death certificates. Again there is no statistically significant difference in the number of deaths above age 100 recorded in the death certificates and the MBR. The standard error for the 42 Hispanic deaths reported at age 100 and older from the MBR is 6.5, with a confidence interval of 29 to 55 deaths. This range includes the 49 deaths above age 100 recorded on the death certificates. Again, the difference is not statistically significant.

Thus, it can be concluded that the accuracy of death certificate ages differs over age and by race. For blacks, deaths at ages up to 84 were overreported and at ages 85 to 94 (and possibly later) underreported on death certificates. Given the differences between Kestenbaum (1992) and Preston et al. (1996), adjusting the data by using either ratio estimate is problematic. Neither match study showed that age reporting above age 100 on the death certificate is statistically different from reporting in the other data components.

The analysis of the two match studies suggests that it is not unreasonable to use death certificate data to calculate age-specific probabilities of death (q_x's) for U.S. white and nonwhite males and females using extinct cohort methods. In this method, the numerator of each q_x is the number of deaths recorded on death certificates for that age. The denominator is the sum of deaths reported on the death certificate at age x, plus deaths reported on death certificates for each subsequent year for each subsequent age. This specification of the denominator is not standard, but it can reduce the effects of certain types of errors in death certificate reports of age at death. For example, if there is a constant ratio of the number of deaths recorded on death certificates to the true number of deaths beyond age x, then the numerator and denominator used to calculate q_x have the same relative error; errors will cancel out, and an accurate estimate of q_x will be produced. This may be the case for nonwhite deaths for ages 85 to 99 recorded on death certificates. In Table 3-2 the downward bias in the denominator for ages

80 to 84 will produce overestimates of q_x's even though the numerator is correct. The near constancy of ratios from ages 70 to 84 means that bias will decline over this range. Thus, using extinct cohort methods to calculate life expectancy should show a slight downward bias in life expectancy for nonwhites relative to whites (if white data are not subject to error, say, to age 95). The q_x's for male cohorts aged 70, 75, and 80 in 1962, followed to 1990, are given in Figure 3-2. Female results are shown in Figure 3-3.

For both genders, nonwhite q_x drops below that for whites at age 81 (i.e., about 5 years below the crossover age observed by Kestenbaum, 1992, in Medicare data for 1987; Figures 3-2 and 3-3 were *not* adjusted to reflect data in Table 3-2). At late ages, rates are variable owing to small numbers. Since we used death certificate data from 1960 to 1990, we had to estimate the number of deaths above ages 98, 103, and 108, the highest ages observed for the three cohorts. We did this by using the data from the cohort 5 years older to fill in the mortality experience at ages higher than we observed in the younger cohort. We excluded deaths above age 118 from all computations. This minimizes between-cohort differences for the younger cohorts, since the experience used to close out tables is identical to that of older cohorts, cohorts likely to be initially smaller and to have higher mortality to late ages (Manton and Stallard, 1996; Stallard and Manton, 1995).

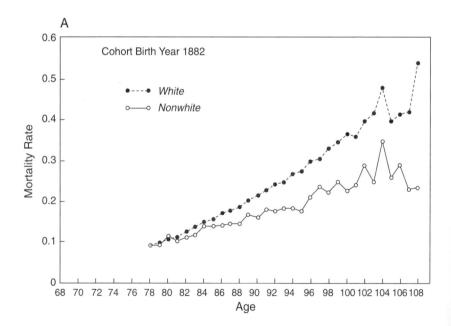

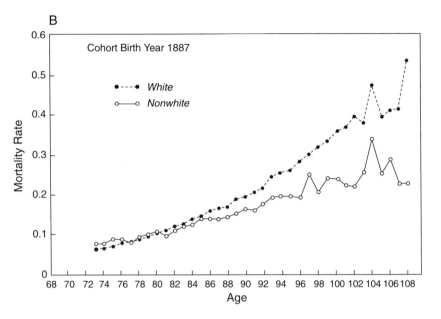

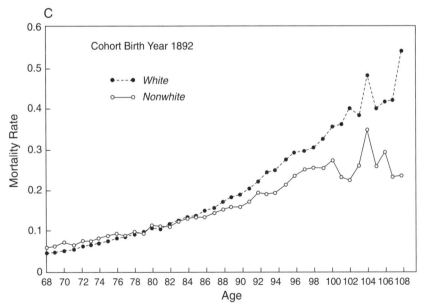

FIGURE 3-2 Mortality rates (q_x) for three male cohorts. SOURCE: Duke University Demographic Studies, analysis of 1960-1990 U.S. death certificate files.

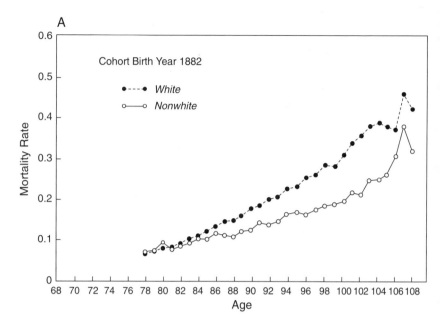

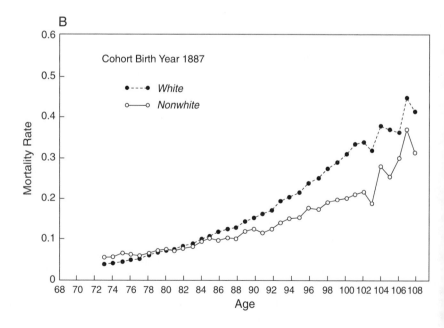

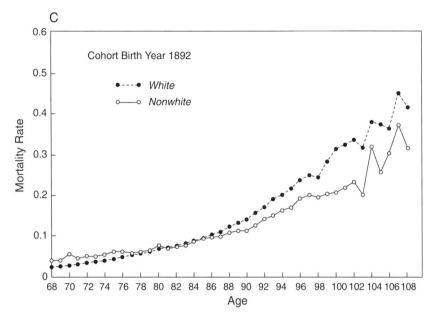

FIGURE 3-3 Mortality rates (q_x) for three female cohorts. SOURCE: Duke University Demographic Studies, analysis of 1960-1990 U.S. death certificate files.

Table 3-3 shows gender-specific ratios of white to nonwhite mortality at every 5th year of age for cohorts aged 70, 75, 80, 85, 90, and 95 in 1962. For both genders the gap for younger cohorts in the age range 80 to 90 narrows owing to declining white, and relatively stable nonwhite, mortality. For the cohort aged 70 in 1962, the white mortality excess at 85 is estimated to be 1.1 percent for females and 3.9 percent for males; at 95 the excess is 28 percent for both genders. The 28 percent white excess converts to a 22 percent nonwhite deficit, too large to be accounted for by any of the death certificate undercount ratios in Table 3-2. The ratios are sufficient to account for the 5-year difference in the crossover age in Kestenbaum (1992) and in the extinct cohort mortality rates in Figures 3-2 and 3-3.

Having examined racial differences in cohort mortality, we then examined cross-sectional (1992) data on several causes of death to see at what ages the peak differences in mortality relative risks occur. Figure 3-4 shows the black to white relative risks for males and females for total and cause-specific mortality. The peak black risk for cancer occurs at age 35 to 44 for females (1.5 to 1) and 45 to 54 for males (2 to 1). For heart disease the peak occurs at age 25 to 34 for males (2.8 to 1) and 35 to 44 for females (3.9 to 1). For both males and females the peak black stroke risk occurs at age 35 to 44 (about 4.5 to 1 and 4.0 to 1, respectively). For total mortality in 1992 the peak black risk occurs at age 35 to 44 (2.5 to 1 for

TABLE 3-3   Mortality Ratios at Specific Ages for Each Cohort

Age Within Cohort	Cohort Birth Year and Age of Cohort in 1962[a]					
	1892 70	1887 75	1882 80	1877 85	1872 90	1867 95
Ratio of White to Nonwhite Male Mortality						
70	0.6983					
75	0.8571	0.8186				
80	0.9490	0.9565	0.9240			
85	1.0385	1.0524	1.1063	1.0523		
90	1.1895	1.1943	1.3228	1.1887	1.2694	
95	1.2838	1.3313	1.5508	1.4682	1.4885	1.6370
100	1.3081	1.4867	1.6141	1.5889	2.1253	2.0077
105	1.5502	1.5502	1.5502	1.9322	1.4089	2.4400
Ratio of White to Nonwhite Female Mortality						
70	0.5111					
75	0.7210	0.6877				
80	0.8990	0.9275	0.8319			
85	1.0106	1.0777	1.1906	1.0674		
90	1.2350	1.2201	1.4155	1.2626	1.0797	
95	1.2811	1.4039	1.3728	1.5326	1.7350	1.5852
100	1.5133	1.5481	1.5900	1.7415	2.2598	2.1098
105	1.4531	1.4531	1.4531	1.6129	1.7305	1.6270

[a]Age of cohort in 1990 was as follows: 98 for birth year 1892; 103 for 1887; 108 for 1882; 113 for 1877; 118 for 1872; and 123 for 1867.
SOURCE: Duke University Center for Demographic Studies, analysis of 1960-1990 U.S. death certificate files.

males and 2.7 to 1 for females). For all causes (except cancer) and total mortality, there is a decline by age 85 to a mortality ratio less than 1.0. Thus, the mortality patterns show declines in black-white ratios beginning no later than age 45 to 54 (National Center for Health Statistics, 1994).

Because of concerns about data quality, no U.S. analysis of racial survival based solely on population data is likely to resolve the issue of whether there is a black-white mortality crossover. However, there are several ways to increase the credibility of results. First, one can determine if population mortality analyses are consistent with differences in the age dependence of mechanisms causing morbidity (and subsequently, mortality) in Hispanics, blacks, and whites in epidemiological studies. Thus, the validity of the population results must be assessed in terms of the substance of the disease mechanisms whose mortality outcomes are observed in the population. As discussed in prior sections, there is ample evidence that the age trajectories of specific diseases for racial groups are not proportional and that certain mechanisms favor the largest mortality disad-

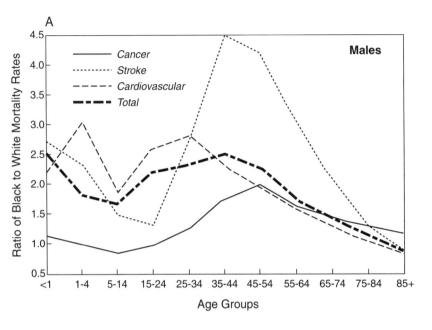

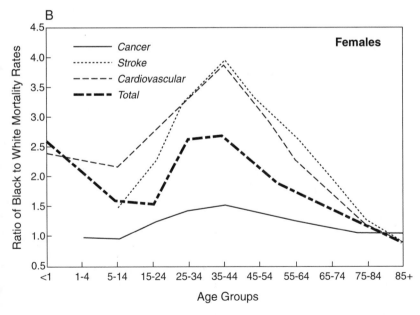

FIGURE 3-4 Ratios of black to white mortality rates, by age, cause of death, and gender.
SOURCE: Data from Kochanek and Hudson, 1994:Table 8.

vantage for blacks in middle and late-middle ages, as found in Figure 3-4. Both mortality selection of frail persons and differences in the age dependence of the mechanisms of disease (which are documented in the section on morbidity) could cause the age trajectory of mortality for whites and nonwhites to cross over. A second way to validate population results is to compare them against national surveys where cause-specific and total mortality risks are assessed through independent data collection mechanisms.

The National Longitudinal Mortality Survey (NLMS) examined black-white differences in mortality. The NLMS used 10 samples (for 1978 to 1985) from the Census Bureau's Current Population Survey, which has a response rate of 96 percent. The NLMS samples covered 500,000 whites and 50,000 blacks aged 25 and above. Linkage to the National Death Index identified 32,508 deaths. The relative (black to white) risks for total mortality declined with age. For males the relative risks were 2.13, 1.67, and 1.04 for ages 25 to 44, 45 to 64, and 65 and above. For women the relative risks were 2.33, 1.82, and 1.16 for the same ages. Adjustments for income reduced male relative risks to 1.74, 1.30, and 0.98 and reduced female relative risks to 1.93, 1.48, and 1.16. For cause-specific mortality, cardiovascular disease showed the same age pattern of relative risk as total mortality (2.06, 1.59, and 0.93 for males; 4.07, 2.09, and 1.16 for females). For cancer there was no convergence for blacks up to age 65; there was a moderate convergence for black females after age 65. For all other causes of death there was a convergence for both genders. Income-adjusted relative risks for total mortality declined by 5-year categories from age 25 to age 85 and above, with convergence, then crossover, by age 60 for males and by 80 to 85 for females (Sorlie et al., 1992).

A similar study was done of Hispanic mortality using 12 Current Population Surveys. Of 700,000 persons aged 25 and above, 40,000 were Hispanic with 1,562 Hispanic deaths. The age patterns are different for Hispanics in that the age-adjusted standardized risk ratios for Hispanics to non-Hispanics were 0.74 for males and 0.82 for females. Age-specific risk ratios for total mortality were 0.97 (age 25 to 44), 0.73 (age 45 to 64), and 0.83 (age 65 and above). Risk ratios for cardiovascular disease declined with age for men (0.77 to 0.59) and increased moderately for females (0.72 to 0.84). Hispanic cancer ratios were lower at all ages (0.46, 0.52, and 0.76 for males; 0.46, 0.68, and 0.55 for females). This was confirmed in age-adjusted rates of cancer incidence, where the relative risk for white Hispanic males was 88 percent of that for white non-Hispanic males. The risk for black Hispanic males was only 71 percent of that for black non-Hispanic males. The cancer risk for black Hispanic males was only 85 percent of that for white Hispanic males (Trapido et al., 1994a). For females, both black and white Hispanic cancer risks were about 70 percent of that for black and white non-Hispanics, with black Hispanic risk about 78.5 percent that of white Hispanics (Trapido et al., 1994b). When the age-specific total mortality risks were adjusted for income, they dropped further: to 0.81 (age 25 to 44), 0.67 (age 45 to 64), and

0.66 (age 65 and above) for males; 0.64 (age 25 to 44), 0.74 (age 45 to 64), and 0.83 (age 65 and above) for females. One explanation of the Hispanic mortality advantage is their recent migrant status. Other explanations may involve differences in risk factors for specific diseases (e.g., while diabetes prevalence is high in Hispanics, so are HDL levels).

A final source of validating data is longitudinal studies of mortality in closed cohorts. Lew and Garfinkel (1990) assessed the mortality of 49,469 people passing age 75 from 1960 to 1987. There were 7,911 person-years of exposure for black males and 7,412 person-years of exposure for black females. Black male mortality rates dropped below white rates at about age 80 to 84. For females the crossover occurred between ages 85 to 89 and 90 to 94. In 4,107 people aged 65 and above in 1986 and followed for 5 years, Guralnik et al. (1993) found higher life and active life expectancies for black men and women above age 75.

WHITE-NONWHITE DIFFERENCES IN DISABILITY AND ACTIVE LIFE EXPECTANCY

Morbidity and disability are both powerful determinants of the age trajectory of mortality. As discussed above, hypertension, stroke, diabetes, renal disease, certain types of heart disease, and some cancers may create higher mortality for blacks in middle age. We compared the age dependence of race-specific disease mechanisms to total and cause-specific age patterns of mortality in several types of data in the preceding section. These represent two of three pairwise relations needed to evaluate the model in Figure 3-1. Here we evaluate the third linkage: the age relation of disability and mortality. We examined this using the 1982, 1984, and 1989 National Long Term Care Surveys (NLTCS) linked to Medicare mortality records for the period 1982 to 1991.

The NLTCS was used because large list samples of individuals were drawn from Medicare enrollment files and followed for up to 9.5 years. There are 30,308 distinct persons, not households, in the 1982, 1984, and 1989 longitudinal file; a total of 60,232 assessments were attempted, with 57,290 completed, an overall response rate of 95.1 percent. The Medicare list sample (which represents 98.4% or more of the U.S. elderly population) allows 100 percent of the sample to be followed for mortality. Both community and institutional persons are represented. In the three surveys, 16,485 detailed community interviews were completed. In 1984 and 1989, 3,100 detailed institutional interviews were done. About 11,000 deaths were recorded from 1982 to 1991 so there are a large number of deaths and person-years of exposure to assess—especially since people had to be aged 65 and older to be in the sample. Replenishment samples of about 4,900 people were drawn in 1984 and 1989 to replace the 65- to 66-year-olds (1984) or the 65- to 69-year-olds (1989) who would otherwise be missing owing to the aging of the original sample of those aged 65 and older. Age is recorded both from Medicare records and as reported by the sample person. If a sample person is too impaired to complete an in-person interview, the interview is conducted with a proxy. The date of birth is also recorded on the interview. Ages can be checked for temporal consistency for people who were interviewed on more than one date. A problem identified by Kestenbaum (1992), timely reporting of age at death, was handled by updating the Medicare mortality records 6 to 12 months after the time of the interview. Age reporting in NLTCS records should be of better quality than standard Medicare records because of validation by direct survey contact and the possibility of tracking people over time.

We analyzed these data in two steps. First, we examined the distribution of disability for whites and nonwhites, stratified by education to control for differences in socioeconomic status. These results are presented in Table 3-4; stratifications by age are found in Table 3-5. After examining white-nonwhite differences in the distribution of disability at specific ages, we modeled the dependence of mortality on disability.

As Table 3-4 shows, the proportion of nondisabled community residents declined 1.03 percent for white nongraduates, but increased 0.61 percent for nonwhite nongraduates from 1982 to 1989. For graduates the proportion of nondisabled whites increased 2.41 percent; for nonwhites it declined 0.41 percent. In general the proportion receiving help with three or more activities of daily living is higher for nongraduates. Stratified by education, race, and age, sample sizes for some estimates are small.

There were sizable changes from 1982 to 1989 in the age distribution of the population aged 65 and older. In Table 3-5, we present age-specific changes in disability for the education groups. There are large changes in the age distribution of disability across education. For whites aged 65 to 74 in 1982 there was little difference in disability between education groups. For nonwhites, the disabled group was 5.0 percent larger in 1982 for nongraduates. From 1982 to 1989, disability declined for white graduates. Whereas white nondisabled nongraduates increased 0.4 percent at age 65 to 74, white nondisabled graduates increased 2.9 percent from 1982 to 1989. Nonwhite, nondisabled graduates increased 1.3 percent.

For age 75 to 84, education effects were larger. For white graduates, the nondisabled proportion was 5.0 percent higher in 1982, 5.1 percent in 1989. For nonwhite graduates the nondisabled proportion was higher: 14.5 percent higher in 1982; 6.7 percent in 1989.

For whites aged 85 and older, disability increased 2.1 percent for graduates versus nongraduates in 1982—based on few (eight) cases. By 1989, with 30 persons in the disabled group, the effect reversed; disability declined 6.8 percent for white graduates, and there was a larger proportion (55.3%) nondisabled. For nonwhites, 85 and older who were graduates, sample sizes are small and estimates unstable.

To link disability to survival, we first identified dimensions of disability and

TABLE 3-4   Disability Status of White and Nonwhite High School Graduates and Nongraduates Living in the Community, 1982-1989

	High School Nongraduate		High School Graduate	
Disability Level[a]	White	Nonwhite	White	Nonwhite
Percentage Distribution (weighted counts)				
1982				
Nondisabled	80.62	78.10	82.86	84.33
1 or more IADLs	5.80	6.61	5.10	5.32
1-2 ADLs	7.11	7.08	6.31	4.01
3-4 ADLs	2.79	3.41	2.67	2.83
5-6 ADLs	3.68	4.79	3.06	3.51
1989				
Nondisabled	79.59	78.71	85.27	83.92
1 or more IADLs	5.37	5.96	3.57	3.88
1-2 ADLs	7.85	6.86	5.75	5.74
3-4 ADLs	3.96	4.47	3.30	2.97
5-6 ADLs	3.23	4.02	2.12	3.51
Sample Size[b,c]				
1982				
Nondisabled	321	48	162	9
Disabled	3,188	594	1,500	89
1989				
Nondisabled	465	77	373	15
Disabled	1,839	411	1,124	61

[a]Disabled persons are defined as receiving help on any of six activities of daily living (ADLs) or nine instrumental activities of daily living (IADLs). The ADLs are eating, getting in or out of bed, getting about inside, dressing, bathing, and toileting. The IADLs are heavy housework, light housework, laundry, cooking, grocery shopping, getting about outside, traveling, managing money, and telephoning.

[b]For the nondisabled, sample size is the unweighed number of persons represented in the percentage distribution above it. For the disabled, the sample size is the unweighted number of persons represented by the sum of four categories—IADLs, 1-2 ADLs, 3-4 ADLs, and 5-6 ADLs—in the percentage distribution above it. In 1982, the disabled sample is about 10 times the size of the nondisabled sample; in 1989, about 4 times.

[c]If we assume a Poisson distribution, coefficients of variation (CV) can be estimated for size n: CV = $1/\sqrt{n}$; for $n = 1$, CV = 100%: for $n = 4$, CV = 50%; for $n = 9$, CV= 33.3%; for $n = 16$, CV = 25%; for $n = 20\%$; for $n = 100$, CV = 10%; and for $n = 400$, CV = 5%. Sample sizes for nonwhite, nondisabled graduates are small; this implies that their estimates in Tables 3-4 and 3-5 have low precision.

SOURCE: Duke University Center for Demographic Studies, analysis of the 1982, 1984, and 1989 National Long Term Care Surveys.

TABLE 3-5   Disability Status of White and Nonwhite Community Residents, Stratified by Age and Education, for 1982 and 1989

Disability[a] Level	Age 65-74		Age 75-84		Age 85+	
	White	Nonwhite	White	Nonwhite	White	Nonwhite
Percentage Distribution (weighted)						
High school nongraduate 1982						
Nondisabled	88.03	84.44	73.31	70.45	49.88	53.66
1 < IADLs	4.19	5.36	7.83	9.26	10.59	7.96
1-2 ADLs	4.11	4.49	10.12	10.64	19.41	15.73
3-4 ADLs	1.58	2.68	3.86	3.93	8.30	7.35
5-6 ADLs	2.10	3.03	4.87	5.71	11.82	15.31
High school graduate 1982						
Nondisabled	87.86	89.44	78.35	84.95	47.80	0.00
1 < IADLs	3.78	4.02	6.94	4.73	10.99	30.86
1-2 ADLs	4.51	2.62	7.52	3.84	20.92	26.86
3-4 ADLs	1.80	2.07	3.40	3.42	9.11	9.10
5-6 ADLs	2.04	1.85	3.79	3.05	11.18	33.18
High school nongraduate 1989						
Nondisabled	88.42	88.21	74.61	68.45	48.53	26.67
1 < IADLs	3.65	3.82	6.78	9.55	9.65	13.94
1-2 ADLs	4.63	3.99	9.83	10.14	18.53	23.94
3-4 ADLs	1.70	2.12	5.13	6.22	12.36	19.00
5-6 ADLs	1.61	1.86	3.65	5.65	10.92	17.45
High school graduate 1989						
Nondisabled	90.77	90.70	79.71	75.17	55.34	32.00
1 < IADLs	2.45	3.57	5.19	4.86	7.27	2.96
1-2 ADLs	3.60	2.73	7.89	11.02	17.67	21.15
3-4 ADLs	1.96	1.42	4.29	3.94	12.27	20.30
5-6 ADLs	1.23	1.57	2.91	5.02	7.46	23.59
Sample Size[b, c]						
High school nongraduate 1982						
Nondisabled	189	30	110	13	22	5
Disabled	1,208	275	1,386	212	594	107
High school graduate 1982						
Nondisabled	104	6	50	3	8	0
Disabled	700	36	540	31	259	22
High school nongraduate 1989						
Nondisabled	190	37	223	35	52	5

TABLE 3-5   Continued

Disability[a] Level	Age 65-74		Age 75-84		Age 85+	
	White	Nonwhite	White	Nonwhite	White	Nonwhite
Disabled	464	123	891	183	484	105
High school graduate 1989						
Nondisabled	182	9	161	5	30	1
Disabled	387	22	487	25	232	14

[a]Disabled persons are defined as receeiving help on any of six activities of daily living (ADLs) or nine instrumental activities of daily living (IADLs). The ADLs are eating, getting in or out of bed, getting about inside, dressing, bathing, and toileting. The IADLs are heavy housework, light housework, laundry, cooking, grocery shopping, getting about outside, traveling, managing money, and telephoning.

[b]For the nondisabled, sample size is the unweighed number of persons represented in the percentage distribution above it. For the disabled, the sample size is the unweighted number of persons represented by the sum of four categories—IADLs, 1-2 ADLs, 3-4 ADLs, and 5-6 ADLS—in the percentage distribution above it. In 1982, the disabled sample is about 10 times the size of the nondisabled sample; in 1989, about 4 times.

[c]If we assume a Poisson distribution, coefficients of variation (CV) can be estimated for size n: CV = $1/\sqrt{n}$; for $n = 1$, CV = 100%: for $n = 4$, CV = 50%; for $n = 9$, CV= 33.3%; for $n = 16$, CV = 25%; for $n = 20$%; for $n = 100$, CV = 10%; and for $n = 400$, CV = 5%. Sample sizes for nonwhite, nondisabled graduates are small; this implies that their estimates in Tables 3-4 and 3-5 have low precision.

SOURCE: Duke University Center for Demographic Studies, analysis of the 1982, 1984, and 1989 National Long Term Care Surveys.

then estimated individual scores on these dimensions. We identified the dimensions from multivariate analyses of 27 items in the 1982, 1984, and 1989 NLTCS (Manton et al., 1995). In the analysis, all years were pooled so that the dimensions identified describe the distribution of cases for any survey year. The analysis produced two types of coefficients. The coefficients describing the relation of the 27 variables to the six disability dimensions are listed in Table 3-6. In addition, we estimated scores for each person in the community sample each time he or she was interviewed. For persons with more than one interview, changes in the scores on the six dimensions can be assessed directly. Scores are estimated so that they sum to 1.0 across the six dimensions for each person at each time; that is, a person may be a partial member of multiple groups.

The six dimensions define six groups that can be characterized by examining which coefficients in Table 3-6 are large. The six groups are as follows:

1. *Nondisabled, with modest physical limitations*, a group with no impair-

TABLE 3-6 Prevalence Rates for Select Functional Disabilities for Six Groups Identified in the 1982, 1984, and 1989 National Long Term Care Survey

Functional Disability	Community Sample Frequency (%)	GROUP					
		1 Nondisabled, Modest Physical Limitations (%)	2 Active (%)	3 IADL Impaired with Performance Limitations (%)	4 IADL Impaired (%)	5 ADL Impaired (%)	6 Frail
Needs help:							
Eating	7.0	0.0	0.0	0.0	0.0	0.0	55.2
Getting in/out of chairs/bed	26.2	0.0	0.0	0.0	0.0	75.4	100.0
Getting about inside	39.9	0.0	0.0	0.0	0.0	100.0	100.0
Dressing	19.4	0.0	0.0	0.0	0.0	0.0	100.0
Bathing	43.1	0.0	0.0	17.6	0.0	100.0	100.0
Toileting	21.7	0.0	0.0	0.0	0.0	49.9	100.0
Heavy housework	71.9	100.0	14.5	100.0	100.0	100.0	100.0
Light housework	22.6	0.0	0.0	0.0	36.2	0.0	100.0
Laundry	41.5	0.0	0.0	100.0	100.0	36.2	100.0
Cooking	29.8	0.0	0.0	0.0	100.0	0.0	100.0
Grocery shopping	56.9	0.0	0.0	100.0	100.0	100.0	100.0
Getting about outside	59.1	0.0	0.0	100.0	61.1	100.0	100.0
Traveling	52.9	0.0	0.0	100.0	100.0	100.0	80.3
Managing money	26.8	0.0	0.0	0.0	100.0	0.0	100.0
Taking medicine	23.5	0.0	0.0	0.0	100.0	0.0	100.0
Telephoning	16.0	0.0	0.0	0.0	87.4	0.0	85.5

Is bedfast	0.8	0.0	0.0	0.0	0.0	0.0	5.6
No inside activity	1.5	0.0	0.0	0.0	0.0	0.0	10.2
Wheelchair-fast	7.0	0.0	0.0	0.0	19.9	0.0	25.8

Has difficulty:

Climbing one flight of stairs

No	18.6	0.0	53.4	0.0	0.0	0.0	0.0
Some	29.1	33.9	46.6	0.0	0.0	88.2	0.0
Very	31.4	66.1	0.0	50.9	73.0	11.8	10.8
Cannot	21.0	0.0	0.0	49.1	27.0	0.0	89.2

Bending for socks

No	43.5	0.0	100.0	0.0	100.0	100.0	0.0
Some	27.9	100.0	0.0	0.0	0.0	0.0	0.0
Very	18.0	0.0	0.0	100.0	0.0	0.0	0.0
Cannot	10.6	0.0	0.0	0.0	0.0	0.0	100.0

Holding 10 lb. package

No	29.6	0.0	84.2	0.0	0.0	0.0	0.0
Some	18.1	39.0	15.9	0.0	25.5	58.1	0.0
Very	15.9	61.1	0.0	0.0	30.7	41.9	0.0
Cannot	36.4	0.0	0.0	100.0	44.7	0.0	100.0

Reaching over head

No	56.1	0.0	100.0	0.0	100.0	100.0	0.0
Some	21.2	100.0	0.0	0.0	0.0	0.0	34.3
Very	13.9	0.0	0.0	76.6	0.0	0.0	14.5
Cannot	8.8	0.0	0.0	23.4	0.0	0.0	51.2

Combing hair

No	71.6	0.0	100.0	0.0	100.0	100.0	0.0
Some	16.0	100.0	0.0	43.0	0.0	0.0	33.5
Very	7.0	0.0	0.0	57.0	0.0	0.0	11.7
Cannot	5.4	0.0	0.0	0.0	0.0	0.0	54.8

Continued on following page

TABLE 3-6 Continued

Functional Disability	Community Sample Frequency (%)	GROUP						
		1 Nondisabled, Modest Physical Limitations (%)	2 Active (%)	3 IADL Impaired with Performance Limitations (%)	4 IADL Impaired (%)	5 ADL Impaired (%)	6 Frail
Washing hair							
No	55.8	0.0	100.0	0.0	100.0	100.0	0.0
Some	14.8	100.0	0.0	0.0	0.0	0.0	0.0
Very	9.4	0.0	0.0	100.0	0.0	0.0	0.0
Cannot	20.0	0.0	0.0	0.0	0.0	0.0	100.0
Grasping small objects							
No	66.0	0.0	100.0	0.0	100.0	100.0	24.6
Some	20.3	100.0	0.0	0.0	0.0	0.0	34.3
Very	10.1	0.0	0.0	95.4	0.0	0.0	14.9
Cannot	3.6	0.0	0.0	4.6	0.0	0.0	26.2
See well enough to read newspaper	74.3	100.0	100.0	100.0	0.0	100.0	45.4

Note: ADL = activity of daily living; IADL = instrumental activity of daily living.
SOURCE: Data from Duke University Center for Demographic Studies, analysis of the 1982, 1984, and 1989 National Long Term Care Surveys.

ments in activities of daily living or instrumental activities of daily living (except heavy housework) and only moderate difficulty doing a few physical tasks.

2. *Active*, a group with no impairments in activities of daily living or instrumental activities of daily living and few physical impairments.

3. *IADL impaired with performance limitation*, a group with a number of impairments in instrumental activities of daily living (but none in the activities of daily living except bathing) and significant physical impairment.

4. *IADL impaired*, a group with many impairments in the instrumental activities of daily living, including those related to cognitive performance (but none in the activities of daily living). Physical performance, however, is less impaired than group 3.

5. *ADL impaired*, a group with impairments in four of the six activities of daily living, impairment in many of the instrumental activities of daily living, and moderate physical impairment.

6. *Frail*, a group with impairments in almost all activities of daily living and instrumental activities of daily living.

This analysis produced six scores for each of the 16,485 community interviews conducted in 1982, 1984, and 1989. To generate scores for all 30,308 people in the longitudinal file, we made two additional calculations. First, there were about 35,700 people who screened out on one or more of the three surveys. These people had no chronic disabilities in activities of daily living or instrumental activities of daily living (the reason for screening out) for that time. Thus, they were assigned a score of 1.0 on the first dimension (i.e., were put into the nondisabled group). A plausible alternative would be to assign them a score of 1.0 on the second dimension (i.e., put them into the active group). We dealt with this uncertainty by combining the first two groups into a single "active/non-disabled" group, which appears later in Table 3-9 and Figure 3-7. Second, there were about 5,100 people in institutions in total in 1982, 1984, and 1989. Because the 1984 and 1989 detailed institutional surveys indicated that the average resident had 4.8 impairments in activities of daily living (no institutional interview was done for 1,992 institutionalized people in 1982), we created a seventh category for institutionalized people. Institutionalized persons received a 1.0 on this seventh category (and 0.0 on all other dimensions).

With these scores and mortality records for 1982 to 1991, we estimated two types of equations. First, we calculated the changes in the disability scores by (1) interpolating monthly values of the disability scores for people with interviews at the beginning and end of an interval, and (2) using a "nearest neighbor" match for people who died in an interval to determine the monthly rate of change for the person most like the decedent. In addition, we weighted cases by replicating each case by the ratio of its sample weight to the base weight. When this was done we calculated a monthly transition matrix,

$$g_i(t + 1) = C_t g_i(t) + e_i(t + 1) \tag{1}$$

where $g_i(t)$ is the seven-element vector of disability scores for the ith individual at age t; $g_i(t + 1)$ is the corresponding vector at age $t + 1$; C_t is the 7×7 matrix of coefficients describing changes in the disability scores from age t to $t + 1$; and $e_i(t + 1)$ is the error in prediction of $g_i(t + 1)$.

A second equation describes mortality as a quadratic function of the current scores $(g_i(t))$ and a term reflecting the dependence of mortality on age net of the changes in disability, that is,

$$\mu(g_i(t)) = \tfrac{1}{2}[g_i(t)]^T B[g_i(t)] \cdot e^{\theta t} \tag{2}$$

The 7×7 matrix B contains hazard coefficients describing how the pairwise interactions of the $g_{ik}(t)$, $k = 1,..., 7$, affect mortality. Those effects are multiplied by the exponential term $e^{\theta t}$, which represents the average effects of unobserved variables on mortality over age. As the $g_{ik}(t)$ become more informative the effects of unobserved factors will decrease. This will decrease the value of θ. The matrix B_t is calculated for age t, as $B_t = B \cdot e^{\theta t}$, making the hazard function age dependent.

With the dynamic and hazard equations estimated, difference equations can use the coefficients from these equations to calculate life-table parameters, for each age t, by applying first the mortality equation to the distribution of the $g_{ik}(t)$, and then the dynamic equations (Manton et al., 1994).

Mortality coefficients for disability scores estimated for white and nonwhite females are given in Table 3-7. Disability-specific mortality is roughly similar for white and nonwhite females (the confidence bounds of nonwhite coefficients were broader). There is a consistently higher level of mortality for nonwhite institutionalized females, and there are fairly large differences for terms involving group 4. The exponent θ, indicating the annual percentage increase in mortality, conditional on the time-variable disability profile, is higher (6.9%) for white females than for nonwhite females (4.3%). The higher age rate of mortality increase for white females will produce a convergence of white and nonwhite female mortality although white females start with lower mortality at age 65.

Table 3-8 shows mortality coefficients for white and nonwhite males. There are more differences in the coefficients for white and nonwhite males (e.g., 12.5 vs. 6.4 for the effect of group 3, with whites disadvantaged; 11.9 vs. 26.0 for group 4, with nonwhite males disadvantaged; 3.75 vs. 4.62 for active males) than for females. The θ for males differs for whites and nonwhites (i.e., conditional on disability, white male mortality increases 7.14% per year vs. 3.73% per year for nonwhites). The ratio of 1.91 for the male θ's (vs. 1.59 for females) suggests that the convergence of mortality with age is more rapid for males.

Figure 3-5 plots the white and nonwhite, male and female, age-specific

TABLE 3-7 White and Nonwhite Female Quadratic Mortality Coefficients

		GROUP						
Group	Race	1 Nondisabled, Modest Physical Limitations	2 Active	3 IADL Impaired with Performance Limitations	4 IADL Impaired	5 ADL Impaired	6 Frail	7 Institutional
1. Nondisabled, modest physical limitations	W	1.98	2.05	4.20	4.65	2.92	3.89	3.66
	NW	2.09	2.23	4.55	5.74	3.74	4.14	4.29
2. Active	W		2.12	4.35	4.81	3.02	4.02	3.78
	NW		2.38	4.85	6.11	3.98	4.41	4.57
3. IADL impaired with performance limitations	W			8.90	9.86	6.19	9.24	7.75
	NW			9.90	12.47	8.13	9.00	9.34
4. IADL impaired	W				10.92	6.86	9.13	8.58
	NW				15.71	10.24	11.33	11.76
5. ADL impaired	W					4.30	5.73	5.39
	NW					6.67	7.38	7.66
6. Frail	W						7.62	7.17
	NW						8.17	8.48
7. Institutional	W							6.74
	NW							8.81
Time-varying age exponent	W	0.06870						
	NW	0.04320						
χ^2	W	2868.15						
	NW	218.99						

Note: ADL = activity of daily living; IADL = instrumental activity of daily living; W = white; NW = nonwhite.
SOURCE: Data from Duke University Center for Demographic Studies, analysis of the 1982, 1984, and 1989 National Long Term Care Surveys.

TABLE 3-8 White and Nonwhite Male Quadratic Mortality Coefficients

Group	Race	GROUP 1 Nondisabled, Modest Physical Limitations	2 Active	3 IADL Impaired with Performance Limitations	4 IADL Impaired	5 ADL Impaired	6 Frail	7 Institutional
1. Nondisabled, modest physical limitations	W	3.75	4.23	6.83	6.68	5.89	6.83	5.84
	NW	4.62	4.61	5.42	10.96	5.51	8.25	6.23
2. Active	W		4.77	7.71	7.54	6.65	7.70	6.59
	NW		4.60	5.41	10.94	5.50	8.23	6.21
3. IADL impaired with performance limitations	W			12.46	12.19	10.74	12.45	10.65
	NW			6.37	12.88	6.48	9.69	7.32
4. IADL impaired	W				11.92	10.50	12.17	10.42
	NW				26.03	13.10	19.59	14.79
5. ADL impaired	W					9.26	10.73	9.18
	NW					6.59	9.85	7.44
6. Frail	W						12.43	10.64
	NW						14.74	11.13
7. Institutional	W							9.11
	NW							8.40
Time-varying age exponent	W	0.07140						
	NW	0.03730						
χ^2	W	1473.13						
	NW	90.33						

Note: ADL = activity of daily living; IADL = instrumental activity of daily living; W = white; NW = nonwhite.
SOURCE: Data from Duke University Center for Demographic Studies, analysis of the 1982, 1984, and 1989 National Long Term Care Surveys.

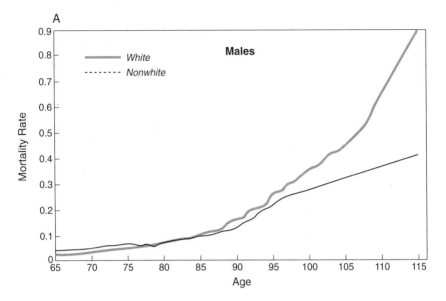

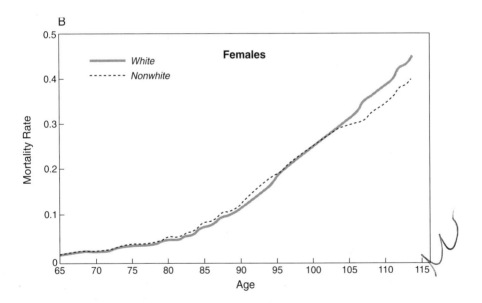

FIGURE 3-5 Estimates of age-specific mortality rates for whites and nonwhites, by gender. SOURCE: Duke University Demographic Studies, analysis of 1982, 1984, and 1989 National Long Term Care Surveys.

probabilities of death calculated from equation (2). Female probabilities of death converge. A crossover is evident only at late ages. For males the crossover occurs about age 83—or roughly halfway between the extinct cohort estimate (age 81) and Kestenbaum's (1992) estimate (age 86).

Figure 3-6 shows male and female survival probabilities (l_t's) normed to 100,000 at age 65. For males, l_t's converge at age 92-93. For females, although l_t's converge, there is no crossover.

The age trajectories of the mean scores (i.e., $\overline{g}_k(t)$) for the first two groups (active and nondisabled with modest physical limitations) for white and nonwhite males and females are shown in Figure 3-7. For both nonwhite males and females, disability (lower functioning) is greater. This is reasonable if (1) the survival of higher proportions of nonwhites to late ages implies their greater survival at higher disability levels, and (2) acute diseases cause mortality to increase more rapidly with age for whites. This may be explicated by examining Table 3-4, where the functioning of white high school graduates improved from 1982 to 1989. In contrast, the disability of nonwhite graduates increased while that of nonwhite nongraduates decreased. This could be due to differences in mortality; that is, nonwhite graduates could appear to be less functional if greater proportions of them survive to higher ages.

Such differences suggest the existence of acute disease mortality, not represented by disability dynamics, but by the age dependence coefficients (θ). The average score in the active/nondisabled group is higher for whites than for nonwhites and, after a long decline to age 95, begins to increase, owing to whites' higher θ's (6.9% and 7.3%), which may cause impaired whites to die off at late ages more rapidly than disability sets in. In nonwhites, θ is smaller (i.e., 4.3% and 3.7%) so there is a relatively slower mortality increase in impaired groups. Another possibly important factor in the higher disability of nonwhites is body mass index, which is higher in black women and is strongly related to mobility disability in the NHANES I follow-up study (Launer et al., 1994). High past and current body mass indexes (> 27) were significant risk factors for incident disability in the young old, possibly because of effects on osteoarthritis. Current weight loss and past high body mass index (> 28) (but not current high body mass index) were significant for the incidence of disability in the oldest old. Thus, different age changes in function for whites and nonwhites can result from mortality interactions with several age-dependent factors.

Table 3-9 presents life tables and average disability scores for white and nonwhite males aged 65, 75, 85, 95, and 105 calculated using the dynamic (1) and mortality (2) equations. Whites have higher life expectancies and higher proportions active/nondisabled at age 65 than nonwhites. Nonwhite survival rates eventually converge with those for whites. At late ages the average active/nondisabled score is lower for nonwhites than for whites. Mortality is higher for whites at late ages owing to their larger θ's so that mortality selection at late ages tends to preserve, or slightly increase, the aggregate level of functioning for whites. A

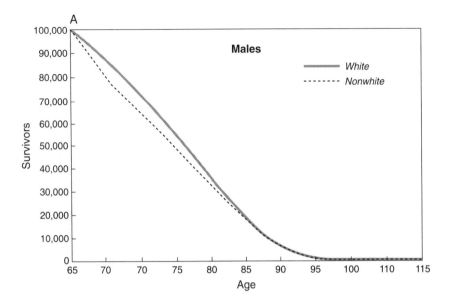

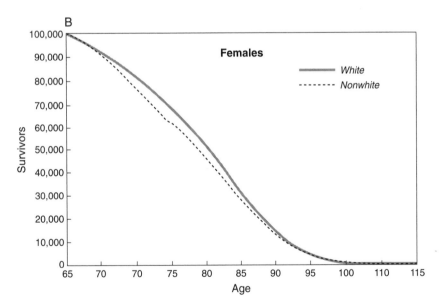

FIGURE 3-6 Race-specific numbers of survivors at estimates of each age by gender if we assume 100,000 males and 100,000 females alive at age 65. SOURCE: Duke University Demographic Studies, analysis of 1982, 1984, and 1989 National Long Term Care Surveys.

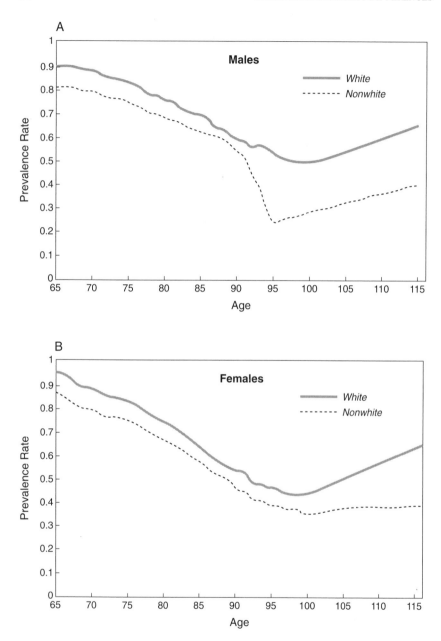

FIGURE 3-7 Estimates of race-specific prevalence rates for active/nondisabled groups (groups 1 and 2 combined) at each age by gender. SOURCE: Duke University Demographic Studies, analysis of 1982, 1984, and 1989 National Long Term Care Surveys.

larger θ generates higher mortality for nondisabled white persons producing life expectancies close to those in Social Security Administration (1992) cohort life tables. The column marked $l_t \times [\overline{g}_1(t) + \overline{g}_2(t)]$ gives survival-weighted activity levels for the $g_{ik}(t)$ summed for the first two groups; that is, survival and functioning are summarized in a single trajectory. Higher white activity levels occur in disability changes observed over a total of seven years, (i.e., from 1982 to 1989). During that time, while the overall prevalence of chronic disability declined in the United States (Manton et al., 1993), the declines in disability were larger for whites than for blacks (Clark and Wolinsky, 1996; Clark et al., 1996). Since the disability declines over the seven years of follow-up occur for most age groups represented in 1982, the life-table calculations in Table 3-9 represent the splicing together of disability and survival experience of distinct cohorts. The trajectories of disability score changes are representative of the changes manifest in the distinct cohort trajectories—as well as the changes between the cross-sectional distributions of disability observed in 1982 and 1989.

SUMMARY

We examined race-specific and ethnic-specific age patterns of health and mortality changes in three ways. First, we examined epidemiological data on racial and ethnic differences in the age dependence of the risk of several diseases. The diseases examined were osteoporosis, heart disease and stroke, cancers, and diabetes; they represent 70 percent of all U.S. mortality above age 65. Not represented were chronic pulmonary conditions, pneumonia and influenza, externally caused deaths (except hip fracture), and liver and selected other conditions. Since a number of major risk factors (diabetes, hypertension, atherosclerosis, anemia, osteoporosis) were examined, the conditions examined probably affect more than 70 percent of deaths above age 65. For example, pneumonia and influenza often cause mortality in persons with other chronic diseases; cardiac problems may affect pulmonary function, and diabetes and hypertension can affect many organs such as the kidney, liver, and brain. There are over 35 types of cancer, so we selected several to represent racial and ethnic differences in risk. For example, prostate and breast cancer are the most frequently diagnosed U.S. cancers; black males have a 20 percent greater incidence of prostate cancer than whites, and white females have a 30 percent greater incidence of breast cancer (NCHS, 1994).

First, we reviewed disease mechanisms. Both the accelerating effect of hypertension and diabetes on black mortality and the stimulating effect of atherosclerosis and other factors on white mortality at late ages suggest the plausibility of a physiological basis for mortality convergences and crossover. We did not discuss specific nonlethal diseases (e.g., osteoarthritis), although their chronic effects on health at later ages are reflected in the disability and mortality linkages.

Second, we examined both the quality of data used to determine the age

TABLE 3-9   Projected Survival Function (l_t), Life Expectancy (e_t), Active Survival $(l_t[\bar{g}_1[t]+\bar{g}_2[t]])$, and Group Prevalence Rates $(\bar{g}_k[t])$ by Age, Race, and Gender

Group	Survival Function $l_t \times 100{,}000$	Life Expectancy e_t	Active/ Nondisabled Survival $l_t[\bar{g}_1[t] + \bar{g}_2[t]]$	Group Prevalence Rates, $\bar{g}_k[t]$ 1 Nondisabled, Modest Physical Limitations
White males	100,000	16.30	0.9364	0.9122
Nonwhite males	100,000	14.28	0.8256	0.7597
White females	100,000	20.88	0.9597	0.9487
Nonwhite females	100,000	18.91	0.9168	0.9049
White males	73,339	10.28	0.6626	0.8059
Nonwhite males	61,228	10.17	0.4909	0.6696
White females	84,265	13.76	0.7746	0.8523
Nonwhite females	79,089	12.49	0.6391	0.6900
White males	35,578	5.72	0.2785	0.6701
Nonwhite males	27,889	6.56	0.2002	0.5678
White females	55,967	7.95	0.4260	0.6443
Nonwhite females	47,248	7.39	0.2782	0.4372
White males	5,820	3.06	0.0380	0.5197
Nonwhite males	6,301	3.62	0.0160	0.2271
White females	18,021	4.40	0.1034	0.4669
Nonwhite females	13,406	4.33	0.0517	0.2737
White males	133	1.79	0.0009	0.5479
Nonwhite males	331	2.68	0.0012	0.3270
White females	1,573	2.91	0.0097	0.5125
Nonwhite females	1,140	3.05	0.0038	0.2247

SOURCE: Duke University Center for Demographic Studies, analysis of the 1982, 1984, and 1989 National Long Term Care Surveys.

trajectory of total and cause-specific mortality and the ages of maximum black-white mortality differences. For cancer, heart disease, and stroke, the peak relative risk occurred in middle age, with declines in relative risk beginning before age 55. This was consistent with the morbidity review.

2 Active	3 IADL Impaired with Performance Limitations	4 IADL Impaired	5 ADL Impaired	6 Frail	7 Institutional
Age 65					
0.0242	0.0095	0.0023	0.0285	0.0231	0.0003
0.0659	0.1292	0.0452	0.0000	0.0000	0.0000
0.0110	0.0101	0.0040	0.0099	0.0076	0.0086
0.0119	0.0111	0.0045	0.0455	0.0221	0.0078
Age 75					
0.0976	0.0092	0.0130	0.0248	0.0234	0.0262
0.1321	0.0346	0.0333	0.0486	0.0447	0.0371
0.0670	0.0125	0.0102	0.0214	0.0142	0.0224
0.1181	0.0349	0.0236	0.0422	0.0616	0.0297
Age 85					
0.1128	0.0142	0.0248	0.0402	0.0521	0.0858
0.1501	0.0307	0.0504	0.0329	0.0734	0.0947
0.1169	0.0201	0.0252	0.0549	0.0379	0.1008
0.1516	0.0552	0.0601	0.1075	0.0886	0.0998
Age 95					
0.1331	0.0159	0.0327	0.0724	0.0976	0.1285
0.0276	0.0635	0.1171	0.0887	0.0961	0.3798
0.1069	0.0149	0.0409	0.0556	0.0676	0.2473
0.1122	0.0435	0.0570	0.0661	0.2045	0.2429
Age 105					
0.1185	0.0048	0.0131	0.2047	0.0356	0.0753
0.0367	0.1030	0.1467	0.0938	0.1456	0.1472
0.1069	0.0080	0.0358	0.0438	0.0548	0.2382
0.1049	0.0236	0.0883	0.0637	0.2163	0.2784

Third, we examined the linkage of disability with mortality at late ages. In a model describing the interaction of disability and mortality, there was a more rapid increase in mortality with age for whites than for blacks. This occurred for both males and females and was consistent with the higher disability found in blacks at later ages. The age at crossover in the NLTCS data was similar to ages found in extinct cohort analyses of death certificate data and Kestenbaum's (1992) matched record study.

Thus, we were able to examine three data elements (age trajectory of morbidity, mortality-morbidity linkages, and disability-mortality linkages) to develop a picture of U.S. racial differences in the age dependence of mortality, morbidity, and disability to extreme ages.

REFERENCES

Aronson, M.K., W.L. Ooi, H. Morgenstern, A. Hafner, D. Masur, H. Crystal, W.H., Frishman, D. Fisher, and R. Katzman
  1990   Women, myocardial infarction, and dementia in the very old. *Neurology* 40:1102-1106.
Ayanian, J.Z.
  1994   Race, class, and the quality of medical care. *Journal of the American Medical Association* 271(15):1207-1208.
Barker, D.J.P., K.M. Godfrey, C. Osmond, and A. Bul
  1992   The relation of fetal length, ponderal index and head circumference to blood pressure and the risk of hypertension in adult life. *Pediatric and Perinatal Epidemiology* 6:35-44.
Barker, D.J.P., T.W. Meade, C.H.D. Fall, A. Lee, C. Osmond, K. Phipps, and T. Stirling
  1992   Relation of fetal and infant growth to plasma fibrinogen and factor VII concentrations in adult life. *British Medical Journal* 304:148-152.
Becker, T.M., C.M. Wheeler, N.S. McGough, C.A. Stidley, C.A. Parmenter, M.H. Dorin, and S.W. Jordan
  1994   Contraceptive and reproductive risk for cervical dysplasia in Southwestern Hispanic and non-Hispanic white women. *International Journal of Epidemiology* 23(5):913-922.
Bild, D.E., A. Fitzpatrick, L.P. Fried, N.D. Wong, M.N. Hann, M. Lyles, E. Bovill, J.F. Polak, and R. Schulz
  1993   Age-related trends in cardiovascular morbidity and physical functioning in the elderly: The cardiovascular health study. *Journal of the American Geriatrics Society* 41:1047-1056.
Boult, C., R.L. Kane, T.A. Louis, and J.G. Ibrahim
  1991   Forecasting the number of future disabled elderly using Markovian and mathematical models. *Journal of Clinical Epidemiology* 44:973-980.
Bowden, M., J. Crawford, H.J. Cohen, and O. Noyama
  1993   A comparative study of monoclonal gammopathies and immunoglobulin levels in Japanese and United States elderly. *Journal of the American Geriatrics Society* 41:11-14.
Browner, W.S., A.R. Pressman, M.C. Nevitt, J.A. Cauley, and S.R. Cummings
  1993   Association between low bone density and stroke in elderly women: The study of osteoporotic fractures. *Stroke* 24:940-946.
Browner, W.S., D.G. Seeley, T.M. Vogt, and S.R. Cummings
  1991   Non-trauma mortality in elderly women with low bone density. *Lancet* 338:355-358.
Campbell, A.J., W.J. Busby, and C. Robertson
  1993   Over 80 years and no evidence of coronary heart disease: Characteristics of a survivor group. *Journal of the American Geriatrics Society* 41:1333-1338.
Carmelli, D., D. Robinette, and R. Fabsitz
  1994   Concordance, discordance and prevalence of hypertension in World War II male veteran twins. *Journal of Hypertension* 12:323-328.

Cauley, J.A., J.P. Gutai, L.H. Kuller, J. Scott, and M.C. Nevitt
  1994   Black-white differences in serum sex hormones and bone mineral density. *American Journal of Epidemiology* 139(10):1035-1046.
Caulfield, M., P. Lavender, M. Farrall, P. Munroe, M. Lawson, P. Turner, and A. Clark
  1994   Linkage of the angiotensinogen gene to essential hypertension. *New England Journal of Medicine* 330(23):1629-1633.
Centers for Disease Control and Prevention
  1994   Mortality from congestive heart failure—United States 1980-1990. *Journal of the American Medical Association* 271(11):813-814.
Chan, J., C. Cockram, M. Nicholls, C. Cheung, and R. Swaminathan
  1992   Comparison of enalapril and nifedipine in treating non-insulin dependent diabetes associated with hypertension: One year analysis. *British Medical Journal* 305:981-985.
Chapuy, M.C., M.E. Arlot, P.D. Delmas, and P.J. Meunier
  1994   Effect of calcium and cholecalciferol treatment for three years on hip fractures in elderly women. *British Medical Journal* 308:1081-1082.
Clark, D.O., T. Stump, and F. Wolinsky
  1996   Race and gender specific replication of five dimensions of health and disability. *American Journal of Public Health.*
Clark, D.O., and F. Wolinsky
  1996   Trends in disability and institutionalization among older blacks and whites. In review at *American Journal of Public Health.*
Colantonio, A., S.V. Kasl, and A.M. Ostfeld
  1992   Level of function predicts first stroke in the elderly. *Stroke* 23(9):1355-1357.
Cooper, R., and C. Rotimi
  1994   Hypertension in populations of West African origin: Is there a genetic predisposition? *Journal of Hypertension* 12:215-227.
Corder, E.H., H.A. Guess, B.S. Hulka, G.D. Friedman, M. Sadler, R.T. Vollmer, B. Lobaugh, M.K. Dreznar, J.H. Vogelman, and N. Orenteigh
  1993   Vitamin D and prostate cancer: A prediagnostic study with stored sera. *Cancer Epidemiology Biomarkers Prevention* 2:467-472.
Couderc, R., F. Mahieux, S. Bailleul, G. Fenelon, R. Mary, and J. Fermanian
  1993   Prevalence of apolipoprotein E phenotypes in ischemic cerebrovascular disease: A case-control study. *Stroke* 24(5):661-664.
Cowie, C.C., M.I. Harris, R.E. Silverman, E.W. Johnson, and K.F. Rust
  1993   Effect of multiple risk factors on differences between blacks and whites in the prevalence of non-insulin-dependent diabetes mellitus in the United States. *American Journal of Epidemiology* 137(7):719-732.
DeStefano, F., R.K. Merritt, R.F. Anda, M.L. Casper, and E.D. Eaker
  1993   Trends in nonfatal coronary heart disease in the United States, 1980 through 1989. *Archives of Internal Medicine* 153:2489-2494.
Dzau, V.
  1994   Cell biology and genetics of angiotensin in cardiovascular disease. *Journal of Hypertension* 12(suppl. 4):S3-S10.
Dzau, V., and R. Re
  1994   Tissue angiotensin system in cardiovascular medicine: A paradigm shift. *Circulation* 89(1):493-498.
Eastell, R., A.L. Yergery, N.E. Vieira, S.L. Cedel, R. Kumar, and B.L. Riggs
  1991   Interrelationship among vitamin D metabolism, true calcium absorption, parathyroid function, and age in women: Evidence of an age-related intestinal resistance to 1-25 dihydroxyvitamin A action. *Journal of Bone Mineral Research* 6:125.

Edelstein, S.L., and E. Barrett-Connor
1993   Relation between body size and bone mineral density in elderly and women. *American Journal of Epidemiology* 138(3):160-169.
Eggen, D.A., and L.A. Solberg
1968   Variation of atherosclerosis with age. *Laboratory Investigations* 18:571-579.
Eggen, D.A., J.P. Strong, and H.C. McGill
1965   Coronary calcification: Relationship to clinically significant coronary lesions and race, sex, and topographic distribution. *Circulation* 32:948-955.
Elledge, R.M., G.M. Clark, G.C. Chamness, and C.K. Osbourne
1994   Tumor biologic factors and breast cancer prognosis among white, Hispanic, and black women in the United States. *Journal of the National Cancer Institute* 86(9):705-712.
Ferrières, J., C.F. Sing, M. Roy, J. Davignon, and S. Lussier-Cacan
1994   Apolipoprotein E polymorphism and heterozygous familial hypercholesterolemia: Sex-specific effects. *Arteriosclerosis and Thrombosis* 14:1553-1560.
Feskens, E.J.M., and D. Kromhout
1994   Hyperinsulinemia, risk factors, and coronary heart disease: The Zutphen Elderly Study. *Arteriosclerosis and Thrombosis* 14:1641-1647.
Flegal, K., T.M. Ezzati, M.I. Harris
1991   Prevalence of diabetes in Mexican Americans, Cubans, and Puerto Ricans from the Hispanic Health and Nutrition Examination Survey, 1982-1989. *Diabetes Care* 14(suppl. 3):628-638.
Fogel, R.W.
1994   Economic growth, population theory, and physiology: The bearing of long-term processes on the making of economic policy. *American Economic Review* 84:369-395.
Fontbonne, A.
1991   Insulin: A sex hormone for cardiovascular risk? *Circulation* 84(3):1442-1444.
Fontbonne, A., G. Tchobroutsky, E. Eschwège, J.L. Richard, J.R. Claude, and G.E. Rosselin
1988   Coronary heart disease mortality risk: Plasma insulin level is a more sensitive marker than hypertension or abnormal glucose tolerance in overweight males. The Paris Prospective Study. *International Journal of Obesity* 12:557-565.
Gann, P.H., C.H. Hennekens, F.M. Sacks, F. Grodstein, E.L. Giovannucci, and M.J. Stampfer
1994   Prospective study of plasma fatty acids and risk of prostate cancer. *Journal of the National Cancer Institute* 86:281-286.
Gayton, J.R., G. Dahlen, W. Patsch, J.A. Kautz, and A.M. Gotto
1985   Relationship of plasma lipoprotein Lp(a) levels to race and to apolipoprotein B. *Arteriosclerosis* 5:265-272.
Ghali, J.K., R. Cooper, and E. Ford
1990   Trends in hospitalization rates for heart failure in the United States, 1973-1986. *Archives of Internal Medicine* 150:769-776.
Griendling, K., T. Murphy, and R. Alexander
1993   Molecular biology of the renin-angiotensin system. *Circulation* 87(6):1816-1828.
Grisso, J.A., J.L. Kelsey, B.L. Strom, L.A. O'Brien, G. Maislin, K. LaPann, L. Samelson, and S. Hoffman
1994   Risk factors for hip fracture in black women. *New England Journal of Medicine* 330(22):1555-1559.
Guccione, A.A., D.T. Felson, J.J. Anderson, J.M. Anthony, Y. Zhang, P.W.F. Wilson, M. Kelly-Hayes, P.A. Wolf, B.E. Kreger, and W.B. Kannel
1994   The effects of specific medical conditions on the functional limitations of elders in the Framingham Study. *American Journal of Public Health* 84:351-358.
Guralnik, J.M., K.C. Land, D. Blazer, G.G. Fillenbaum, and L.G. Branch
1993   Educational status and active life expectancy among older blacks and whites. *New England Journal of Medicine* 329(2):110-116.

Guzmán, M.A., C.A. McMahan, H.C. McGill, J.P. Strong, C. Tejada, C. Restrepo, D.A. Eggen, W.B. Robertson, and L.A. Solberg
1968 Selected methodologic aspects of the International Atherosclerosis Project. *Laboratory Investigations* 18:479-497.

Haffner, S.M., H.P. Hazuda, M.P. Stern, J.K. Patterson, W.A.J. Van Heuven, and D. Fong
1989 Effect of socioeconomic status on hyperglycemia and retinopathy levels in Mexican-Americans with NIDDM. *Diabetes Care* 12:128-134.

Harris, M.I., R. Klein, T.A. Welborn, and M.W. Knuiman
1992 Onset of NIDDM occurs at least 4 to 7 years before clinical diagnosis. *Diabetes Care* 15:815-819.

Heller, D.A., U. de Faire, N.L. Pedersen, G. Dahlén, and G.E. McClearn
1993 Genetic and environmental influences on serum lipid levels in twins. *New England Journal of Medicine* 328(16):1150-1156.

Helmhold, M., J. Bigge, R. Muche, J. Mainoo, J. Thiery, D. Seidel, and V.W. Armstrong
1991 Contribution of the apo(a) phenotype to plasma Lp(a) concentrations shows considerable ethnic variation. *Journal of Lipid Research* 32:1919-1928.

Hunter, C.P, C.K. Redmond, V.W. Chen, D.F. Austin, R.S. Greenberg, P. Correa, H.B. Muss, M.R. Forman, M.N. Wesley, R.S. Blacklow, R.J. Kurman, J.J. Dignam, B.K. Edwards, and S. Shapiro
1993 Breast cancer: Factors associated with stage at diagnosis in black and white women. *Journal of the National Cancer Institute* 85(14):1129-1137.

Jeunemaitre, X., F. Soubrier, Y.V. Kotelevstev, R.P. Lifton, C.S. Williams, A. Charru, S.C. Hunt, P.N. Hopkins, R.R. Williams, J.-M. Lalouel, and P. Corvol
1992 Molecular basis of human hypertension: Role of angiotensinogen. *Cell* 71:169-180.

Joffe, B.I., V.R. Panz, J.R. Wing, F.J. Raal, and H.C. Seftel
1992 Pathogenesis of non-insulin-dependent diabetes mellitus in the black population of southern Africa. *Lancet* 340:460-462.

Kahn, K.L., M.L. Pearson, E.R. Harrison, K.A. Desmond, W.H. Rogers, L.V. Rubenstein, R.H. Brook, and E.B. Keeler
1994 Health care for black and poor hospitalized Medicare patients. *Journal of the American Medical Association* 271(15):1169-1174.

Kaul, L., M.Y. Heshmat, J. Kovi, M.A. Jackson, A.G. Jackson, G.W. Jones, M. Edson, J.P. Enterline, R.G. Worrell, and S.L. Perry.
1987 The role of diet in prostate cancer. *Nutritional Cancer* 9:123-128.

Keene, G.S.
1993 Mortality and morbidity after hip fractures. *British Medical Journal* 307:1248-1250.

Keil, J.E., S.E. Sutherland, R.G. Knapp, D.T. Lackland, P.C. Gazes, and H.A. Tyroler
1993 Mortality rates and risk factors for coronary disease in black as compared with white men and women. *New England Journal of Medicine* 329:73-78.

Kellie, S.E., and J.A. Brody
1990 Sex specific and race specific hip fracture rates. *American Journal of Public Health* 80:326-380.

Kestenbaum, B.
1992 A description of the extreme aged population based on improved Medicare enrollment data. *Demography* 29(4):565-581.

Kiechl, S., F. Aichner, F. Gerstenbrand, G. Egger, A. Mair, G. Rungger, F. Spögler, E. Jarosch, F. Oberhollenzer, and J. Willeit
1994 Body iron stores and presence of carotid atherosclerosis: Results from the Bruneck Study. *Arteriosclerosis and Thrombosis* 14:1625-1630.

Knapp, R.G., S.E. Sutherland, J.E. Keil, P.F. Rust, and D.T. Lackland
1992 A comparison of the effects of cholesterol on CHD mortality in black and white women: Twenty-eight years of follow-up in the Charleston Heart Study. *Journal of Clinical Epidemiology* 45(10):1119-1129.

Ko, W., J.P. Gold, R, Lazzaro, J.A. Zelano, S. Lang, O.W. Isom, and K.H. Kreiger
   1992   Survival analysis of octogenarian patients with coronary artery disease managed by elec-
          tive coronary artery bypass surgery versus conventional medical treatment. *Circulation*
          86(suppl. II):191-197.
Kochanek, M.A., and B.L. Hudson
   1994   Advance report of final mortality statistics, 1992. *Monthly Vital Statistics Report* 43(6).
          Hyattsville, MD: National Center for Health Statistics.
Lakka, T.A., K. Nyyssonen, and J.T. Salonen
   1994   Higher levels of conditioning leisure time physical activity are associated with reduced
          levels of stored iron in Finnish men. *American Journal of Epidemiology* 140(2):148-160.
Launer, L.J., T. Harris, C. Rumpel, and J. Madans
   1994   Body mass index, weight change, and risk of mobility disability in middle-aged and older
          women. *Journal of the American Medical Association* 271(14):1093-1098.
Lew, E.A., and L. Garfinkel
   1990   Mortality after age 76 and older in the Cancer Prevention Study (CPSI). *CA: A Cancer
          Journal for Clinicians* 40:211-224.
Lin, R.S., W.C. Lee, Y.T. Lee, P. Chou, and C. Chung-Fu
   1994   Maternal role in type 2 diabetes mellitus: Indirect evidence for a mitochondrial inherit-
          ance. *International Journal of Epidemiology* 23(5):886-890.
Lindpaintner, K.
   1994   Genes, hypertension, and cardiac hypertrophy. *New England Journal of Medicine*
          330(23):1678-1679.
Lipton, R.B., Y. Liao, G. Cao, R.S. Cooper, and D. McGee
   1993   Determinants of incident non-insulin-dependent diabetes mellitus among blacks and
          whites in a national survey: The NHANES I epidemiologic follow-up study. *American
          Journal of Epidemiology* 138(10):826-839.
Löwick, M.R.H., J. Odink, F.J. Kok, and T. Ockhuizen
   1992   Hematocrit and cardiovascular risk factors among elderly men and women. *Gerontology*
          38:205-213.
MacMahon, B., P. Cole, and J. Brown
   1973   Etiology of human breast cancer: A review. *Journal of the National Cancer Institute*
          50:21-42.
Manton, K.G., L. Corder, and E. Stallard
   1993   Estimates of change in chronic disability and institutional incidence and prevalence rates
          in the U.S. elderly population from the 1982, 1984, and 1989 National Long Term Care
          Survey. *Journal of Gerontology Social Sciences* 47(4):S153-S166.
Manton, K.G., C.H. Patrick, and K. Johnson
   1987   Health differentials between blacks and whites: Recent trends in mortality and morbidity.
          Milbank Quarterly 65:129-199.
Manton, K.G., and E. Stallard
   1992   Demographics (1950-1987) of breast cancer in birth cohorts of older women. *Journal of
          Gerontology* 47(special issue):32-42.
   1996   Longevity in the U.S.: Age and sex specific evidence on life span limits from mortality
          patterns, 1960-1990. *Journal of Gerontology: Biological Sciences* 51A:B362-B375.
Manton, K.G., E. Stallard, and B. Singer
   1994   Projecting the future size and health status of the U.S. elderly population. Pp. 41-77 in
          Statistics of the Economics of Aging, D. Wise, ed., Chicago: University of Chicago Press.
Manton, K.G., E. Stallard, and M.A. Woodbury
   1995   Home health and skilled nursing facilities use: 1982 to 1990. *Health Care Financing
          Review* 16:155-186.

Manton, K.G., M.A. Woodbury, J.M. Wrigley, and H.J. Cohen
1991 Multivariate procedures to describe clinical staging of melanoma. *Methods of Information in Medicine* 30:111-116.

Marcovina, S.M., J.J. Albers, D.R. Jacobs, L.L. Perkins, C.E. Lewis, B.V. Howard, and P. Savage
1993 Lipoprotein[a] concentrations and apolipoprotein[a] phenotypes in Caucasians and Africans: The CARDIA study. *Arteriosclerosis and Thrombosis* 13:1037-1045.

Marenberg, M.E., N. Risch, L.F. Berkman, B. Floderus, and U. de Faire
1994 Genetic susceptibility to death from coronary heart disease in a study of twins. *New England Journal of Medicine* 330(15):1041-1046.

Mariotti, S., P. Sansoni, G. Barbesino, P. Caturegli, D. Monti, A. Cossarizza, T. Giacomelli, G. Passeri, U. Fagiolo, A. Pinchera, and C. Franceschi
1992 Thyroid and other organ-specific autoantibodies in healthy centenarians. *Lancet* 339:1506-1508.

Marshall, J.A., R.F. Hamman, J. Baxter, E.J. Mayer, D.L. Fulton, M. Orleans, M. Rewers, and R.H. Jones
1993 Ethnic differences in risk factors associated with the prevalence of non-insulin-dependent diabetes mellitus. *American Journal of Epidemiology* 137(7):706-718.

Materson, B., D. Reda, W. Cushman, B. Massie, E. Freis, M. Kochar, R. Hamburger, C. Fye, R. Lakshman, J. Gottdiener, E. Ramirez, and W. Henderson
1993 Single-drug therapy for hypertension in men: A comparison of six antihypertensive agents with placebo. *New England Journal of Medicine* 328(13):914-921.

Mathiesen, E., E. Hommel, J. Giese, and H. Parving
1991 Efficacy of captopril in postponing nephropathy in normotensive insulin dependent diabetic patients with microalbuminuria. *British Medical Journal* 303:81-87.

Matthews, K.A., R.R. Wing, L.H. Kuller, E.N. Meilahn, and P. Plantinga
1994 Influence of the perimenopause on cardiovascular risk factors and symptoms of middle-aged healthy women. *Archives of Internal Medicine* 154:2349-2355.

Mayberry, R., and C. Stoddard-Wright
1992 Breast cancer risk factors among black women and white women: Similarities and differences. *American Journal of Epidemiology* 136(12):1445-1456.

McCance, D., D. Pettitt, R. Hanson, L. Jacobsson, W. Knowler, and P. Bennett
1994 Birth weight and non-insulin dependent diabetes: Thrifty genotype, thrifty phenotype, or surviving small baby genotype? *British Medical Journal* 308:942-945.

McKeigue, P., A. Laws, Y. Chen, M. Marmot, and G. Reaven
1993 Relation of plasma triglyceride and Apo B levels to insulin-mediated suppression of nonesterified fatty acids: Possible explanation for sex differences in lipoprotein pattern. *Arteriosclerosis and Thrombosis* 13(8):1187-1192.

McKeigue, P.M., B. Shah, and M.G. Marmot
1991 Relation of central obesity and insulin resistance with high diabetes prevalence and cardiovascular risk in South Asians. *Lancet* 337:382-386.

Melby, C.L., M.L. Toohey, and J. Cebrick
1994 Blood pressure and blood lipids among vegetarian, semivegetarian, and nonvegetarian African Americans. *American Journal of Clinical Nutrition* 59:103-109.

Modan, M., H. Halkin, J. Or, A. Karaski, Y. Drory, Z. Fuchs, A. Lusky, and A. Chetrit
1991 Hyperinsulinemia, gender and risk of atherosclerotic cardiovascular disease. *Circulation* 84:1165-1175.

Moon, J., B. Bandy, and A. Davison
1992 Hypothesis: Etiology of atherosclerosis and osteoporosis: Are imbalances in the calciferol endocrine system implicated? *Journal of the American College of Nutrition* 11(5):567-583.

National Center for Health Statistics.
    1994   *Health, United States, 1994*. Hyattsville, MD: Public Health Service.
Okamoto, Y.
    1992   Health care for the elderly in Japan: Medicine and welfare in an aging society facing a
            crisis in long term care. *British Medical Journal* 305:403-405.
Ornish, D., S.E. Brown, L.W. Scherwitz, J.H. Billings, W.T. Armstrong, T.A. Ports, S.M.
McLanahan, R.L. Kirkeeide, R.J. Brand, and K.L. Gould
    1990   Can lifestyle changes reverse coronary heart disease? The Lifestyle Heart Trial. *Lancet*
            336:129-133.
Parra, H-J., I. Luyéré, C. Bouramoué, C. Demarquilly, and J-C. Fruchart
    1987   Black-white differences in serum Lp(a) lipoprotein levels. *Clinica Chimica Acta* 168:27-
            31.
Pathobiological Determinants of Atherosclerosis in Youth Research Group
    1993   Natural history of aortic and coronary atherosclerotic lesions in youth: Findings from the
            PDAY Study. *Arteriosclerosis and Thrombosis* 13(9):1291-1298.
Perez-Stable, E.J., R. Otero-Sabogal, F. Sabogal, S.J. McPhee, and R.A. Hiatt
    1994   Self-reported use of cancer screening tests among Latinos and Anglos in a prepaid health
            plan. *Archives of Internal Medicine* 154:1073-1081.
Perneger, T., M. Klag, H. Feldman, and P. Whelton
    1993   Projections of hypertension-related renal disease in middle-aged residents of the United
            States. *Journal of the American Medical Association* 269(10):1272-1277.
Perry, H., D. Miller, J. Morley, M. Horowitz, F, Kaiser, H. Perry Jr., J. Jensen, J. Bentley, S. Boyd,
and D. Kraenzle
    1993   A preliminary report of vitamin D and calcium metabolism in older Africans Americans.
            Journal of the American Geriatrics Society 41(6):612-616.
Peterson, E.D., S.M. Wright, J. Daley, and G.E. Thibault
    1994   Racial variation in cardiac procedure use and survival following acute myocardial infarc-
            tion in the Department of Veterans Affairs. *Journal of the American Medical Association*
            271:1175-1180.
Pollitzer, W.S., and J.B. Anderson
    1989   Ethnic and genetic differences in bone mass: A review with a hereditary vs. environmen-
            tal perspective. *American Journal of Clinical Nutrition* 50:1244.
Preston, S.H., I.T. Elo, I. Rosenwaike, and M. Hill
    1996   African-American mortality at older ages: Results of a matching study. *Demography*
            33:193-209.
Psaty, B., P. Savage, G. Tell, J. Polak, C. Hirsch, J. Gardin, and R. McDonald
    1993   Temporal patterns of antihypertensive medication use among elderly patients: The Car-
            diovascular Health Study. *Journal of the American Medical Association* 270(15):1837-
            1841.
Qualheim, R., S. Rostand, K. Kirk, and R. Luke
    1991   Changing patterns of end-stage renal disease due to hypertension. *American Journal of
            Kidney Disease* 18:336-343.
Radl, J., J.M. Sepers, F. Skvaril, A. Morell, and W. Hijmans
    1975   Immunoglobulin patterns in humans over 95 years of age. *Clinical Experimental Immu-
            nology* 22:84-90.
Ragland, K., S. Selvin, and D. Merrill
    1991   Black-white differences in stage-specific cancer survival: Analysis of seven selected
            sites. *American Journal of Epidemiology* 133:672-682.
Reed, T., J. Quiroga, J.V. Selby, D. Carmelli, J.C. Christian, R.R. Fabsitz, and C.E. Grim
    1991   Concordance of ischemic heart disease in the NHLBI twin study after 14-18 years of
            follow-up. *Journal of Clinical Epidemiology* 44:797-805.

Riggs, B.L., and L.J. Melton III
   1992   Drug therapy: The prevention and treatment of osteoporosis. *New England Journal of Medicine* 327(9):620-627.

Ross, R.K., and B.E. Henderson
   1994   Do diet and androgens alter prostate cancer risk via a common etiologic pathway? *Journal of the National Cancer Institute* 86(4):252-254.

Rotimi, C., R. Cooper, G. Cao, C. Sundarum, and D. McGee
   1994   Familial aggregation of cardiovascular diseases in African-American pedigrees. *Genetic Epidemiology* 11:397-407.

Rutan, G., L. Kuller, J. Neaton, D.N. Wentworth, R.H. McDonald, and W. McFate-Smith
   1988   Mortality associated with diastolic hypertension and isolated systolic hypertension among men screened for the Multiple Risk Factor Intervention Trial. *Circulation* 77(3):504-514.

Salive, M.E., J. Cornoni-Huntley, C.L. Philips, R.B. Wallace, A.M. Ostfeld, and H.J. Cohen
   1992   Anemia and hemoglobin levels in older persons: Relationship with age, gender, and health status. *Journal of the American Geriatrics Society* 40:489-496.

Salonen, J., K. Nyyssonen, H. Korpela, J. Tuomilehto, R. Seppanen, and R. Salonen
   1992   High stored iron levels are associated with excess risk of myocardial infarction in eastern Finnish men. *Circulation* 86(3):803-811.

Sandholzer, C., D.M. Hallman, N. Saha, G. Sigurdsson, C. Lackner, A. Császár, E. Boerwinkle, and G. Utermann
   1991   Effects of apolipoprotein(a) size polymorphism on the lipoprotein(a) concentration in 7 ethnic groups. *Human Genetics* 86:607-614.

Schaefer, E., S. Lamon-Fava, S. Johnson, J. Ordovas, M. Schaefer, W. Castelli, and P. Wilson
   1994   Effects of gender and menopausal status on the association of apolipoprotein E phenotype with plasma lipoprotein levels: Results from the Framingham Offspring Study. *Arteriosclerosis and Thrombosis* 14:1105-1113.

Schunkert, H., H.W. Hense, S.R. Holmer, M. Stender, S. Perz, U. Keil, B.H. Lovell, and G.A.Riegger
   1994   Association between a deletion polymorphism of the angiotensin-converting-enzyme gene and left ventricular hypertrophy. *New England Journal of Medicine* 330:1634-1638.

Seelig, M.S.
   1969   Vitamin D and cardiovascular, renal, and brain damage in infancy and childhood. *Annals of the New York Academy of Sciences* 147:537-582.

Selby, J.V., M.A. Austin, C. Sandholzer, C.P. Quesenberry, D. Zhang, E. Mayer, and G. Utermann
   1994   Environmental and behavioral influences on plasma lipoprotein(a) concentration in women twins. *Preventive Medicine* 23:345-353.

Sempos, C.T., J.I. Cleeman, M.D. Carroll, C.L. Johnson, P.S. Bachorik, D.J. Gordon, V.L. Burt, R.R. Briefel, C.D. Brown, K. Lippel, and B.M. Rifkind
   1993   Prevalence of high blood cholesterol among US adults: An update based on guidelines from the second report of the National Cholesterol Education Program adult treatment panel. *Journal of the American Medical Association* 269(23):3009-3014.

Sempos, C.T., R. Cooper, M.G. Kovar, and M. McMillen
   1988   Divergence of the recent trends in coronary mortality for the four major race-sex groups in the United States. *American Journal of Public Health* 78:1422-1427.

Sheu, W.H.H., S.M. Sheigh, M.M.T. Fuh, D.D.C. Shen, C.Y. Jeng, Y.D.I. Chen, and G.M. Reaven
   1993   Insulin resistance, glucose intolerance, and hyperinsulinemia: Hypertriglyceridemia versus hypercholesterolemia. *Arteriosclerosis and Thrombosis* 13(3):367-370.

Shintani, S., S. Kikuchi, H. Hamaguchi, and T. Shiigai
   1993   High serum lipoprotein(a) levels are an independent risk factor for cerebral infarction. *Stroke* 24(7):965-969.

Singh, J., A.W. Dudley, and K.A. Kulig

1990   Increased incidence of monoclonal gammopathy of undetermined significance in blacks and its age-related differences with whites on the basis of a study of 397 men and 1 woman in a hospital setting. *Journal of Laboratory Clinical Medicine* 116:785-789.

Singh, G.K., K.D. Kochanek, and M.F. McDonan

1996   Advance report of final mortality statistics, 1994. *Monthly Vital Statistics Report* 45(3 supp.). Hyattsville, MD: National Center for Health Statistics.

Skoog, I., L. Nilsson, B. Palmertz, L. Andreasson, and A. Svanborg

1993   A population-based study of dementia in 85-year-olds. *New England Journal of Medicine* 328(3):153-158.

Smith, S., S. Julius, K. Jamerson, J. Amerena, and N. Schork

1994   Hematocrit levels and physiologic factors in relationship to cardiovascular risk in Tecumseh, Michigan. *Journal of Hypertension* 12:455-462.

Social Security Administration

1992   *Life Tables for the United States Social Security Area 1900-2080.* Actuarial Study 107. SSA publication 11-11536. August. Baltimore, MD:Social Security Administration.

SOLVD Investigators

1991   Effect of enalapril on survival in patients with reduced left ventricular ejection fractions and congestive heart failure. *New England Journal of Medicine* 325(5):293-302.

Sorlie, P., E. Rogot, R. Anderson, N.J. Johnson, and E. Backlund

1992   Black-white mortality differences by family income. *Lancet* 340:346-350.

Srinivasan, S.R., G.H. Dahlen, R.A. Jarpa, L.S. Webber, and G.S. Berenson

1991   Racial (black-white) differences in serum lipoprotein(a) distribution and its relation to parental myocardial infarction in children: Bogalusa Heart Study. *Circulation* 84:160-167.

Stallard, E., and K.G. Manton

1995   The trajectory of mortality from age 80 to 110. Presented at the Southern Demographic Association Annual Meeting, October 19-20, 1995, Richmond, VA.

Strong, J.P.

1972   Atherosclerosis in human population. *Atherosclerosis* 16:193-201.

Strong, J.P., and H.C. McGill

1963   The natural history of aortic atherosclerosis: Relationship to race, sex, and coronary lesions in New Orleans. *Exploratory Molecular Pathology* (suppl.):15-27.

Sullivan, J.L.

1989   The iron paradigm of ischemic heart disease. *American Heart Journal* 117:1177-1188.

Sutherland, S., P. Gazes, J. Keil, G. Gilbert, and R. Knapp

1993   Electrocardiographic abnormalities and 30-year mortality among white and black men of the Charleston Heart Study. *Circulation* 88(6):2685-2692.

Svetkey, L.P., L.K. George, B.M. Burchett, P.A. Mortan, and D.G. Blazer

1993   Black/white differences in hypertension in the elderly: An epidemiologic analysis in central North Carolina. *American Journal of Epidemiology* 137:64-73.

Takata, H., M. Suzuki, T. Ishii, S. Sekiguchi, and H. Iri

1987   Influence of major histocompatability complex region genes on human longevity among Okinawan-Japanese centenarians and nonagenarians. *Lancet* 2:824-826.

Taussig, H.B.

1966   Possible injury to the cardiovascular system from vitamin D. *Annals of Internal Medicine* 65:1195-1200.

Taylor, H.A., B.R. Chaitman, W.J. Rogers, M.J. Kern, M.L. Terrin, F.V. Aguirre, G. Sopko, R. McMachon, R.N. Ross, E.C. Bovill, and TIMI investigators

1993   Race and prognosis after myocardial infarction: Results of the Thrombolysis in Myocardial Infarction (TIMI), phase II trial. *Circulation* 88:1484-1494.

Tiret, L., P. de Knijff, H.-J. Menzel, C. Ehnholm, V. Nicaud, and L.M. Havekes (for the EARS Group)
1994 ApoE polymorphism and predisposition to coronary heart disease in youths of different European populations: The EARS study. *Arteriosclerosis and Thrombosis* 14:1617-1624.

Trapido, E.J., F. Chen, K. Davis, N. Lewis, and J.A. MacKinnon
1994a Cancer among Hispanic males in south Florida. *Archives of Internal Medicine* 154:177-185.

Trapido, E., F. Chen, K. Davis, N. Lewis, J. MacKinnon, and P. Strait
1994b Cancer in south Florida Hispanic women: A 9-year assessment. *Archives of Internal Medicine* 154:1083-1088.

Trapido, E., C. McCoy, N. Stein, S. Engel, J. Zavertnik, and M. Comerford
1990 Epidemiology of cancer among Hispanic males. *Cancer* 65:1657-1662.

Valentine, R., P. Grayburn, G. Vega, and S. Grundy
1994 Lp(a) lipoprotein is an independent, discriminating risk factor for premature peripheral atherosclerosis among white men. *Archives of Internal Medicine* 154:801-806.

Wallace, D.C.
1992 Mitochondrial genetics: A paradigm for aging and degenerative diseases. *Science* 256:628-632.

White, P.
1994 Disorders of aldosterone biosynthesis and action. *New England Journal of Medicine* 331(4):250-258.

Williams, G.
1994 Management of non-insulin-dependent diabetes mellitus. *Lancet* 343:95-100.

Witteman, J., D. Grobbee, H. Valkenburg, A. van Hemert, T. Stijnen, H. Burger, and A. Hofman
1994 J-shaped relation between change in diastolic blood pressure and progression of aortic atherosclerosis. *Lancet* 343:504-507.

Yantani, R., I. Chigusa, K. Akazaki, G.N. Stemmermann, R.A. Welsh, and P. Correa
1982 Geographic pathology of latent prostatic carcinoma. *International Journal of Cancer* 29:611-616.

Yki-Järvinen, H.
1994 Pathogenesis of non-insulin-dependent diabetes mellitus. *Lancet* 343:91-94.

4

Race, Socioeconomic Status, and Health in Late Life

James P. Smith and Raynard S. Kington

INTRODUCTION

For over a hundred years, medical and social scientists have studied differences in health status among racial groups in the United States. The resulting literature has focused on comparisons between the health of white Americans and that of African Americans, a reflection of the historical and continued prominence of the debates over the status of African Americans in this society. In response to the growth of other racial and ethnic groups, comparisons have been broadened in recent years to include a growing literature addressing the relative health status of Hispanic, Asian, and Native American populations, but the literature remains dominated by black-white comparisons.

In the last 20 years, scientific inquiry has shifted from describing gross health disparities between the races to explaining the underlying factors that account for these differences. Understanding these underlying causes requires disentangling the complex web of factors connecting the nexus between race, socioeconomic status, and health. The more recent literature that has described this nexus has typically posed the research question as, "How much of the racial difference in health is directly accounted for by differences in socioeconomic status between populations?"

This paper has two interrelated goals. First, it examines racial and ethnic disparities in health outcomes among older Americans using two important new data sets: the Health and Retirement Survey (HRS) and the Asset and Health Dynamics Among the Oldest Old (AHEAD). Second, our research attempts to shed light on the central issue of the underlying causes of the strong relationship between socioeconomic status and health outcomes. The rest of this paper is divided into seven main sections. The first sketches the implications of the principal economic model that has been used to analyze health outcomes. The second section presents a brief review of the existing empirical literature on the relation of racial health disparities to socioeconomic status. Using HRS and AHEAD, the third section describes racial differences in a variety of health outcomes. A brief summary of the income and wealth/health gradients obtained from these data is provided in the fourth section. Using these same data, the fifth section highlights both racial and ethnic differences in health risks. The sixth and major section of the paper summarizes a series of empirical models of self-assessed health status. In particular, these models focus on understanding the reasons underlying the strong correlation between income and health and on the implications of that correlation for racial and ethnic health disparities. The final section presents conclusions.

THE THEORY OF HEALTH PRODUCTION AND ITS RELEVANCE TO SOCIOECONOMIC STATUS-RACE-HEALTH RESEARCH

Most of the research addressing the relationship of socioeconomic status, race, and health has been grounded in a theoretical framework based in sociology. In this framework, social class or socioeconomic status is a way of ranking relative position in a society based on class, status, and power (Liberatos et al., 1988). Only relatively recently have there been significant efforts to explain the well-known differences in health across socioeconomic groups explicitly based on the economic model of health, especially to non-economists (Selden, 1993; DaVanzo and Gertler, 1990; Dardanoni and Wagstaff, 1987; Wagstaff, 1986; Muurinen and Le Grand, 1985). Rarely have these analyses been extended to address the relationships among socioeconomic status, health, and race.

The standard economic model of health is based on a few key principles, largely developed by Grossman (1972). In the economic model, health is considered to be a commodity or "good" that can be viewed as a durable capital stock that produces a flow of services over time, depreciates, and can be increased with investment. Each individual begins life with a genetic health endowment. Choices made over the lifetime, such as the use of preventive medical services or smoking, can decrease or increase the health capital stock, but there are diminishing returns to investment in health. This capital can also be affected by random events that are not under the control of individuals.

There are a few important and distinct relationships that form the core of this model. First, there is the relationship between various inputs and the stock or commodity "health" (H_t). The inputs might include one's genetic or background endowment (G_o), health promoting activities and other behaviors such as smoking (B_t), use of medical care (MC_t), a vector of family education levels (ED), and environmental factors (E_t) such as the air pollution level. This relationship is described as the health production function:

$$H_t = f(H_{t-1}, G_o, B_t, MC_t, ED, E_t) \qquad (1)$$

Health changes over the life course, and the trajectory of these changes, are the result of a number of factors. In its most simple form, health in time period t, H_t, is the result of the stock of health in the period time period $t-1$, H_{t-1}, depreciation over the previous time period, and investments to improve health in the previous time period. This production function, which summarizes the transformation of these inputs into health outputs, is typically governed by biological considerations. Health is produced by a number of different inputs, including a wide variety of purchased medical inputs, the adoption of good personal health behaviors (exercise), and the avoidance of bad ones (smoking, excessive drinking).

These inputs, such as the demand for medical care, are "derived" demands: not valued directly but valued only because of their impact on health. Because the purchase of these inputs or the adoption of these health-related behaviors is a choice individuals or families can make, they are, in the parlance of economics, "endogenous" variables. In addition to purchased inputs and health behaviors, the stock of health may enter into the health production function. To put it simply, individuals in better health may be more able to translate other inputs into more productive health investments. Therefore, today's investments are influenced by today's health status and produce tomorrow's health status.

Education may enter this production function because it may affect the way individuals can transform inputs into good health. For example, more educated households may choose more qualified doctors, be more aware of the harmful health effects of behaviors such as smoking or environmental risks, or be better able to provide self-care to prevent illness or to mitigate its more harmful effects. Since some family members may be more adept at performing these functions than others, a vector of education levels of all family members is included in the production function.

Family background or genetic endowments (G_o), which are typically unobserved by the researcher, have played an important role in contemporary research on this topic. Rosenzweig and Schultz (1983) have argued that the existence of these unobserved background factors, which can often be traced to early childhood, may seriously bias estimates of this production function. For example, a person who has been generally sickly throughout life may require more medical care. If we do not control for this persistent unhealthiness, a regression of current health on medical services will understate the efficacy of medical care.[1]

---

[1]We do not deal with the important issue of family background effects in this paper. For a recent evaluation of the importance of family background on latter life health outcomes, see Smith and Kington (1996).

Another fundamental insight of the household production approach is that health is a stock. The current inputs and behaviors chosen are investments that produce increments to the stock of health. If these increments are affected by current inputs and current behaviors, today's stock of health is determined by the entire history of current and past inputs and behaviors. A corollary implication is that additional current economic resources are unlikely to have a quantitatively large impact on the current stock of health, especially in the age groups that are the focus of this research. Additional economic resources may increase health care utilization or induce good health behaviors, but these sorts of behavioral changes may be slow to be adopted. Even if these behaviors were altered instantaneously, they can have a direct impact only on health investments and not on health capital.

A second relationship describes the process underlying the behavioral choices that affect health. These choices are guided by a utility function (U) measured at the individual or household level. Health (H_t) is one commodity in the function, and X_t represents all other commodities that go into this utility function, U:

$$U = \int_0^T U_t e^{-rt} \text{ where } U_t = f(H_t, X_t) \tag{2}$$

Individuals or households maximize lifetime utility subject to a lifetime budget constraint. Thus, total expenditures across all periods on health- and non-health-related activities must not exceed total lifetime financial resources, Y; P is a vector of prices for non-health-related activities, P_H is a vector of health-related prices, and H_X is a vector of health-related activities:

$$Y = \int_0^T (W_t + R_t + T_t)e^{-rt} + A_o = \int_0^T (P * X_t + P_{Ht} * H_{Xt})e^{-rt} \tag{3}$$

Health is desired for two different but related purposes. Health has both consumption benefits (i.e., the benefit of feeling good) and production benefits (i.e., allowing one to engage in activities that produce income). Under utility maximization, individuals will invest in health until the gain in benefits from more health equals associated costs in terms of time or money.

Equation 3 highlights another central insight of this model. The budget constraint that limits household choices is a lifetime budget summarizing the discounted sum of lifetime income and current asset income. In general, households are not limited solely by their current-period resources. Financial resources in any period consist of the earnings W_t of all household members, retirement-related income R_t, government transfers T_t, and asset income A_t. Over the lifetime, these resources are spent on medical services and other desired commodities.[2]

---

[2]There is a similar constraint in time devoted to various activities. In order to maintain focus on the essential points, this equation is not discussed in the text.

An important consideration is that to different degrees and in different ways, each of these income sources may be affected by the stock of health. For example, earnings (W_t) in each period are a function of an individual's human capital and a set of local labor market demand and supply conditions (d_t). In this formulation, human capital is broadly defined to include health (H_t) and other forms of skills (K_t), including those formed in school and acquired during on-the-job training. Most directly, healthier people can work longer hours in any given week and more weeks during a year, which leads to higher earnings. Similarly, poor health may trigger the receipt of means-tested government transfer income, inducing a causation from health to income.

$$W_t = w(H_t, K_t, d_t) \qquad (4)$$

Equations 3 and 4 illustrate our central point that health enters into the model in two ways, producing a two-way causation between health and income. We have already seen that people desire good health as an outcome and that higher income enables them to purchase more of it. Current health also affects a person's ability to earn in some quite fundamental ways. As we have stated, healthier people can work longer hours in any given week and more weeks during a year. This "labor supply" effect leads to higher earnings. Similarly, healthier people may have more incentive to invest in other forms of human capital and therefore command higher wages in the labor market. While good health may facilitate the receipt of some income sources (earnings), it may discourage the receipt of others (transfers). Most of the applied health literature has emphasized the first pathway from income to health, but we will present evidence in this paper that the reverse pathway from health to income cannot be ignored.

Another relationship that flows from this approach is a series of derived demand functions for each input into the health production function. These input demand functions have as arguments all the input prices and the underlying determinants of the level of health demand, including household income and tastes. For example, the demand for medical care is a function of its own price (P_{mc}), the price of other inputs (P_o), education of each family member (ED), household resources (Y) and tastes (T).

$$MC = M(P_{mc}, P_o, ED, Y, T) \qquad (5)$$

As with all goods, an increase in the price of medical care will reduce the demand for it; however, as the price of other inputs change, the demand for medical care will increase or decline depending on whether these other goods are substitutes for medical care or complements to it. Education enters into these demand functions in part because it may affect the efficiency with which households can transform inputs into good health. Finally, household income acts as a scaler expanding the demand for health and thereby increasing the demand for the inputs used to produce good health. Whereas in most applications, the arguments in these input demand functions are taken to be exogenous, an important exception in our case is household income, which we have already argued has an important feedback relation from health to income.

The final equation in this system is the reduced-form demand function for health. The purpose of the reduced form is to solve out for the endogenous variables in the system by expressing health as a function of all the exogenous variables.

$$H_t = H^*(H_{t-1}, P_{mc}, P_o, ED, E_t, R_t, T_t, A_t, G_o) \qquad (6)$$

Equation 6 expresses current health as a function of all input prices and total household income. While this is a frequent expression of a reduced form, there are two issues with equation 6 that raise a concern. The first issue results from the inclusion of lagged health in the function. Last period's health is determined by last period's set of prices, so that current health is more correctly a function of all past prices. Secondly, there may exist important feedback relations from health to income. This second possibility is the central focus of this paper.

A reformulation of equation 6 highlights the empirical difficulties in uncovering the relation between socioeconomic status and health. Sequentially solving current health can be expressed as a function of all past prices and past incomes. This argument implies that equation 6 can be solved sequentially as

$$H_t = H^*(\tilde{P}_{mc}, \tilde{P}_o, ED, \tilde{E}_t, \tilde{R}_t, T_t, \tilde{A}_t, G_o) \qquad (7)$$

where the ~ indicates a time series vector of values.

Even this simple formulation highlights the extreme demands placed on data, especially cross-sectional surveys. To monitor the evolution of health outcomes over the life cycle, we would ideally like to know the entire lifetime sequence of health stocks, health behaviors, prices, and components of incomes and wealth. Although eventually the longitudinal nature of HRS and AHEAD will be an important step in that direction for an older population, such data do not currently exist. Consistent with the limitations imposed by current data, our aim here is a more modest but important step in the direction of understanding the reasons for the demographic and economic correlates of health outcomes at older ages. This step rests on the distinction between contemporaneous (current period) feedbacks from health to economic status and health behaviors and the full lifetime sequence of such feedback relationships. The full lifetime sequence of interactions between health and socioeconomic status is beyond the scope of our inquiry in this paper, and we concentrate instead on informing the nature of the possible contemporaneous feedbacks.

The Socioeconomic Status-Health Gradient

In the theoretical framework outlined above, socioeconomic status may affect health and health-related behaviors in many ways. At the most basic level, income and wealth determine the budget constraint: those who are poor have fewer resources to devote to health. As a result, they may purchase fewer medical services or be less able to afford medical insurance. From this view, health is no different than any other commodity such as housing, food, or entertainment— the more well-to-do consume more. If this were all there is, knowing the socioeconomic status-health gradient would require only the estimation of the wealth elasticity of health. In the computation of that elasticity, economic status should be defined as broadly as possible to include all income sources of all household members and wealth.

That is not all there is, largely owing to the real possibility of reverse causality or simultaneity bias. A large amount of the literature that has addressed the relationship between health and socioeconomic status has been based on cross-sectional data. Thus, these data have not allowed a simple but important question to be addressed: To what extent does low socioeconomic status lead to poor health rather than poor health's leading to low socioeconomic status? The ambiguity of the association between contemporaneous health and socioeconomic status is most obvious when income is the measure of socioeconomic status, and a classic example of the analytic issue illustrates the problem. There are two plausible explanations for the relationship between contemporaneously measured low income and poor health. First, low income may lead to poor health by, for example, limiting the use of preventive health care services as predicted in the economic model of health production. An alternate plausible explanation, however, is that poor health may lead to lower socioeconomic status by, for example, limiting an individual's ability to work or the wage he or she can earn.[3]

The statistical conditions for identification of the causal pathways are relatively easy to state and quite difficult to implement. For example, to statistically identify the pathway from health to income requires having exogenous variables that affect income only through their effect on health (that is, these variables have no direct effect on income). In this case, the health-income correlation induced by this variable only reflects a causal pathway from health to income. To use one illustration, a lower price of health care can directly affect health status through increased utilization of health care. Because health status is altered, there may also be subsequent alterations in household income. However, this lower price of health care should not have any direct impact on household income (outside of its

---

[3]The analogous statistical conceptualization of this problem is called simultaneity bias. Namely, estimation of relationships using standard statistical techniques may be biased if explanatory variables can be a consequence as well as a cause of the dependent variable such as health (Garber, 1989).

influence on health care). In this case, variation in the price of health care can be used to identify the causal pathway from health to income.[4]

Unfortunately, our current data sources do not contain the type of statistical variation that would allow us to formally identify the causal pathways. Consistent with the limitations imposed by current data, our aim here involves a more modest but important step toward understanding the health-socioeconomic status nexus. This step rests first on a distinction between contemporaneous (current period) feedbacks from health to economic status and health behaviors and the full lifetime sequence of such feedback relationships. While our cross-sectional data imply that unraveling the full lifetime interrelated sequences is beyond our scope, our rich array of economic, demographic, health behavior and outcome data allows us to make progress on the contemporaneous relationships.

Our research strategy begins with a separation of household income into its important components. We argue a priori that some of these income components largely reflect causation from health to income. After these contaminated components are separated out, it is more likely that the other income components will reflect a pathway from income to health. At a minimum, this empirical strategy can serve as an important diagnostic device about the relative importance of the two pathways that connect income and health. For example, both HRS and AHEAD allow us to separate income into its distinct components. Some of these income components are strongly affected by contemporaneous feedbacks from health to economic status. Past the retirement age, other income components are largely free of these feedbacks so that, at a minimum, we are able to mitigate the contemporaneous feedbacks from health to income.

There are a number of other possible sources of bias that complicate the estimation of the effect of socioeconomic status on health. For example, financial status may also determine where one lives, which may be related to a range of exogenous factors from the quality of health providers to exposure to air pollution and toxic waste to public expenditures on prevention of communicable diseases. Although environmental factors are often considered to be exogenous, in fact residence may also be a choice partly determined by such factors as regional health risks (Preston and Taubman, 1994).

Financial status may also affect one's choices for such activities as smoking or exercise by determining opportunity sets for the trade-offs between alternative utility-increasing or utility-decreasing activities and the associated increases or decreases in health risk (Muurinen and Le Grand, 1985). For example, individuals clearly derive some benefit from smoking. A person with limited alternative resources to satisfy such needs may be more willing to accept the health risks associated with smoking. Uncertainty may also play a role in explaining differences in investments in health across socioeconomic groups. Early models of

---

[4]A completely symmetrical argument exists for the identification of the pathway from income to health.

investment suggested that the poor may invest less in prevention, because greater risk aversion among the poor may push them away from relatively riskier investments in health capital (Dardanoni and Wagstaff, 1987). However, more recent extensions of the models suggest that there may be a countervailing incentive for the poor to invest in health because they are less able to afford losses in income because of ill health (Selden, 1993).

Measurement of Socioeconomic Status

In studies of the impact of socioeconomic status on health, education, occupation, and financial resources have typically been used as proxies. How each is defined may affect analyses of the race-socioeconomic status-health nexus in late life. If these variables are imprecisely measured, incorrect conclusions may be drawn about the relationships among the variables (Garber, 1989). In this section, we briefly discuss some of the major issues that arise with each proxy.

Education

Education is an important explanatory variable in both economic and sociological-based empirical models of the socioeconomic status-health relationship. As is demonstrated in the theoretical model outlined above, education may affect health status through a number of channels. First, schooling is an important determinant of economic status. Individuals with more schooling in general have significantly higher lifetime wealth than those with less schooling. In addition, schooling may alter the efficiency of health production—that is, the efficiency of the process by which the various inputs are transformed into health. For example, better educated individuals may have more information at their disposal about the effect of nutrition on health and may thus make healthier choices in eating habits.

An often-cited advantage of education as a proxy for socioeconomic status is that decisions about education are usually completed by early adulthood. This temporal ordering is taken to imply that schooling is free of reverse causality (i.e., not a result of poor health). While there is some truth to this argument, it applies only for health conditions that are unanticipated at the time schooling decisions are made. If poor health conditions are known, they will generally influence investments in schooling since future work effort will be lower owing to poor health. Socioeconomic status may also be related to so-called third factors affecting health investments (e.g., preventive activities). For example, education may be related to one's willingness to invest in health now by giving up something else in order to have an improvement in health in the future (Fuchs, 1982).

The imprecise measurement of education may be especially relevant when race is added to the relationship.[5] In the United States, simple counts of years of educational attainment present problems because historically there have been large differences in the content and quality of education between races. These differences are probably greatest among the current generation of elderly, many of whom were born into a rigidly segregated society with large racial differences in public investment in education (Smith, 1984).

Financial Resources

The measurement of financial resources presents even more challenges. Most studies in the health literature have measured financial resources with some form of individual or household/family income in the year of or the year before a cross-sectional survey, sometimes called contemporaneous income. There are several potential problems with the use of contemporaneous income as a measure of financial resources. First, income in a single year may not adequately measure the financial resources available to an individual over the lifetime in which decisions affecting health are made. This timing issue is different from the reverse causation question and may be even more important in late life. It may be especially important in assessing the comparative health status of currently older blacks versus whites because of the large changes in the relative income of blacks versus whites that have occurred over their lifetimes.

Second, income may not be the best measure of economic resources among older individuals, especially those who are retired. Instead, wealth may be a far better proxy for their command over economic resources. Income is typically lower after retirement than before. In the extreme, an older person may be worth a million dollars and simply live off this principal with no income. Wealth captures an important dimension of financial resources because it may be a indicator of long-run income. The distinction between income and wealth may be especially critical for understanding racial health disparities because racial differences in wealth are even greater than in income.[6]

Some studies have simplified the measurement of financial resources by translating contemporaneous income into a dichotomous variable indicating whether a household's income is above or below the federally defined poverty line. This is in general a mistake because it substitutes a political concept for a scientific construct. One potential problem with this practice is that income effects are known to extend across the spectrum of income even into high-income

---

[5]Education is generally measured in years of education attained. The effects of education on such outcomes as income are typically not linear. Analogously, flexibility in the form of the effect of education on health should be permitted. For example, attainment could be expressed in categories such as high school graduate, college graduate, and so forth.

[6]Finally, regional differences in costs of living (Liberatos et al., 1988) also have an impact on the significance of income. To the extent to which there are racial differences in geographic distribution, failure to control for geographic location may bias estimates of the racial differences in the relationships among race, socioeconomic status, and health.

ranges. Dichotomizing income may lead to incorrect conclusions about the relationships among race, health, and income. For example, blacks are much more likely to have income near the poverty level. Thus, a multivariate analysis that simply includes a poverty dummy may result in a still significant race dummy effect even in the absence of a real racial difference because the range of upper level income and the corresponding variation in health in the wealthier white population are not accounted for.

Occupation

A final measure of socioeconomic status that has been commonly used, especially by sociologists, is occupation.[7] One reason for this is that occupation is arguably a better measure of long-run economic status than current income is. Whatever the traditional merit of this argument, it is certainly mitigated when data sets contain measures of wealth and long-run time series on income. There are some other problems that may affect the interpretation of occupation. In comparisons across racial and ethnic groups with different status rankings of occupations, a particular occupation may translate into a different status in a community depending on the racial composition of the community. Second, broad groupings of occupation may not capture significant variation within occupational categories. Third, there is controversy over how one measures occupation in late life. For example, for many important occupational health exposures (e.g., the relationship between asbestos and lung cancers), the temporal relationship between the exposure and the outcome is distant. Thus, for studies of racial differences in the relationship between health and occupation in late life, it is especially unclear which occupation is most appropriate. Occupational categories may also present added problems in the context of the socioeconomic status-race-health analysis because there may be differences between races in exposures and treatment of persons in the same occupational category.

The Race Connection

The Role of Race

Typically, race per se has not been explicitly analyzed in the context of an economic model of health production. The reasons for the failure to explicitly incorporate race into this framework remain unclear. In one standard textbook of

---

[7]Although occupation has historically been an important measure of socioeconomic status for sociological studies, it has been relatively less important in the economic literature on health. Occupation is related to a number of important factors in health in late life. First, occupation is related to occupational injuries and exposures that have an impact on health. Second, occupation is related to both education and income.

health economics, for example, the author concludes that so-called cultural-demographic variables are not typically the focus of economic models of health because they do not change rapidly in a population and are not the instrument of public policy (Feldstein, 1983). Clearly, government policy cannot change race, as, for example, government taxation policy can change the income distribution. But race directly or indirectly is often used to target government policies in health care. For example, *Healthy People 2000* (U.S. Department of Health and Human Services, 1990), the federal government's most comprehensive statement on health objectives for the country, includes numerous race-specific health objectives. Furthermore, race may have indirectly many of the same effects that socioeconomic status has directly, and the government has a major role in policies that affect race-based behaviors such as job discrimination. For example, racial discrimination in hiring may affect job choices that are in turn associated with risks of injury or toxic exposure, and prevention of racial discrimination in hiring is very much a government policy.

The economic model may serve as a framework for assessing many aspects of the relationships among race, socioeconomic status, and health. For example, race may affect the health production function per se independently of any race-related genetic or biological predispositions to certain diseases. Studies have described subtle racial differences in the effectiveness of certain drugs in the treatment of hypertension, possibly related to racial differences in the pathophysiology of hypertension (see review in Kaplan, 1994). These differences might lead one to predict differences in the demand for these treatments by race by affecting the trade-off between marginal benefits and marginal costs of treatment. Although the actual physiological differences may be minimal, racial differences in the perceptions of efficacy of treatment may lead to similar results.

Race remains an important factor in residential patterns in the United States (Massey and Denton, 1989). Area of residence may in turn determine a range of health-related factors such as supply of and distance to health providers and environmental pollution. Race and racial discrimination may also play a role in other factors such as time preferences and risk aversion, which may in turn affect investments in health. Clearly, the application of an economic framework may provide new, complementary insights into the relationships among race, socioeconomic status, and health.

The race-health relationship is distinguished from the socioeconomic status-health relationship in two ways. First, legitimately or not, race is often assumed to include at least some biological or genetic component. Most researchers no longer consider genetic or biological differences to be important factors in explaining differences in health among groups of varying socioeconomic status. In support of the position that genetics and biological factors do not play a large role in explaining race differences in health, researchers (Williams et al., 1984; Krieger et al., 1993) point to the literature that has suggested that racial classifications account for only small amounts of the human genetic diversity (e.g., Lewontin, 1972; see also Neel, this volume). A frequently mentioned example of a disease that has a genetically based difference in rates between races is sickle cell anemia, but even this example may be flawed. Sickle cell anemia is in fact well described in white populations (Serjeant, 1985), and the higher rates in blacks may have more to do with geography than genetics per se (e.g., Williams, 1994).

The second important distinction is that race has meant more than just socioeconomic status in the United States in light of the extensive degree to which race has determined an individual's set of life opportunities independently of socioeconomic status as traditionally defined. For example, for many older African Americans, high education and even high income did not necessarily translate into differences in how one was treated in daily life in large sections of the country; this might have implications for health via proposed influences of stress. Thus, there are added dimensions to the race-health relationship that are often difficult to measure.

To add an additional layer of complexity to the socioeconomic status-health-race literature, there may be important cohort differences in what race has meant in this country. During the life course of the current population of older African Americans, there have been dramatic changes in the opportunities for and the treatment of African Americans in this society. These changes have produced potentially important cohort effects that may confound other factors—especially age—important to understanding racial differences in health.

Measurement of Race

Over the last several years there has been growing interest in the health literature on how researchers measure race (Williams et al., 1984; LaViest, 1994; Hahn, 1992; Osborne and Feit, 1992; Jones et al., 1991; Cooper, 1986). There are two general methods of measuring race: self-report and observation. Most categorizations typically distinguish between race (usually African American, white, Asian) and ethnicity (usually Hispanic or not). Although there are theoretical arguments that may support the use of self-reports versus observational measures, the number of discordant classifications is probably minimal for data on blacks and whites. Furthermore, the importance of the measurement of race as a potential source of bias may change as the number of acknowledged interracial births grows and the life experiences and attitudes of individuals become more diverse with respect to racial identity (e.g., young people who would be traditionally classified as "black" being raised in entirely white communities and who may or may not identify as black and whose experiences may differ from those of most blacks in terms of stress, etc.).

In the next section we review recent major studies that have addressed the relationship among health, race, and socioeconomic status and present new findings from analyses of data from the HRS and the AHEAD surveys.

RACE, SOCIOECONOMIC STATUS, AND HEALTH STATUS: EXISTING EMPIRICAL EVIDENCE

In this section, we briefly review key studies that have specifically addressed the role of socioeconomic status in explaining racial differences in health, with a focus on health in late life. Any review of this issue is complicated because health status is multifaceted. Because mortality is among the broadest and most studied traditional measures of health status, this literature is summarized first. We then review relevant studies that have used other measures of health status in assessing the role of socioeconomic status in explaining racial differences in health. Finally, our findings from analyses of recently available data on health status from the HRS and the AHEAD surveys are presented.

Mortality

The literature on racial comparisons of mortality in the United States dates to over a hundred years ago. In almost every study, African Americans have been shown to have higher rates of mortality than white Americans (Ewbank, 1987).[8] Although even the earliest research proposed socioeconomic status as a major factor explaining racial health disparities, only within the last two decades have there been high-quality longitudinal data sets that provide important information on the temporal relationship between ill health or death and socioeconomic status. Table 4-1 summarizes the results of some key studies that over the last decade have assessed the contribution of socioeconomic status to racial differences in mortality. All except one are based on longitudinal data. This research varies widely along several dimensions, but the conclusions are similar. Most if not all of the racial differences in mortality appear to be related to differences in socioeconomic status.[9] In several studies in fact, there was no statistically significant racial difference once socioeconomic status was controlled for (Kaplan et al., 1987; Keil et al., 1992; Rogers, 1992; Zick and Smith, 1991).

The uniformity of this conclusion is impressive in light of the enormous diversity in study samples and in measures of socioeconomic status. For example, several data sets were restricted to a single geographic area,[10] and among those with national samples, only one controlled for geographic region and

---

[8]Almost all of the early studies used census data.

[9]It was not always possible to estimate from the published results a measure of how much of the racial variation was accounted for by socioeconomic status, but when this was published explicitly, the percentage explained was over 60 percent.

[10]North Carolina in Guralnik et al., 1993b; Charleston, South Carolina, in Keil et al., 1992; Alameda County, California, in Kaplan et al., 1987.

TABLE 4-1 Race, Socioeconomic Status and Health in Late Life: Selected Studies of Total Mortality and Life Expectancy

Author/Year	Data Set	Outcome/ Statistical Method	Explanatory Variables	Racial Differences Explained
Guralnik et al. (1993b)	PHSE 1986-1988; N = 4,057 55% black; age $\geq$ 65 yrs. at baseline	Total life expectancy; multistate life tables stratified	Age, education, gender	Most
Menchik (1993)	NLSMM 1966-1983; N = ~4,000[a] male; mean age 51 yrs. at baseline	Total mortality; logistic regression	Age, marital status, parent education, net worth (1966), no. of yrs. in poverty region, urban, health status (1966)	75%
Keil et al. (1992)	CHS 1960-1988; N = 1,088 40% black; age 35-74 yrs. at baseline	Total mortality; age-adjusted deaths/1,000 person-years stratified	Age, high/low SES (education and occupation)	100%
Rogers (1992)	Merged NHIS 1986; N = 37,917 and NMFS 1986; N = 18,733 ~11% black; age $\geq$ 25 yrs.	Total mortality 1986; logistic regression	Age, gender, marital status, family size, family income (categories)	100%
Sorlie et al. (1992)	NLMS 1978-1985; N = ~ 550,000 10% black; age $\geq$ 25 yrs. at baseline	Total mortality; Cox proportional hazards by age, gender	Age, sex, labor force participation, family income (categories)	$\geq$ age 65, 100%
Berman et al. (1991)	RHS 1969-1976; N = 1,384 50% black; age 58-63 yrs. at baseline	Total mortality; several alternative hazard models	Age, education, marital status, personal income (1977), social security benefits, SSI, dependent children	60-80%

TABLE 4-1   Continued

Author/Year	Data Set	Outcome/ Statistical Method	Explanatory Variables	Racial Differences Explained
Zick and Smith (1991)	PSID 1968-1984; ~7-8% black; N = 1,990 mean age ~50 yrs. (among person years)	Total mortality; logistic regression	Age, education, sex, employed, marital status, poverty	No race difference in multi-variate analysis (race not focus of study)
Otten et al. (1990)	NHANES I 1971-1984; N = 8,806 14% black; age 25-77 yrs. at baseline	Total mortality; Cox proportional hazard	Age, sex, family income, risk factors: smoking, alcohol, BP, DM, cholesterol, BMI	69% (income and risk factors)
Kaplan et al. (1987) [also Haan and Kaplan (1985)]	HPL's Alameda County Study 1965-1982; N = 4,174[a] age 60-94 yrs. at baseline	Total mortality; Cox proportional hazard	Age, sex, household size, adjusted total income	No racial difference adjusted or unadjusted

[a]Unable to determine percentage by race in sample
Note: PHSE = Piedmont Health Survey of Elderly; NLSMM = National Longitudinal Survey of Mature Men; CHS = Charleston Heart Study; NHIS = National Health Interview Survey; NMFS = National Mortality Followback Survey; NLMS = National Longitudinal Mortality Study; SSI = Supplemental Security Income; RHS = Retirement History Survey; PSID = Panel Study of Income Dynamics; NHANES I = National Health and Nutrition Examination Survey I; BP = Blood Pressure; BMI = Body Mass Index; DM = diabetes mellitus; HPL = Human Population Laboratory; SES = socioeconomic status.

urbanicity (Menchik, 1993). Most projects had total sample sizes of over 1,000, with the percentage black (when it was reported) ranging from 10 percent to over 50 percent. However, the time span covered varied from 1 to 18 years, with the earliest period of observation beginning in 1960. Similarly, these representative research projects differed considerably in how they defined socioeconomic status. While all controlled for at least age, gender,[11] and education, there was considerable variation in proxies for socioeconomic status beyond that. Two studies (Guralnik et al., 1993b; Keil et al., 1992) had no measure of financial

---

[11]Two analyses were restricted to men (Keil et al., 1992; Menchik, 1993).

resources and only one (Menchik, 1993) included net worth at baseline as a proxy for wealth.

Contemporaneous income for the baseline year computed at the family or household level was the typical income construct (Kaplan et al., 1987; Rogers, 1992; Sorlie et al., 1992; Otten et al., 1990), but some studies apparently used individual incomes (e.g., Menchik, 1993). There was further variation in the measurement of contemporaneous income. For example, some authors adjusted family income by size of household (e.g., Kaplan et al., 1987), while Berman et al. (1991) defined several variables, including personal income, the receipt of Social Security benefits, and the receipt of Supplemental Security Income. However, this diversity in study populations and explanatory variables did not produce great differences in the primary finding across studies confirming the prominent role of socioeconomic status in explaining racial differences in total mortality.

General Health Status, Functional Status, and Morbidity

Mortality is at best a crude indicator of the health status of a population because it fails to capture the overall burden of poor health. This limitation may be especially significant for older populations, where rates of poor functional status may be very high. Measures of general health status fall into three broad categories: (1) self-reports of general health or specific dimensions of health or function, (2) observed indicators of health and function, and (3) the presence of disease (morbidity). Each captures a different dimension of health and raises a unique set of issues. For example, one potential problem with self-reported health is that people may implicitly compare their health with that of those around them. Thus, people who live in communities with poor health may rate their health higher than people with the same general health status in a different community with better average health. Research comparing the health status of different racial groups has used a wide variety of outcome measures, but probably the most common measure of health status is self-reported general health on a scale of excellent, very good, good, fair, and poor. In this review, we focus on self-reported measures of general health and function in discussing the relative contribution of socioeconomic status to racial differences in health.

By most measures of general health status, blacks in late life have worse health than whites. For example, analysis of the 1986 National Health Interview Survey (NHIS) revealed that blacks over age 65 were more likely to report their health as poor or fair.[12] Comparing black and white elderly in functional status points to similar conclusions. For example, fewer blacks than whites remain independent in activities of daily living and instrumental activities of daily living;

---

[12]The percentages were 44.7 percent and 46.9 percent for black males and females, respectively, and 29.8 percent and 28.8 percent for white males and females, respectively (Mermelstein et al., 1993).

this was true for both men and women above age 65 (Furner, 1993). Among community residents, black elderly report a larger number of functional impairments (Macken, 1986; Manton et al., 1987; Kington and Smith, in press).

The relative health and functional status of black and white elderly is not uniform across older populations. Gibson reviewed several national studies of racial differences in the health of older adults and noted the frequent finding that the black disadvantage in health and function was greater among younger elderly than among older elderly (Gibson, 1991). For example, using data from the 1982 National Long Term Care Survey, Manton and colleagues found that the black-white ratio for total disability was 1.81 among persons 65 to 74 but only 1.22 among persons 74-84 (Manton et al., 1987). Several potential explanations have been proposed for this race-age interaction, including selective survival of healthier blacks (e.g., see the discussion in Gibson, 1991), but the patterns suggest a more complex story than simply worse health for older blacks compared with whites.

Compared with white elderly, black elderly also have worse health in terms of morbidity. Black elderly have higher rates of several important causes of poor health and poor functioning such as hypertension, diabetes, and arthritis (Furner, 1993; Blesch and Furner, 1993). For some conditions, however, black elderly have lower rates than white elderly. For example, a lower rate for broken hips among black women, possibly related to lower rates of osteoporosis among black women, is well described (Kellie and Brody, 1990). A recent analysis of stroke incidence over a year found lower rates for blacks over 75 and higher rates below 75 (Broderick et al., 1992), while prevalence studies have found higher rates of stroke or "cerebrovascular disease" among older blacks (e.g., Schoenberg et al., 1986).

Relatively few studies have attempted to describe explicitly the amount of variation among racial groups in health and functional status that is accounted for by socioeconomic status. Table 4-2 summarizes results from several studies that have assessed the contribution of socioeconomic status to observed racial differences in function and, like the analyses we present in later sections, are based on cross-sectional data.

The range of measures of general health and function compared with mortality makes it more difficult to summarize these findings succinctly. For example, the variation explained by socioeconomic status often depended on how health status was measured. This research also exhibited diversity along other dimensions, including the measurement of financial resources, the age groups considered, and geographic scope. In general, the literature suggests that a significant amount, but definitely not all, of racial differences in health status are attributable to differences in socioeconomic status.[13]

---

[13]Unlike the mortality studies, few of these studies were presented in such a way as to allow easy estimation of the amount of the variation that was accounted for by socioeconomic status when a race residual effect remained.

TABLE 4-2   Race, Socioeconomic Status, and Health in Late Life: Selected
Cross-Sectional Studies of General Health and Functional Status

Author/Year	Data Set	Outcome/ Statistical Method	Explanatory Variables	Racial Differences Explained
Mutchler and Burr (1991)	SIPP 1984; $N = 9,803$ 9% black; age $\geq$ 55 yrs.	Self-reported general health, mobility index; ADLs, bed days, logistic and Tobit regressions	Age, sex, education, income (for couple if married), and net worth (logged), region	100% for mobility index; ADLs, bed days; less for general health
House et al. (1990)	ACL 1986; $N = 3,617$ age $\geq$ 25 yrs.[a] (oversampled blacks, $\geq$ 60 yrs.) NHIS 1985: $N = 55,690$ age $\geq$ 25 yrs.[a]	ACL: chronic medical conditions; functional status index; self-rated health limitations NHIS: chronic conditions; limitations on major activities scale; ordinary least squares regressions	Age, sex, marital status, education, income	ACL: 100% for functional status index; less for medical conditions; no unadjusted difference in limitations NHIS: reported "similar" results (regressions not presented)
Ferraro (1987)	CPS subsample of SLIAD 1973; $N = 3,183$ 10% black; age $\geq$ 65 yrs. (low and middle income only)	Self-reported general health; physical disability index; OLS regressions	Age, sex, education, chronic conditions, serious illness	Blacks worse health after controls
Satariano (1986)	Survey Alameda County, CA 1979-1980; $N = 906$ 35% blacks; age $\geq$ 20 yrs. (27% $\geq$ 60 yrs.)	Self-reported general health index; ANOVA	Age, sex, occupation, education, family income (categories)	100% with income adjustment

TABLE 4-2   Continued

Author/Year	Data Set	Outcome/ Statistical Method	Explanatory Variables	Racial Differences Explained
Dowd and Bengtson (1978)	Survey Los Angeles County, CA 1974; $N = 1,269$ age ≥ 45 yrs.; 32% black, 35% Mexican American	Self-reported general health; Multiple Classification Analysis	Age, sex, occupational prestige (Duncan), family income (categories)	Blacks, Mexican Americans in worse health after controls

[a]Unable to determine percentage by race in sample.

Note: SIPP = Survey of Income and Program Participation; ADL = Activity of Daily Living; ACL = Americans Changing Lives Survey; NHIS = National Health Interview Survey; CPS = Current Population Survey; OLS = ordinary least squares; ANOVA = analysis of variance; SLIAD = Survey of Low-Income Aged and Disabled; SES = socioeconomic status.

Several national studies are especially noteworthy. First, Mutchler and Burr (1991), using data from the 1984 Survey of Income and Program Participation (SIPP) for people over age 55, compared self-reported general health, limitations in activities of daily living, and a multi-item mobility index for blacks and whites. Age, sex, education, income (defined at the couple level if the person surveyed was married), and net worth accounted for almost all of the racial difference with the exception of general health perceptions. This analysis was unusual because it is one of the few studies of racial differences in general health status that controlled for wealth. Using 1973 data on a sample of people over 65 years old, Ferraro (1987) found persistent racial differences in subjective health and disability after controlling for age, education, illness, and chronic conditions.

Other notable studies in this area have covered the full range of adults from young age to old age. House and colleagues (1990) analyzed data from the 1986 Americans' Changing Lives (ACL) survey. When age, sex, education, marital status, and income were controlled, among adults over age 25, race was not a significant predictor of functional status or limitation in daily activities, but was associated with a larger number of chronic conditions. Satariano (1986), however, found that racial differences in the health status of a sample from Alameda County, California, above age 20 were entirely explained by age, occupation, sex, education, and family income.

A growing number of longitudinal studies of functional status have found that varying amounts of the racial differences in function are explained by socioeconomic status. Several studies have found that most of the racial disparity is explained by socioeconomic status (Mor et al., 1989; Clark and Maddox, 1992; Guralnik, Land, et al., 1993), while other studies have found that significant

TABLE 4-3   Distribution of Population by Self-Assessed Health Status

Self-Assessed Health Status	Men White (%)	Black (%)	Women White (%)	Black (%)
	HRS (Ages 51-61)			
Excellent	23.3	13.5	25.1	9.8
Very good	27.9	20.8	29.5	22.4
Good	28.8	30.6	25.8	33.1
Fair	12.3	22.5	14.3	22.7
Poor	7.7	12.6	6.7	12.0
	AHEAD (Ages 70 and Over)			
Excellent	11.7	7.6	11.5	4.8
Very good	22.9	14.0	24.4	18.1
Good	32.0	28.0	30.1	27.6
Fair	21.0	30.0	22.5	29.7
Poor	12.5	20.4	11.5	19.7

SOURCE: Health and Retirement Survey (HRS) data for 1993 and data from Assets and Health Dynamics of the Oldest Old (AHEAD) for 1994.

differences in functional status remain even after accounting for socioeconomic status (Guralnik and Kaplan, 1989; Clark et al., 1993; Guralnik et al., 1993b).

RACIAL HEALTH DISPARITIES

In this section, we describe some racial differences in health outcomes using recent HRS and AHEAD data. To start this comparison, Table 4-3 displays self-reported health status by gender and race. Not surprisingly, people self-rate themselves in better health in the younger HRS sample. As a quick generalization, twice as many HRS respondents in each race-sex group are in excellent health compared with the older AHEAD sample. In both surveys, blacks are considerably more likely to report much poorer health. For example, while almost half of black AHEAD households place themselves in fair or poor health, only one in three white households so respond. More than a third of whites are in excellent or very good health compared with a fifth of black respondents.

Respondents in these surveys were also asked a series of questions about the presence of chronic medical conditions and symptoms and about the use of selected medical services related to specific conditions. Tables 4-4 and 4-5 contrast the responses to these questions for black and whites by gender. The emerging racial patterns in disease prevalence are mostly consistent with other published data. In both AHEAD and HRS, blacks had substantially higher rates of hypertension, stroke, and diabetes and lower rates for diseases of the lung and for a heart attack within the previous 5 years (men only). For hip fracture, black women had lower rates (data were collected only in AHEAD). In AHEAD,

TABLE 4-4 Prevalence of Medical Conditions by Race and Sex, HRS Sample (Ages 51-61)

	Men		Women	
Medical Condition	White (%)	Black (%)	White (%)	Black (%)
High blood pressure	39.1	53.3	30.7	55.6
Diabetes	10.0	17.2	7.5	17.9
Cancer	3.8	3.4	7.8	5.4
Diseases of the lung	8.8	4.5	8.2	7.7
Heart condition	16.9	15.2	9.8	12.8
Heart attack in last 5 years	9.3	8.5	2.5	4.8
Heart surgery	4.8	2.6	0.9	1.3
Stroke	3.1	6.7	1.9	3.2
Emotional or psychiatric problems	7.4	6.5	13.1	12.5
Arthritis, rheumatism in last year	33.2	33.5	40.7	45.8
Asthma	5.2	6.7	6.7	7.7
Back problems	34.2	30.5	35.8	33.6
Kidney, bladder	8.2	12.2	11.4	13.1
Stomach ulcers	8.9	11.6	8.5	11.8
High cholesterol	23.1	15.2	24.7	23.0
Eyeglasses	92.8	73.8	93.9	88.8

SOURCE: Health and Retirement Survey (HRS) data for 1993.

blacks had a higher rate of arthritis, while in HRS, the rate was higher only for black women.[14] There were minimal racial differences in rates of several conditions for both surveys including emotional/psychiatric problems and angina.

These relative prevalence rates are influenced by several factors that influence the interpretation of racial differences. These factors include whether a physician was seen for a specific condition, how symptoms are attributed to specific medical diagnoses, and treatment modalities for specific conditions. Prevalence rates derived from self-reported conditions, for example, may confound true health differences with other behaviors, including frequency of contact with physicians and health care utilization. Blacks reported lower rates of cataract surgery, which may reflect lower rates of access to health care rather than lower rates of cataracts. Analysis of data from the Baltimore Eye Survey found

---

[14]Some differences between the two surveys may reflect differences in the wording of the questions. For example, AHEAD asked whether the respondent had ever been told that he or she had arthritis or rheumatism, while the HRS survey asked about seeing a doctor in the previous 12 months specifically because of arthritis or rheumatism.

TABLE 4-5   Prevalence of Medical Conditions by Race and Sex, AHEAD
Sample (Ages 70 and Over)

Medical Condition	Men		Women	
	White (%)	Black (%)	White (%)	Black (%)
High blood pressure	42.2	59.7	50.8	67.2
Diabetes	12.8	21.0	10.0	22.9
Cancer	16.4	14.8	13.3	7.0
Diseases of the lung	14.3	10.8	10.5	4.4
Heart condition	37.2	25.5	28.1	26.1
Heart attack in last 5 years	9.2	4.5	5.2	7.4
Stroke	9.3	13.9	7.3	8.8
Emotional or psychiatric problems	8.4	8.8	12.4	12.2
Arthritis, rheumatism in last year	17.3	30.6	25.5	40.9
Broken hip	3.2	5.4	6.0	4.0
Cataract surgery	23.3	20.4	29.0	26.4
Often bothered by pain	27.4	31.2	35.1	36.3
Pain keeps person from activities	53.0	58.5	59.9	59.7

SOURCE: Health and Retirement Survey (HRS) data for 1993.

that the age-adjusted risk of unoperated cataracts among older blacks was 5.25
times that of whites (Sommer et al., 1991).

Although biological and genetic factors may have a part, socioeconomic
status may also play a role in accounting for racial differences in many of these
conditions. For example, stress has long been raised as a potential reason for
racial differences in hypertension rates (James et al., 1987). A recent analysis of
longitudinal data on health and occupational position found that although both
blacks and whites who remained in low occupational classes over approximately
a 10-year period were more likely to develop uncontrolled hypertension, the odds
of developing hypertension for blacks were twice the odds for whites (Waitzman
and Smith, 1994).

Perhaps obesity is the most important underlying factor that may be both
mediated by socioeconomic status and associated with the incidence of three
conditions found in higher rates among blacks (hypertension, diabetes, and arthritis). Racial and ethnic differences in obesity among women are profound.[15]
Low socioeconomic status is also clearly associated with a greater likelihood of

---

[15]Data in the third National Health and Nutrition Examination Survey (NHANES III) revealed an
age-adjusted prevalence of overweight of 48.5 percent among non-Hispanic black women between
ages 20 and 74 years, while for non-Hispanic and Mexican American white women the prevalence
was 32 percent, and for Mexican-American women it was 47.2 percent. The rates for non-Hispanic
black, non-Hispanic white and Mexican American men aged 20 to 74 years were 31 percent, 32
percent, and 39.1 percent, respectively (Kuczmarski et al., 1994).

obesity (Sobal and Stunkard, 1989). The higher prevalence of strokes among blacks possibly also may be mediated by socioeconomic status through such risk factors as hypertension and diabetes. Differences in access to health care may also explain other patterns seen in these data. For example, black women have a similar or lower rate of breast cancer after age 40 compared with white women (Krieger, 1990). Black women, however, are more likely to have breast cancer diagnosed at a later stage and to have shorter survival rates as a result (e.g., Eley et al., 1994). This difference is believed to be related to lower mammography screening rates among black women (Caplan et al., 1992). The differential survival may lead to lower prevalence rates for conditions such as cancer in the face of similar incidence rates.

HEALTH AND WEALTH

A key risk to successful aging rests in the complex two-way interactions among income, wealth, and good health. Debates about the direction of causation have made conclusions about the relation of the wealth and health of older populations difficult to pin down. We know that healthier households are wealthier ones. Is that simply because higher incomes lead to better health? Or does poor health restrict a family's ability to accumulate assets by limiting the ability to work or through rising medical expenses? Or perhaps neither direction of influence is important, and the association merely reflects some unobserved factor that makes some people healthier and wealthier. Even to try to answer such questions requires panel data (to average out individual differences) and good health and wealth information to isolate the reasons for the association. With HRS and AHEAD, answering this sort of fundamental scientific question may now be feasible.

Table 4-6 displays the relation between total household income and the health of respondents in both HRS and AHEAD. Confirming a number of prior studies, this relationship is largely uniform and quantitatively strong. As a gauge of the quantitative importance of this relationship, Table 4-7 arrays median household net worth[16] by self-reported health status in both the HRS and the AHEAD samples. The magnitude and consistency of these results are impressive. In virtually every case, each step up in health status is associated with a large increment in household wealth. For example, in the HRS sample, the median middle-aged white man in excellent health possessed $184,000 in wealth compared with $37,250 for the median middle-aged white man in poor health. Al-

---

[16]In addition to housing, household net worth is built up from the following 11 categories: other real estate; vehicles; business equity; individual retirement account or Keogh; stocks, trusts, or mutual funds; checking, savings, or money market funds; certificates of deposit; government savings bonds or Treasury bills; other bonds; other savings and assets; and other debt. Because of extensive missing values in assets, an innovative method of imputing missing values was developed. For a summary of the details underlying this imputation algorithm, see Smith (1995, in press).

TABLE 4-6   Median Household Income by Self-Reported Health Status

Self-Reported Health Status	Men's Median Net Worth		Women's Median Net Worth	
	White ($)	Black ($)	White ($)	Black ($)
	(%) HRS (Ages 51-61)			
Excellent	55,740	42,150	51,260	33,000
Very good	49,950	38,788	43,000	31,000
Good	41,500	32,950	36,700	25,000
Fair	31,200	25,530	26,300	16,512
Poor	23,900	13,166	16,372	9,106
	AHEAD (Ages 70 and Over)			
Excellent	26,892	12,342	21,888	11,512
Very good	24,977	17,145	19,212	10,134
Good	21,295	16,423	15,850	9,380
Fair	19,531	13,598	13,252	8,651
Poor	16,223	10,798	10,117	7,386

SOURCE: Health and Retirement Survey (HRS) data for 1993 and data from Assets and Health Dynamics of the Oldest Old (AHEAD) for 1994.

TABLE 4-7   Median Net Worth by Self-Reported Health Status

Self-Reported Health Status	Men		Women	
	White ($)	Black ($)	White ($)	Black ($)
	HRS (Ages 51-61)			
Excellent	184,000	72,500	183,950	69,075
Very good	156,000	61,500	141,000	53,750
Good	120,000	41,000	100,300	35,800
Fair	86,000	26,875	59,975	12,750
Poor	37,250	2,150	25,000	23
	AHEAD (Ages 70 and Over)			
Excellent	194,500	29,000	141,000	21,000
Very good	162,500	50,000	124,900	32,600
Good	135,000	38,000	100,000	20,900
Fair	97,500	32,100	65,000	11,150
Poor	74,500	18,000	33,892	1,500

SOURCE: Health and Retirement Survey (HRS) data for 1993 and data from Assets and Health Dynamics of the Oldest Old (AHEAD) for 1994.

though the size of the wealth-health gradient is quite large in both samples, the AHEAD data in Table 4-7 may suggest some attenuation among older Americans compared with their middle-aged counterparts. While blacks have lower wealth levels than whites in all health categories, the wealth-health gradient may even be quantitatively larger in African-American households, especially when our reference points are households in poor health. In the HRS sample, for example, black male respondents in poor health had only about $2,000 of wealth, one-thirty-sixth of the wealth of black male respondents in excellent health. For white men, the wealth of those in excellent health exceeds that of those in poor health only by a factor of five. The gradients of these wealth-health relationships are much larger than those previously displayed for income and health.

The real value of these surveys in understanding the health-wealth nexus will be realized only in subsequent rounds as the dynamics of the process unfolds. However, some clues may be gleaned from the baseline by combining information on current status with a question about how health status compares with health a year ago. Table 4-8 provides the results from that combination.[17] The patterns in this table are remarkably consistent. Whatever the ultimate resolution of the thorny issue of causality, baseline HRS and AHEAD data confirm earlier findings that the association between contemporaneous health and wealth is not trivial. The relationship is monotonic and quantitatively large—each step down in current health status significantly reduces net worth. In addition, current HRS and AHEAD assets are correlated both with current health levels and with changes in health. Virtually all transitions in Table 4-8 associated with improved health had higher assets while transitions into poorer health had lower assets.

Another unique advantage of HRS and AHEAD is that the detailed health module was given to both spouses. Although owing to data limitations, household outcomes are typically related only to the health of one spouse, this is no more justified than defining household income by using only one member's income. Episodes of poor health of either spouse may deplete family resources. In addition, families may be better able to cope with the care-giving requirements for a person in fair or poor health if the spouse is in very good or excellent health.

To examine this joint distribution, Table 4-9 arrays household net worth for married couples by the health of each spouse. Although not without the odd exception, the pattern is remarkably consistent—an increase in the health of either spouse has a strong positive correlation with household net worth. This relationship is also quantitatively strong. Arrayed only against the health of the

---

[17]For the purposes of this table, we assumed that health would move across only one threshold during a year. For example, those currently in good health with deteriorating health over the last year were considered to be in very good health last year. Similarly, those currently in good health whose health improved during the year were considered to be in fair health last year.

TABLE 4-8   Mean Net Worth by Changing Health Status, HRS and AHEAD

Last Year	Current Year	Median Net Worth ($)
	HRS	
Excellent	Excellent	370,842
Excellent	Very good	224,083
Very good	Excellent	316,274
Very good	Very good	269,267
Very good	Good	200,645
Good	Very good	266,434
Good	Good	199,555
Good	Fair	160,338
Fair	Good	189,008
Fair	Fair	136,656
Fair	Poor	51,281
Poor	Fair	165,525
Poor	Poor	93,658
	AHEAD	
Excellent	Excellent	285,213
Excellent	Very good	216,551
Very good	Excellent	157,703
Very good	Very good	226,881
Very good	Good	148,890
Good	Very good	188,836
Good	Good	166,962
Good	Fair	98,334
Fair	Good	154,512
Fair	Fair	108,880
Fair	Poor	85,360
Poor	Fair	92,411
Poor	Poor	77,405

SOURCE: Health and Retirement Survey (HRS) data for 1993 and data from Assets and Health Dynamics of the Oldest Old (AHEAD) for 1994.

TABLE 4-9   Mean and Median HRS Net Worth by Health Status of Spouses

Health of Financial Respondent	Health of Spouse				
	Excellent ($)	Very Good ($)	Good ($)	Fair ($)	Poor ($)
			Mean		
Excellent	220,250	201,000	149,500	90,000	121,500
Very good	218,000	164,110	128,800	84,000	46,400
Good	175,070	135,000	97,800	83,075	37,369
Fair	146,000	116,600	69,900	63,200	61,650
Poor	99,250	55,800	40,550	34,030	19,000
			Median		
Excellent	330,000	220,200	170,000	192,000	115,000
Very good	189,750	220,750	168,500	131,000	123,900
Good	201,000	185,000	143,800	127,000	63,000
Fair	319,000	142,600	90,000	66,500	60,500
Poor	121,225	101,000	115,000	35,500	41,000

SOURCE: Health and Retirement Survey (HRS) data for 1993 and data from Assets and Health Dynamics of the Oldest Old (AHEAD) for 1994.

financial respondent, net worth varies by a factor of about 4 to 1 as the health index moves from poor to excellent health. Table 4-9 demonstrates, however, that net worth varies by almost 10 to 1 when our health index moves from both spouses' being in poor health to both being in excellent health.

A critical component of how joint spousal health affects savings behavior depends on the correlation in their health outcomes. For a number of plausible reasons, this correlation is likely to be positive. Not only are spouses more likely to be closer in age (and hence facing similar aging-related health risks), but they have shared similar economic, social, and health environments for some time. Both HRS and AHEAD indicate that this correlation is indeed strongly positive. For example, while only 13 percent of AHEAD financial respondents report themselves in poor health, the odds increase to 1 in 3 if the spouse is also in poor health. On the other extreme on the health spectrum, 1 in 10 AHEAD financial respondents report themselves in good health, a ratio that doubles if the spouse is in excellent health.

One of the most frequently cited reasons for lower savings among the poor is that they have higher time preferences for the present (e.g., shorter horizons). HRS, especially in its panel features, will eventually allow one of the first explicit tests of this hypothesis, but the baseline survey points to its promise. Consistent with persistent speculation, black and Hispanic households are more likely to have very short time horizons. For example, 28 percent of black and Hispanic households, compared with only 17 percent of white households, report a planning horizon of only a few months.

RISK BEHAVIORS

One pathway through which economic status may influence health is behavior typically placed under the label "risk factors." Epidemiological studies have identified the following as important risk factors associated with mortality and morbidity: smoking, alcohol intake, excess weight, and high cholesterol level. While the diseases through which these risk factors mediate vary—for example, smoking (cancer and heart disease), body mass index (heart disease, diabetes), alcohol (injuries, cirrhosis)—all have the potential of mediating through socioeconomic status. If so, they may explain part of the racial disparities in health outcomes. Both HRS and AHEAD have a rich array of such self-reported risk behaviors. HRS measures include smoking, drinking, light and vigorous physical exercise, current and past exposure to occupational health hazards, and current weight and height. A more limited set of risk factors—smoking, drinking, height, and weight—is available in AHEAD.

Tables 4-10 and 4-11 contrast race and sex differences in these health-related risks. Cigarette smoking is perhaps the most well-documented behavioral risk, a leading cause of cancers of the lung. Compared with white men, black men in the HRS age range are more likely to be current smokers and are less successful in quitting smoking: 38 percent of black men in their fifties are current smokers compared with 23 percent of white men. Among those who ever smoked, 7 in 10 white men had quit compared with slightly less than half of black men. At the same time, black men are less likely to engage in heavy smoking. While less than 1 in 20 HRS black men report that they smoked at least a pack a day, 1 in every 10 white men did. Racial differences in smoking behavior among women are much less severe than those just described among men. Women in their fifties smoke less than similarly aged men, but there are trivial racial differences in current or past cigarette smoking or in its intensity.

Although smoking is much less common among all groups in the AHEAD sample (ages 70 and above), similar patterns of racial disparities persist. In AHEAD, current smoking prevalence rates are roughly half of those observed in HRS, but black men still smoke at twice the rate of white men. The percentage of these elderly men who were able to quit smoking is higher than that observed among men in their fifties (86% of white and 70% of black men). While these trends could reflect cohort differences in smoking behavior or differential mortality selection (e.g., higher mortality of smokers excludes more of them from the AHEAD sample range), we see it largely as a life-cycle phenomenon where larger and larger numbers of former smokers cease. Presumably, some of them have been told to do so for health reasons. The reason why a life-cycle interpretation appears plausible is that a roughly similar fraction of each birth cohort ever smoked.

Racial differences in drinking behavior are much smaller. While blacks in both samples are somewhat more commonly quite heavy drinkers (five or more

TABLE 4-10 Risk Behaviors and Factors, by Race and Sex, HRS Sample (Ages 51-61)

Risk Behavior or Factor	Men White (%)	Men Black (%)	Women White (%)	Women Black (%)
Smoking				
Currently smoking	23.1	38.0	25.9	25.6
Formerly smoked	51.3	35.8	27.8	29.7
Never smoked	25.5	26.2	46.3	44.7
(Number of cigarettes per day)				
1-10	5.4	17.3	7.8	16.0
11-20	10.9	16.0	12.1	7.8
21-30	4.3	2.3	3.1	0.7
> 30	6.4	2.2	2.8	0.5
Alcohol (drinks per day)				
0	31.7	36.2	43.5	55.7
< 1	44.7	40.4	47.2	37.2
1-2	14.2	12.7	7.1	5.6
3-4	6.2	6.5	1.9	1.1
5+	3.0	3.9	0.4	0.5
Light physical activity				
Never	9.3	16.2	8.7	16.1
Less than once a month	6.5	5.3	8.2	9.6
1-3 times a month	7.8	7.6	10.1	9.5
1-2 times a week	20.2	17.5	22.6	20.4
3 or more times a week	55.9	53.4	50.3	44.2
Heavy physical activity				
Never	45.6	57.5	49.1	66.5
Less than once a month	19.6	14.7	20.3	16.0
1-3 times a month	8.9	6.4	8.5	5.0
1-2 times a week	10.3	9.3	10.2	6.0
3 or more times a week	15.5	11.8	11.7	6.2
Exposure to hazardous materials at work				
Ever exposed to work hazard	50.5	42.0	23.7	21.6
Years of exposure				
1-10	6.0	6.9	6.3	4.1
11-20	6.0	5.9	4.1	4.3
21+	15.8	11.3	2.8	3.1
Body mass index				
0-23.7	20.5	23.0	35.6	14.3
23.8-26.5	29.4	26.4	22.8	20.8
26.6-29.6	28.5	25.0	18.6	22.3
29.7+	21.6	25.6	23.0	42.6

Note: Some columns do not add to 100 due to rounding.
SOURCE: Health and Retirement Survey (HRS) data for 1993.

TABLE 4-11   Risk Behaviors and Factors by Race and Sex, AHEAD Sample
(Ages 70 and Over)

| | Men | | Women | |
Risk Behavior or Factor	White (%)	Black (%)	White (%)	Black (%)
Smoking				
Currently smoking	11.2	21.6	9.0	8.1
Formerly smoked	65.3	53.3	28.9	28.1
Never smoked	23.4	25.1	62.0	63.8
(Number of cigarettes per day)				
1-10	3.6	13.3	4.1	5.2
11-20	3.9	5.5	3.9	2.5
21 or more	1.5	1.2	0.9	0.1
Alcohol (drinks per day)				
0	42.3	63.6	56.4	78.0
< 1	39.6	25.4	35.8	18.4
1-2	13.9	5.8	6.8	3.2
3-4	3.4	3.4	0.9	0.1
5+	0.7	1.6	0.1	0.3
Body mass index				
1st quartile	17.4	19.2	30.4	14.4
2nd quartile	27.0	23.8	24.6	19.5
3rd quartile	31.3	28.6	20.4	20.7
4th quartile	23.7	25.8	23.4	41.6

Note: Some columns do not add to 100 due to rounding.
SOURCE: Data from Assets and Health Dynamics of the Oldest Old (AHEAD) for 1994.

drinks a day), the real disparities appear among nondrinkers, who are far more
likely to be black. While this finding characterizes each sex in both samples, the
differences are particularly striking among women. In the HRS sample, 56
percent of black women are nondrinkers, 12 percentage points higher than their
white counterparts. This racial discrepancy is even larger among older women,
where almost 4 in 5 black women are teetotalers compared with 3 in 10 older
white women.

Although this problem affects all behaviors contained in these tables, exercise is a risk factor for which it is especially difficult to disentangle cause and
effect. While exercise may lower risks associated with heart disease, it is also
true that individuals in poor health may simply be unable to engage in vigorous
exercise. Whether light or heavy physical exercise is used as the yardstick,
blacks are more likely not to engage in any exercise. To use but one example
from these tables, two-thirds of black women have no episodes of heavy physical
activity compared with only half of white women.

In HRS, respondents were asked whether they ever had been exposed to
dangerous chemicals or other hazards at work as well as the number of years of

such exposure.[18] While many studies are confined to specific occupations or even job tasks, an advantage of the HRS question is that it provides a population-based estimate, at least for a specific cohort. Black men are less likely than white men to report any work-related occupational exposure or to report an exposure of very long duration. Given women's more sporadic history of labor force attachment, not surprisingly, work-related hazards are far less common among women, with little evidence of any significant racial disparity.

Respondents in both surveys gave self-reports of their heights and weights. Obesity is a well-established risk associated with both heart disease and adult onset diabetes. Tables 4-10 and 4-11 confirm that African Americans are more likely to suffer from being overweight, a problem particularly acute among black women. In both surveys, roughly 42 percent of black women are in the top quartile of body mass index for the entire sample, almost twice the rate observed among white women.

EMPIRICAL MODELS OF SELF-REPORTED HEALTH OUTCOMES

In this section, a series of sequential empirical models explores the relationship between a household's economic resources and its health. This section liberally uses material in Smith and Kington (1996). Our central interest in this exploration lies in understanding the reasons underlying the strong correlation between income and health. We begin with an empirical specification that mimics the current standard in the literature. Then, we assess whether this standard can withstand a very aggressive set of tests about the direction of the causal relationship between socioeconomic status and income. All models are estimated with the recent HRS and AHEAD data. While a number of salient health measures are available in these surveys, only a respondent's self-assessed health status is used as an outcome. Since self-assessed health is a ranked categorical response, ordered probit models are used in estimation. The underlying score is estimated as a linear function of the co-variates and a set of cut points. The probability of observing health status i can be expressed as

$$Pr(health = i) = Pr(k_{i-1} < \beta X + u_j < k_i) \tag{8}$$

The model estimates the parameter vector β along with the four cut points (k_i).

To establish a baseline, the first and second columns of Tables 4-12 (for HRS) and 4-13 (for AHEAD) contain a model that incorporates race, ethnic, and gender demographic controls only. In both samples, blacks and Hispanics report consistently lower health outcomes than whites do. Women rank higher than men in their self-assessed health in the HRS age range, but there are no statisti-

---

[18]More precisely, the question was, "Have you ever had to breathe any kinds of dusts, fumes, or vapors, or been exposed to organic solvents or pesticides at work?"

TABLE 4-12   Ordered Probit Analysis of Self-Assessed Health Status, HRS Sample (Ages 51-61)

Co-variate	Parameter	z	Parameter	z	Parameter	z	Parameter	z
Black	−.5278	17.60	−.2977	9.49	−.2402	7.50	−.1763	5.43
Hispanic	−.5037	12.90	−.1774	4.11	−.1626	3.94	−.0810	1.94
Female	.0700	3.67	.0770	4.11	.0489	2.20	.0527	2.39
Marital status								
Never married			.0739	1.18	.0140	0.22	.1577	2.46
Separated			−.0736	1.03	−.1478	2.06	.0419	0.57
Divorced			−.0043	0.11	.0304	0.75	.1007	2.41
Widowed			.0375	0.75	.0483	0.96	.1731	3.37
Education								
Individual education								
12-15 years			.4327	17.50	.3240	12.92	.2568	10.04
16 or more years			.6639	19.01	.4609	12.83	.3880	10.72
Advanced degree			.2106	1.45	.1726	1.18	.1752	1.19
Spousal education								
12-15 years			.1332	5.02	.0828	3.09	.0378	1.39
16 or more years			.1738	5.15	.0983	2.59	.0739	1.93
Advanced degree			−.1280	0.78	−.1848	1.11	−.1666	1.00
Income and wealth[a]								
Total income			.0034	11.30	.0025	8.34		
Income 1st tercile							.0153	7.46
Income 2nd tercile							.0046	3.41
Income 3rd tercile							.0009	2.64
Total wealth			.0003	8.83	.0002	5.80		
Wealth 1st tercile							.0059	7.42
Wealth 2nd tercile							.0009	3.07
Wealth 3rd tercile							.0001	2.73
Cohort								
1935-1937			.1235	4.67	.1217	4.56	.1300	4.86
1938+			.2166	9.63	.2128	9.26	.2289	9.87
Risk factors								
Smoking								
Current smoker					−.0903	2.39	−.0770	2.04
Cigarettes smoked per day					−.0034	2.31	−.0027	1.85

TABLE 4-12   Continued

Co-variate	Parameter	z	Parameter	z	Parameter	z	Parameter	z
Drinking								
< 1 drink per day					.2127	9.69	.1920	8.70
1 or 2					.2560	7.26	.2397	6.77
3 or 4					.2015	3.79	.1874	3.51
5 or more					−.0580	0.72	−.0293	0.36
Light exercise								
3 times per week					.4368	12.10	.4098	11.28
1-2 times per week					.3845	9.74	.3443	8.68
1-3 times per month					.3832	8.31	.3463	7.49
less than once a month					.2786	5.84	.2469	5.22
Vigorous exercise								
3 times per week					.5110	15.45	.4926	14.88
1-2 times per week					.3864	11.01	.3603	10.22
1-3 times per month					.3266	8.72	.3107	8.28
less than once a month					.2774	10.43	.2610	9.74
Occupational hazard								
Ever exposed					−.0805	1.92	−.0721	1.71
Years exposed					−.0046	3.59	−.0049	3.79
Body mass index								
BMl					−.0077	−0.78	−.0126	1.27
BMl^2					−.0034	2.15	−.0003	1.59
Cut point 1	−1.5562		−.8239		−1.0245		−.6471	
Cut point 2	−0.9116		−.1231		−.2701		.1228	
Cut point 3	−0.1110		.7474		.6567		1.0612	
Cut point 4	0.6922		1.6073		1.5624		1.9708	

[a]Expressed in thousand dollar units.
SOURCE: Health and Retirement Survey (HRS) data for 1993.

cally significant gender differences among older Americans in AHEAD. Blacks and Hispanics each trail whites by half a standard normal deviation in HRS and a slightly smaller amount in AHEAD. The advantage women hold over men is considerably smaller in either survey.

The third and fourth columns of Tables 4-12 and 4-13 extend this model by adding a standard list of demographic and economic co-variates; current marital status, education, household income and wealth, birth cohort (or, equivalently, age), and location (in AHEAD). In both surveys, more recent birth cohorts exhibit higher self-reported health. Given the cross-sectional nature of the survey, one cannot distinguish between a life-cycle and a cohort interpretation of this relation. Younger respondents may be healthier simply because they are younger and at an earlier stage in the aging process. Alternatively, as for many

TABLE 4-13   Ordered Probit Analysis of Self-Assessed Health Status, AHEAD Sample (Ages 70 and Over)

Co-variate	Parameter	z	Parameter	z	Parameter	z	Parameter	z
Black	−.4005	9.91	−.1633	3.83	−.1169	2.71	−.0560	1.28
Hispanic	−.4038	6.76	−.1642	2.65	−.1313	2.11	−.0304	0.48
Female	−.0159	0.64	.0592	2.20	.0772	2.65	.0907	3.10
Marital status								
Never married			.1259	1.67	.1007	1.33	.2288	2.96
Separated or divorced			.0524	0.84	.0665	1.06	.2078	3.22
Widowed			.1090	3.17	.1004	2.91	.2137	5.78
Education								
Individual education								
12-15 years			.3011	10.62	.2627	9.18	.1975	6.70
16 or more years			.4876	10.83	.4212	9.26	.3339	7.18
Advanced degree			.1081	0.88	.1225	1.00	.1310	1.07
Spousal education								
12-15 years			.1140	3.07	.0882	2.37	.0654	1.73
16 or more years			.1979	3.48	.1406	2.46	.1347	2.34
Advanced degree			−.0268	0.18	.0052	0.03	.0027	0.18
Income and wealth[a]								
Total income			.0008	2.63	.0009	2.85		
Income 1st tercile							.0126	1.83
Income 2nd tercile							.0023	5.74
Income 3rd tercile							.0005	1.40
Total wealth			.0006	8.32	.0005	7.05		
Wealth 1st tercile							.0050	5.12
Wealth 2nd tercile							.0005	1.20
Wealth 3rd tercile							.0002	2.40
Cohort								
1919-1923			.2053	5.11	.2001	4.84	.1402	3.35
1914-1918			.0490	1.18	.0501	1.19	−.0071	0.17
1909-1913			.0098	0.23	.0109	0.25	−.0226	0.52
Living in a standard metropolitan statistical area			−.0582	1.97	−.0782	2.64	−.0769	2.58
Region								
Northeast			−.0613	1.51	−.0759	1.86	−.0594	1.46
North Central			−.0080	0.22	−.0062	0.17	−.0176	0.48
South			−.1274	3.52	−.0852	2.34	−.0776	2.12

TABLE 4-13   Continued

Co-variate	Parameter	z	Parameter	z	Parameter	z	Parameter	z
Risk factors								
Smoking								
Ever smoked					−.1427	5.08	−.1492	5.30
Currently smoke					−.1285	2.00	−.1191	1.85
Number of cigarettes					−.0057	1.66	−.0058	1.71
Drinking								
< 1 drink per day					.3531	12.82	.3212	11.64
1 or 2 drinks					.4475	9.62	.4167	8.92
3 or 4 drinks					.6192	6.55	.5666	5.98
5 or more drinks					.3551	1.50	.3152	1.41
Body mass index								
BM1					.0873	5.68	.0821	5.34
BM1^2					−.0017	6.09	−.0016	5.71
Cut point 1	−1.2193		−.7866		.361		.6348	
Cut point 2	−.4138		.0316		1.200		1.4832	
Cut point 3	−.3581		.8678		2.054		2.3445	
Cut point 4	1.1845		1.7302		2.931		3.2247	

[a]Expressed in thousand dollar units.
SOURCE: Data from Assets and Health Dynamics of Oldest Old (AHEAD) for 1994.

other forms of human capital, health stocks may be improving for each new generation. At this stage of the analysis, variation in current marital status does not significantly influence current health outcomes.[19] Older residents of standard metropolitan statistical areas and the South have somewhat lower health status than those who live elsewhere.

Three dimensions of economic resources are incorporated into the baseline models in Tables 4-12 and 4-13: schooling, total household income, and household net worth.[20] Education is commonly thought to affect health status through a number of channels. First, schooling is an excellent measure of stable long-term economic status. In addition, more educated respondents may have acquired more knowledge about personal behaviors that enhance health or the timely use of preventive health care to stop small negative health shocks from becoming big ones. Because the schooling occurred before current health, many have argued that it is

---

[19]Somewhat puzzlingly, widows are healthier than those with other marital status in the AHEAD sample.

[20]Net worth is well known to contain a significant amount of measurement error. Therefore, these data were trimmed by eliminating observations with the highest and lowest 1 percent net worth values.

less subject to the confounding effects of reverse causation than other measures of socioeconomic status. While this argument at a minimum is overstated, whatever its substantive interpretation, schooling remains an extremely powerful correlate of current health status.[21] If years of schooling are translated into the additional dollars of household income received, education's effect on health is greater than what can be attributed to this extra income only. The implication is that the beneficial impact of education does not flow only from the additional economic resources that schooling buys. Education must in part mediate through information and behavioral adjustments that promote better health.

While its impact is not quantitatively as large as the effect of a person's own education, spousal schooling also raises self-perceived health status. In this formulation, spousal education should have effects on family income that are symmetrical to the effects of a person's own schooling. Therefore, the smaller impact of spousal education implies that some of the beneficial behavioral adjustments associated with schooling are person specific and do not flow over to other family members. In addition to the resource- and information-based interpretations assigned to the effect of a person's own education, spousal schooling may in part capture positive assortative mating in marriage markets as people in better health marry each other.

Both total household income and wealth are associated with higher health status. In the HRS sample, a dollar of wealth has about one-tenth the effect of a dollar of household income. Since income is a flow and wealth a stock, the relative magnitude of these estimated effects is consistent with a 10 percent real interest rate. While this is a little high, there are no strong reasons to suggest that when income and wealth are appropriately dimensioned, they have differential effects on individual health. In contrast, wealth has a quantitatively larger effect than household income does on health status in the older AHEAD sample. Whereas the influence of wealth is similar in the two samples, the estimated effect of income is much smaller in AHEAD, which is about one-third to one-fourth of the HRS estimate. This may reflect shorter life spans of older Americans and higher discount rates for them.

Collectively, these simple economic controls account for a significant part, but certainly not all, of the racial and ethnic disparities in self-reported health status. If we contrast the first two and the second two columns of Table 4-12, we find that the estimated racial disparity is reduced by 40 percent by these standard demographic and economic co-variates. Socioeconomic status, as proxied by these variables, accounts for a considerably larger proportion of ethnic health disparities in the HRS sample. While the unadjusted racial and ethnic differences are about the same in the first two columns of Table 4-12, the estimated Hispanic disparity is almost half as large as the racial coefficient in the third and fourth

---

[21]Throughout this paper, education is specified as a set of dummy variables indicating less than a high school degree, a high school degree with no or some college, and a college degree.

column.[22] This mimics the result in other applications, such as wages, where observable characteristics such as education explain substantially more of the Hispanic ethnic deficit (Smith, 1994). These standard demographic and economic variables explain slightly more (60%) of the racial and ethnic disparities in the AHEAD age group.

While modeling risk behaviors is problematic from a micro-behavioral perspective, they are included in the model summarized in the fifth and sixth columns of Tables 4-12 and 4-13 to provide comparability with much of the existing health literature. Not surprisingly, health risk factors are powerful co-variates that have statistically significant and well-ordered associations with self-assessed health outcomes. Former smoking (in AHEAD), current smoking, and the intensity of smoking lower self-reported health, while all levels of moderate drinking are positively correlated with health status. Consistent with a growing number of findings in the literature, the "optimal" number of drinks in the HRS sample range is one or two a day, but rises to three or four a day in AHEAD. In these results, we cannot distinguish between those respondents who do not drink at all and those who drink a great deal. Higher regimens of light and heavy physical exercise in HRS are correlated with better current health status in a remarkably well-ordered way. Even though these are self-reported episodes and durations, this analysis provides statistically significant evidence that exposure to work-related health risks as well as the duration of that exposure is associated with lower self-reported health. Finally, obesity is a negative marker of poor health in both samples.

While these HRS risk factors are statistically important, their collective impact on racial and ethnic health disparities is relatively modest. Indeed, Hispanic health deficits in the model with risk factors are almost identical to those estimated without risk behaviors. The racial health disparity is smaller, but only one-sixth of the deficit was eliminated by these risk factors. The dominant risk factor in lowering the racial deficit was the body mass index, which by itself accounted for half the observed reduction in the racial health disparity. The collective influence of the AHEAD risk factors is somewhat larger, reducing the unexplained racial disparity by a third and the Hispanic deficit by less than one-fifth. One mechanism through which these risk factors may operate is socioeconomic status. However, these risk behaviors are largely independent of socioeconomic status. Even in the model with risk factors included, the estimated effects of socioeconomic status are approximately as large as they were without risk factors in the model.

We also estimated one model for married households that adds a set of variables measuring the identical set of risk factors for the spouse. For most of

---

[22]Since male and female education levels are about the same and men and women mostly share similar economic resources, it is not surprising that the sex coefficient is not altered much by the inclusion of these simple economic and demographic variables.

the HRS risk factors—drinking, exercise whether light or vigorous, or the body mass index—we are unable to detect any indirect effect of the spouse's behavior on the respondent's health. The two possible exceptions involve years of exposure to an occupational hazard and smoking. There appears to be a statistically significant effect of spousal occupational exposure, although the mechanism by which this has an impact on the respondent's health is unclear. We do estimate a negative effect of spousal smoking that is 70 percent as large as the direct effect. This estimate has little precision, however, so we are unable to reject the hypothesis that secondhand smoking has no effect on health. The parallel AHEAD results are much easier to summarize. There is no evidence that any of the spousal risk factors have any association with the respondent's self-assessed health status.

The last two columns of Tables 4-12 and 4-13 test for nonlinearity in income and wealth effects on probability scores by including linearly splined terciles of total household income and wealth. In both samples and for both income and wealth, there is strong evidence of nonlinearity. Income and wealth affect self-perceived health status throughout the entire range of the income and wealth distributions. Consequently, one cannot interpret, as is often done, the beneficial effects of income or wealth as differentiating poverty-level families from those who are above the poverty line. However, the size of income and wealth effects on health status does decay as one moves up the income and wealth distribution. For example, in the HRS sample, the estimated effect in the lowest income tercile is 16 times larger than the effect in the highest tercile, and the effect of the lowest wealth tercile is 53 times larger than the effect in the highest tercile. In the AHEAD sample, the lowest tercile's income and wealth coefficients exceed the highest tercile estimates by approximately 25 to 1.

Including only linear terms in income and wealth turns out to be a serious misspecification of the relationship between economic resources and health status. In particular, it results in a quantitatively large overstatement of the unexplained racial and ethnic health disparities. To illustrate, the racial coefficient in the HRS sample is reduced by a quarter and the ethnic coefficient by one-half when nonlinearities are permitted. Even more dramatic results are obtained in the AHEAD sample, where there are now no statistically significant racial or ethnic disparities remaining.[23]

---

[23]There are a number of simple stratifications of these basic models by marital status, sex, and race or ethnicity that are illuminating. Both the unadjusted and the adjusted racial and ethnic disparities in this fully interacted model are smaller among HRS married couples than among HRS nonmarried individuals. However, this ranking is reversed in the AHEAD sample. While there are some exceptions, the general pattern of results that has been just described for the combined sample carries over to both the married and the nonmarried samples separately.

In large part, the conclusions summarized thus far carry over with surprisingly few exceptions to race-ethnic and sex-specific models. In particular, the effects of our socioeconomic status variables—education, household income, and net worth—are quite similar for men and women in HRS,

Measurement of Household Resources

In health outcomes and health services research, total household income is the conventional empirical proxy for aggregate economic resources. It is often the only option available because health surveys typically expend little survey time attempting to measure household resources. If we place a high priority on understanding why socioeconomic status has such a quantitatively strong association with a variety of health outcomes, reliance on such a simple summary statistic as total household income is surely a mistake. One reason is that household income is built up from conceptually unique subcomponents, many of which influence health or are affected by health in distinct ways. For openers, there may be multiple income recipients in a household. While standard economic theory blends all income into an indistinguishable homogeneous amalgam, more recent theoretical models argue that the way in which household resources are spent may be affected by who controls resources. These models suggest that at a minimum, it is essential to distinguish the effect of a person's own income on his or her own health from that of the income of other family members. Secondly, the receipt of some income sources may be consequences rather than determinants of poor health. For example, respondents in the HRS sample who are recipients of either pension or Social Security income are mostly retired. Since early retirees may well have retired because of their poor health, the causality for this component of income more plausibly runs from poor health to income. Similarly, recipients of welfare income are generally in poorer health, and their poor health condition leads to the receipt of this income.

To test these speculations, Table 4-14 summarizes the estimated effects of different types of household income on self-assessed health outcomes.[24] Coefficients of the other co-variates, not listed in Table 4-14, were not significantly altered by the experiments performed in this table. HRS household income is separated into six distinct conceptual components. For each spouse, these components are market earnings,[25] retirement-related income (pensions, Social Secu-

---

but the household income effect may be smaller for women in AHEAD. In the separate estimates for men and women, racial and particularly ethnic deficits are larger among women in HRS whereas there appears to be little gender difference in AHEAD. While the HRS racial health disparity is two-thirds as large among men compared with women, the truly dramatic difference takes place among Hispanics. Whereas there exists a large health disparity between Hispanic and white women, there exists no statistically significant HRS difference between Hispanic and white men. Among the risk factors, obesity appears to be a more salient risk factor for women. The final comparisons are separate runs by race and ethnicity. The major persistent pattern in the two samples is that the beneficial effects of spousal characteristics such as education appear to be confined to the white sample.

[24]The models partially summarized in Table 4-14 contained the same list of co-variates as those presented in Tables 4-12 and 4-13. To highlight the main points, only the coefficients on the income and wealth variables (and the race, ethnic, and gender indicators) are listed in this table.

[25]Current market earnings are the sum of wages and salary, bonuses, overtime, tips, commissions, and self-employment income from all jobs.

TABLE 4-14   Ordered Probit Models with Alternative Measures of Income[a]

Co-variate	Parameter	z	Parameter	z
		HRS Sample (Ages 51-61)		
Individual				
Earnings	.0018	4.41	.0012	2.69
Retirement income	−.0036	2.40	.0100	4.95
Welfare income	−.0347	5.21	−.0220	2.33
Earnings = 0			−.0734	2.86
Retirement income = 0			.2875	7.89
Welfare income = 0			.0788	1.58
Spouse				
Earnings	.0040	8.45	.0013	2.57
Retirement income	−.0087	5.41	.0003	0.14
Welfare income	−.0436	5.78	−.0170	0.92
Earnings = 0			−.3197	11.52
Retirement income = 0			.0604	1.55
Welfare income= 0			.0170	0.29
Household				
Asset income	−.0001	0.19	.0010	1.57
Asset income = 0			.0839	3.86
Wealth				
Wealth 1st tercile	.0070	8.95	.0065	8.26
Wealth 2nd tercile	.0010	3.38	.0013	4.49
Wealth 3rd tercile	.0001	2.67	.0014	3.24
Black	−.1807	5.56	−.1980	−6.07
Hispanic	−.1169	2.81	−.1268	−3.05
Female	.0730	2.99	.0871	3.55
		AHEAD Sample (Ages 70+)		
Individual				
Earnings	.0073	4.90	.0002	0.14
Social Security income	.0083	1.97	.0096	2.01
Retirement income	.0031	1.61	.0024	1.08
Salary = 0			−.3820	8.66
Social Security = 0			.1088	1.62
Retirement income = 0			−.0391	1.28
Spouse				
Earnings	.0037	2.27	.0038	1.95
Social Security income	.0046	0.90	.0078	1.29
Retirement income	.0044	1.96	.0042	1.34
Salary = 0			.0219	0.40
Social Security = 0			.1121	1.38
Retirement income = 0			−.0306	0.75

TABLE 4-14   Continued

Co-variate	Parameter	z	Parameter	z
Household				
Welfare income	−.0444	3.01	.0105	0.53
Welfare = 0			.3219	4.75
Asset income	.0004	0.48	.0002	0.17
Other income			−.0811	2.78
Net worth wealth 1st tercile	.0050	5.14	.0034	3.38
Net worth wealth 2nd tercile	.0010	2.62	.0009	2.33
Net worth wealth 3rd tercile	.0002	1.73	.0002	1.95
Black	−.0490	1.13	−.0328	0.74
Hispanic	−.0095	0.15	.0286	0.08
Female	.0978	2.82	.1087	3.07

^{a}Continuous income and asset coefficients expressed in thousand dollar units.
SOURCE: Health and Retirement Survey (HRS) data for 1993 and data from Assets and Health Dynamics of the Oldest Old (AHEAD) for 1994.

rity, and annuities), and welfare-related income (Supplemental Security Income, unemployment or workers' compensation, and welfare). The seventh component—defined only at the household level—consists of interest and dividends, rent, trusts or royalties, and income from businesses and partnerships. In the AHEAD sample, a slightly different classification is used. For each spouse, earnings remains a distinct category. Because of its fundamental importance within this age range, Social Security and other retirement income (private pensions and annuities) are placed in separate categories. Finally, welfare and asset income are defined at the household level.

The empirical estimates listed in the first two columns of Table 4-14 strongly support our earlier conjectures. While earnings of either spouse are positively correlated with better health in both samples, additional welfare income is actually strongly associated with lower self-assessed health status. Per dollar of income received, the negative effect of welfare income actually exceeds the positive effect of earnings. The most intriguing results occur with retirement income, which has a negative association with health status in the HRS but a strongly positive one in AHEAD. We interpret the negative coefficient in HRS as capturing a causal mechanism from poor health to early retirement. However, virtually all AHEAD respondents are past the normal retirement age so that this possible reverse causation is largely inoperative.

Our arguments are taken a step further in the third and fourth columns of Table 4-14, which add a set of variables indicating zero receipt of each income source. This specification suggests that the effect of each income type is not continuous at zero and that nonreceipt of income is particularly informative about why health and socioeconomic status may be correlated. In both samples, for example, the absence of any earnings is a signal of health problems that constrain a respondent's ability to work. Once again, the more plausible causality runs from poor health to nonwork to non-income. Controlling for positive earnings reduces the positive effect of a person's own earnings on current health status by a third. More dramatically, the entire positive effect of a person's own earnings on self-assessed health in the AHEAD sample is due to this reverse correlation. Similarly, the presence of either HRS or AHEAD welfare income is associated with lower current health status, a causation more readily interpreted from health to income.

A more complex set of results is obtained for the retirement variables, the effect of which varies in a systematic way across the two samples. These differences reflect the quite distinct character of retirement in the two samples. While virtually all AHEAD respondents have retired, retirement in HRS generally implies early retirement. For example, having no retirement income in HRS is positively correlated with current health, but once there is retirement income, additional retirement income is associated with better health status. This combination supports our interpretation that early retirement is in part a consequence of poor health. Rather than capturing any effect of socioeconomic status on health, the receipt of retirement income in this age group is a marker of health problems of respondents. However, given that a household has some such income, wealthier households, through higher accumulations of either Social Security or private pensions, have better self-assessed current health status. In contrast, the positive effects of the retirement variables are largely unaffected by the inclusion of the zero-income controls.

The final step in the decomposition of income involves separating earnings into its wage and labor supply components. The level of work effort is especially vulnerable to reverse causality problems since poor health may be an important limitation on the ability to work for long periods of time. In Table 4-15, the specifications of the HRS section of Table 4-14 are repeated with weekly wages substituted for annual earnings. Because this problem is relevant only for samples in which market work is relatively common, these equations are estimated only with the HRS sample. When the presence of zero for each income component is not controlled for (the first two columns of the table), respondent weekly wages remain positively correlated with self-assessed health status. However, evaluated at a work effort of 50 weeks, the weekly wage coefficient is about half as large as that on annual earnings. Most important, when we control for zero weekly wages in the second column, the weekly wage effect is not significantly different than zero.

In this section, we have demonstrated that conventional estimates of the effects of household income on current health most likely seriously overstate the direct effect of household resources on health outcomes, particularly in working populations. Different sources of household income clearly have quite distinct associations with health. Variation in many of these income components reflects the influence of health on income rather than the influence of socioeconomic

TABLE 4-15   Ordered Probit Models With Alternative Measures of Weekly Wages,[a] HRS Sample (Ages 51-61)

Co-variate	Parameter	z	Parameter	z
Individual				
Weekly wages	.0467	4.39	.0061	0.66
Retirement income	−.0050	3.42	.0108	5.40
Welfare income	−.0355	5.34	−.0184	1.96
Weekly wages = 0			−.3663	13.5
Retirement income = 0			.2915	8.01
Welfare income = 0			.0756	1.51
Spouse				
Weekly wages	−.0032	0.37	−.0199	2.27
Retirement income	−.0118	7.47	−.0022	1.05
Welfare income	−.0479	6.34	−.0442	4.23
Welfare wages= 0			.0549	1.89
Retirement income= 0			.0541	1.39
Welfare income= 0			−.0213	0.37
Household				
Asset income	−.0005	0.93	.0005	0.89
Asset income = 0			.0781	3.59
Wealth				
Wealth 1st tercile	.0072	9.27	.0061	7.82
Wealth 2nd tercile	.0011	3.84	.0014	4.66
Wealth 3rd tercile	.0002	3.57	.0002	3.79
Black	−.1766	5.56	−.1946	−5.96
Hispanic	−.1266	2.81	−.1222	−2.94
Female	.0251	2.99	.0438	1.89

[a]Continuous wage and asset coefficients expressed in thousand dollar units.

status on health. The size of this bias stemming from reverse causation may not be trivial. For example, after the receipt and size of the components of household income are controlled for, the estimated effect in HRS of a person's own earnings on current health status is half as large as the estimated effect of total household income on his or her own health. Moreover, even this estimated effect of a person's own earnings completely disappears when the more appropriate weekly wage measure is used.

Changes in Health Outcomes

The real analytical power of HRS and AHEAD will be realized only when many subsequent waves are available. With multiple health and economic measurements, researchers will be better able to control for unobservable factors that jointly influence both outcomes. However, a tentative step in that direction can be achieved even with the baseline surveys. In both HRS and AHEAD, respondents were asked not only their current health status but also whether it had improved over the last year. By combining these two questions, we can approximate the last and current period's self-assessed health status. In Table 4-16, ordered probit models are summarized where the outcomes range from a great improvement in health over the last year to a great deterioration.[26] In addition to variables measuring previous year's health status, the other co-variates parallel those included in the cross-sectional models with total household income and total household wealth as our measure of economic resources.[27] Table 4-17 contains change models with a decomposition of household income similar to what has been presented in Tables 4-14 and 4-15.

One advantage of this specification is that the analytical spotlight focuses exclusively on changes in health, conditional on the stock of health in the last period. The stock of health at any point is determined by the entire history of past health behaviors (drinking, exercise, smoking) as well as the complete lifetime history of purchased medical services. No data set, including those used in this study, can meet that demanding information requirement. For example, excessive drinking in the past may have led to a deterioration in an individual's health. This health deterioration may in turn have produced a complete cessation of drinking, perhaps under doctor's orders. In this case, an analysis of current health as a function of current drinking would produce quite biased estimates of the health effects of drinking. The change formulation with the past stock of health as a co-variate offers a partial solution to this problem since the past health stock serves as a summary statistic for all past health behaviors and purchased medical inputs.

The empirical estimates summarized in Table 4-16 generally support our interpretation of the change model. All current-period risk factors—smoking, drinking, and exercise—have their predicted impact on changes in health. As expected, their quantitative impact on changes in health is smaller than their accumulated effect on the current health stock. For example, the better health associated with moderate drinking maximizes at one or two drinks a day. But now very heavy drinking is associated with worse outcomes for improvements in health than not drinking at all. This seems a more reasonable result than that observed in the static cross-sectional analysis, suggesting that the previous period's health may well control for some of the biases obtained from not observ-

---

[26]There are five possible categories in HRS (improved a great deal, improved somewhat, stayed the same, deteriorated somewhat, deteriorated a great deal), but only three categories in AHEAD (improved, stayed the same, deteriorated).

[27]We are unable to find any evidence of nonlinearity in the effects of wealth or income in the change in health specification.

ing past values of behavioral or input variables. In a similar vein, those who are currently divorced or separated in HRS have less health improvement than those respondents currently married.

Our principal interest in these change models concerns the economic resource variables, especially total household income. In the models contained in Table 4-16, total household income has a statistically significant positive association with health improvements. However, the strength of this relationship signals some reasons for concern. In addition to the influence of permanent income, income shocks may lead to health changes for two reasons. First, transitory income may affect the ability to purchase health care and lower health. Second, income shocks may revise expectations of permanent income as people see their future lot as better than they did in the past. As with other commodities, this upward revision in wealth may lead to the purchase of additional medical services. For a number of reasons, this is not a very reasonable scenario. First, in the age groups we are analyzing, income shocks are relatively unimportant since lifetime economic prospects have been largely determined. Second, as emphasized earlier, revisions in the health stock are by no means instantaneous, and current investments may take years to alter the stock. While income shocks are diminishing in importance in this age range, health shocks are becoming increasingly common. In contrast to our skepticism on the income side, health shocks may have relatively large and quick effects on income prospects. The estimates contained in Table 4-17 generally confirm the cross-sectional estimates. Estimates of the effects of earnings on changes in health status virtually disappear in both samples when we eliminate labor supply effects. Welfare income also largely mirrors reverse causality from health to income.

When no co-variates are included in these models (the first two and the fifth and sixth column of Table 4-16), there are statistically significant racial and ethnic disparities in health trajectories in both samples. Hispanics and blacks are more likely than nonblacks to experience health declines in either age group. These disparities in health trajectories are remarkably similar in size for blacks and Hispanics within and across the two samples. However, after co-variates are controlled for, there are no significant racial or ethnic effects in the differenced formulation. Given the large racial and ethnic health disparities that exist among these middle-aged or older respondents, there is no further racial and ethnic divergence among "similar" people as they age.

Long-Run Measures of Economic Resources

The results thus far demonstrate that regressing current health status on current economic resources hopelessly confuses cause and effect for working-age samples. The short-run reverse causality from health to socioeconomic status is simply too strong. A more promising avenue to pursue is to model short-run health dynamics as a function of long-term household economic status that pre-

TABLE 4-16 Ordered Probit Analysis of Self-Assessed Health Status Change, HRS and AHEAD Samples

Co-variate	HRS Sample				AHEAD Sample			
	Parameter	z	Parameter	z	Parameter	z	Parameter	z
Black	-.1500	4.42	-.0008	00.02	-.1456	3.21	.0114	0.23
Hispanic	-.1686	3.90	-.0060	0.71	-.1626	3.94	.0424	0.61
Female	.0436	2.04	.0566	2.29	.0172	0.62	.0431	1.31
Marital status								
Never married			-.0182	0.25			.1091	1.28
Separated			-.1672	2.12			.0413	0.59
Divorced			-.0884	1.94				
Widowed			.0026	0.05			.0457	1.17
Individual education								
12-15 years			.1347	4.71			.1533	4.73
16 or more years			.1719	4.25			.1899	3.69
Advanced degree			-.1059	0.67			-.0529	0.39
Spousal education								
12-15 years			.0912	3.01			.0485	1.15
16 or more years			.0730	1.72			.0252	0.39
Advanced degree			-.2611	1.39			.0471	0.28
Income and wealth[a]								
Total income			.00160	5.07			.0007	1.88
Total wealth			.00005	1.23			.0002	2.48
Cohort								
1935-1937[b] (1919-1923)[c]			.0631	2.09			.3164	6.78
1938+ (1914-1918)			.0839	3.24			.2481	5.24
(1909-1923)							.1759	3.62

Risk factors				
Smoking				
Ever smoked	-.0718	2.26	-.1202	1.66
Current smoker	-.0427	1.01	-.0018	0.48
Cigarettes smoked per day	-.0031	1.92		
Drinking				
< 1 drink per day	.0668	2.69	.1558	4.97
1 or 2	.1134	2.85	.0539	1.02
3 or 4	.0869	1.44	.0912	0.86
5 or more	-.1540	1.73	-.2081	0.83
Light exercise				
3 times per week	.5541	13.77		
1-2 times per week	.4554	10.35		
1-3 times per month	.3989	7.72		
less than once a month	.2613	4.90		
Vigorous exercise				
3 times per week	.3721	10.07		
1-2 times per week	.2138	5.37		
1-3 times per month	.2276	5.33		
less than once a month	.1788	5.82		
Occupational hazard				
Ever exposed	-.0266	0.57		
Years exposed	-.0047	3.21		

Continued on following page

TABLE 4-16 Continued

Co-variate	HRS Sample				AHEAD Sample			
	Parameter	z	Parameter	z	Parameter	z	Parameter	z
Body mass index (BM1)								
BM1	.0221	2.01			.0753	4.51		
BM1^2	-.0005	3.17			-.0015	4.92		
Prior year's health								
Excellent	-1.876	35.2	-1.387	28.2	-1.792	26.4	-1.597	24.5
Very good	-1.525	30.7	-1.138	24.3	-1.636	27.2	-1.456	25.0
Good	-1.347	28.0	-1.089	23.5	-1.565	27.2	-1.447	25.7
Fair	-1.201	24.1	-1.084	22.2	-1.485	25.5	-1.423	24.7
Cut point 1	-2.561		-2.509		-1.046		-2.202	
Cut point 2	-1.735		-1.686		1.048		-.153	
Cut point 3	.710		-0.755					
Cut point 4	1.607		1.409					

[a]Expressed in thousand dollar units.
[b]Cohort category for HRS sample.
[c]Cohort category for AHEAD sample.

TABLE 4-17   Ordered Probit Analysis of Health Change with Alternative Measures of Income[a]

Co-variate	Parameter	z	Parameter	z	Parameter	z
	HRS Sample (Ages 51-61)					
Individual						
Earnings	.0018	4.06	.0008	1.58		
Weekly wages					.0084	0.86
Retirement income	−.0011	0.68	.0085	3.84	.0079	3.56
Welfare income	−.0187	2.49	−.0009	0.09	.0029	0.27
Earnings = 0			−.1528	5.35		
Weekly wages = 0					−.1584	3.94
Retirement income = 0	.1723	4.23	.1308	3.20		
Welfare income = 0			.1048	1.88	.0620	1.11
Spouse						
Earnings	.0021	4.16	.0008	1.40		
Weekly wages					−.0134	1.34
Retirement income	−.0007	0.36	.0062	2.63	.0089	3.77
Welfare income	−.0271	3.27	−.0022	1.94	−.0018	1.57
Earnings = 0			−.1675	5.36		
Weekly wages = 0					.1190	2.89
Retirement income = 0	.0704	1.60	.0866	1.96		
Welfare income = 0			.0224	0.35	−.0021	0.03
Asset income	−.0001	0.19	.0012	1.93	.0007	1.07
Asset income = 0			.0502	2.12	.0404	1.70
Wealth	.0001	1.63	.0001	2.42	.0001	2.86
Black	−.0027	0.07	−.0127	−0.35	.0111	0.30
Hispanic	−.0045	0.10	−.0061	−0.13	.0043	0.09
Female	.0643	2.36	.0679	2.47	.0917	3.42
	AHEAD Sample (Ages 70 and Over)					
Individual						
Earnings	.0049	3.01	.0001	0.04		
Social Security	.0042	0.89	.0065	1.21		
Other retirement income	.0020	0.91	.0014	0.55		
Earnings = 0			−.2675	5.37		
Social Security = 0			.1166	1.54		
Other retirement income = 0			−.0280	0.81		
Spouse						
Earnings	−.0001	0.06	−.0009	0.42		
Social Security	.0042	0.72	.0096	1.43		
Retirement income	.0043	1.73	.0028	1.00		
Earnings = 0			−.0236	0.39		
Social Security = 0			.1917	2.09		
Retirement income = 0			−.0491	1.07		

Continued on following page

TABLE 4-17   Continued

Co-variate	Parameter	z	Parameter	z	Parameter	z
Asset income	.0003	0.75	.0003	0.69		
Asset income = 0			−.0184	0.58		
Welfare income			−.0194	0.90		
Welfare income = 0			.2329	3.17		
Wealth	.0001	1.81	.0001	1.63		
Black	.0346	0.71	.0457	0.92		
Hispanic	.1165	1.61	.1376	1.89		
Female	.0476	1.22	.0487	1.22		

[a]All continuous income and wealth coefficients expressed in thousands of dollars.

dates current health transitions. Fortunately, we are able to do this in the part of the HRS sample that is linked to Social Security records. These records contain the complete history of a respondent's Social Security earnings.[28] Two proxies for Social Security wealth are used in this research. The first measures the sum of the household's Social Security earnings up to age 50, the starting age of the HRS sample. The second construct sums household Social Security earnings up to age 40. The advantage of the second measure is that it predates HRS health measurement by at least 10 years, effectively eliminating short-run reverse causality from health to economic status.

The empirical estimates summarized in Table 4-18 do suggest that long-term wealth as measured by Social Security earnings affects health trajectories of mature men and women. This effect is present whether we sum past earnings to age 50 or age 40. While both spouses' Social Security earnings have positive effects, the impact of one's own Social Security is larger. While these estimates are less subject to short-run reverse causality problems, they are not immune from long-run problems. If individuals work and earn less as a result of poorer health in the past, causation may still flow from health to economic status.

CONCLUSIONS

This paper has critically explored the role that socioeconomic status plays in explaining racial and ethnic differences in health outcomes of Americans during their middle and old age. Although our results are consistent with other research suggesting an important role for socioeconomic status as a factor accounting for

---

[28]The use of these data creates a number of issues. First, in only two-thirds of all households did the respondent and spouse agree to the Social Security linkage. All estimates in this section are confined to that subsample. Second, Social Security earnings are capped at the limit.

TABLE 4-18   Ordered Probit Analysis of Health Change with Alternative Measures of Social Security Earnings Histories, HRS Sample (ages 51-61)

Characteristic	Parameter	z	Parameter	z	Parameter	z
	Social Security Earnings to Age 50					
Total income[a]	.0011	2.18	b		b	
Wealth[a]	.0001	1.27	.0001	2.11	.0001	2.12
Social Security Earnings[a]						
Household	.0002	3.95	.0001	2.93		
Respondent					.0002	2.98
Spousal					.0001	1.15
Black	−.0456	0.92	−.0680	−1.30	−.0673	1.34
Hispanic	.0465	0.68	.0403	0.58	.0398	0.57
Female	.0339	1.00	.0324	0.64	.0111	0.26
	Social Security Earnings to Age 40					
Total income	.0012	2.36	b	b		
Wealth	.0001	1.27	.0001	2.14	.0001	2.15
Social Security Earnings						
Household	.0004	4.30	.0003	3.41		
Respondent					.0003	3.25
Spousal					.0002	1.69
Black	−.0413	0.83	−.0639	−1.30	−.0635	1.26
Hispanic	.0533	0.76	.0476	0.68	.0471	0.67
Female	.0392	0.76	.0377	1.00	.0207	0.63

[a]All continuous income and asset coefficients expressed in thousands of dollars.

[b]For last four columns, the model includes all income components and non-receipts of income components.

racial and ethnic differences, our results indicate that the relationship among race and ethnicity, socioeconomic status, and health is far more complex than many current analyses recognize. We focus attention on the complexity involved in accounting for economic status as an underlying factor in health status. First, there are two important dimensions of economic status—income and wealth—each with distinct conceptual and empirical associations with health. Second, the association of some common measures of socioeconomic status with health status is highly nonlinear. For example, the association of both income and wealth with self-reported general health status is strongest among the poorest households and is relatively weak among the most affluent members of our society.

Both of these issues may affect how we account for racial and ethnic differences in health in later life. Finally, there is compelling evidence that the feedbacks from health to current socioeconomic status are quantitatively strong and should not be ignored in empirical investigations. In particular, the entire association between current household income and health among households with a member in his or her fifties appears to reflect causation from health to income rather than from income to health. As new longitudinal data sets with more detailed and varied measures of economic status and health status become available, future research should progress toward a more complete understanding of the pathways linking race and ethnicity, socioeconomic status, and health across the lifespan.

ACKNOWLEDGMENT

This research was supported by Grant 5PO1-AG08291 awarded by the National Institute on Aging, U.S. Department of Health and Human Services, and by Grant 5P50-HD12639 awarded by the National Institute of Child Health and Human Development.

REFERENCES

Berman, J.R., R. Sickles, P. Taubman, and A. Yazbeck
  1991   Black-white mortality inequalities. *Journal of Econometrics* 50:183-203.
Blesch, K., and S. Furner
  1993   Health of Older Black Americans. *Vital and Health Statistics* S2:229-273.
Broderick, J.P., T. Brott, T. Tomsick, G. Huster, and R. Miller
  1992   The risk of subarachnoid and intracerebral hemorrhages in blacks as compared with whites. *New England Journal of Medicine* 326:733-736.
Caplan, L.S., B.L. Wells, and S. Haynes
  1992   Breast cancer screening among older racial/ethnic minorities and whites: Barriers to early detection. *Journal of Gerontology* 47:101-110.
Clark, D.O., and G.L. Maddox
  1992   Racial and social correlates of age-related changes in functioning. *Journal of Gerontology* 47:S222-232.
Clark, D.O., G.L. Maddox, and K. Steinhauser
  1993   Race, aging, and functional health. *Journal of Aging and Health* 5:536-553.
Cooper, R.
  1986   The biological concept of race and its application to public health and epidemiology. *Journal of Health Politics, Policy Law* 11(1):97-116.
Dardanoni, V., and A. Wagstaff
  1987   Uncertainty, inequalities in health and the demand for health. *Journal of Health Economics* 6:283-390.
DaVanzo, J., and P. Gertler
  1990   Household production of health: A microeconomic perspective on health transitions. An unpublished paper presented at workshop on the Measurement of Health Transition Concepts in London, June 7-9, 1989; N-3014-RC. RAND, Santa Monica, CA.
Dowd, J.J., and V.L. Bengtson
  1978   Aging in minority populations: An examination of the double jeopardy hypothesis. *Journal of Gerontology* 33:427-436.

Eley, J.W., H.A. Hill, V.W. Chen, D.F. Austin, M.N., Wesley, H.B. Muss, R.S. Greenberg, R.J. Coates, P. Correa, C.K., Redmond, C.P. Hunter, A.A. Herman, R. Kurman, R. Blacklow, S. Shapiro, and B.K. Edwards
   1994   Racial differences in survival from breast cancer: Results of the National Cancer Institute black/white cancer survival study. *Journal of the American Medical Association* 272:947-954.

Ewbank, D.C.
   1987   History of black mortality and health before 1940. *Milbank Quarterly* 65:100-128.

Feldstein, P.J.
   1983   *Health Care Economics*, 2nd. ed. New York: Wiley Medical Publication.

Ferraro, K.F.
   1987   Double jeopardy to health for black older adults. *Journal of Gerontology* 42:528-533.

Fuchs, V.R.
   1982   Time preference and health: An exploratory study. In *Economic Aspects of Health*, V.R. Fuchs, ed. Chicago: University of Chicago Press.

Furner, S.E.
   1993   Special topics. *Vital and Health Statistics* (29):37-55.

Garber, A.
   1989   Pursuing the links between socioeconomic factors and health: Critique, policy implications, and directions for future research. In *Pathways to Health—The Role of Social Factors*, J.P. Bunker, D.S. Gomby, and B.H. Kehrer, eds. Menlo Park, CA: Henry J. Kaiser Family Foundation.

Gibson, R.C.
   1991   Age-by-race differences in the health and functioning of elderly persons. *Journal of Aging Health* 3:335-351.

Grossman, M.
   1972   *The Demand for Health: A Theoretical and Empirical Investigation*. New York: National Bureau of Economic Research.

Guralnik, J.M., and G.A. Kaplan
   1989   Predictors of health aging: Prospective evidence from the Alameda County Study. *American Journal of Public Health* 79:703-708.

Guralnik, J.M., A.Z. LaCroix, R.D. Abbott, L.F. Berkman, A. Satterfield, D.A. Evans, and R. Wallace
   1993   Maintaining mobility in late life: Demographic characteristics and chronic conditions. *American Journal of Epidemiology* 137:845-857.

Guralnik, J.M., K.C. Land, D. Blazer, G.G. Fillenbaum, and L.G. Branch
   1993   Educational status and active life expectancy among older blacks and whites. *New England Journal of Medicine* 329(2):110-116.

Haan, M.N., and G.A. Kaplan
   1985   The contribution of socioeconomic position to minority health. Report to the NIH Task Force on Black and Minority Health. Bethesda, MD: National Institutes of Health.

Hahn, R.A.
   1992   The state of federal health statistics on racial and ethnic groups. *Journal of the American Medical Association* 267(2):268-271.

House, J.S., R.C. Kessler, A.R. Herzog, R.P. Meto, A.M. Kinney, and M. J. Breslow
   1990   Age, socioeconomic status, and health. *Milbank Quarterly* 68:383-411.

James, S.A., D.S. Strogatz, S.B. Wing, and D.L. Ramsey
   1987   Socioeconomic status, John Henryism, and hypertension in blacks and whites. *American Journal of Epidemiology* 126:664-673.

Jones, C.P., T.A. LaVeist, and M. Lillie-Blanton
   1991   "Race" in the epidemiologic literature: An examination of the American Journal of Epidemiology. *American Journal of Epidemiology* 134(10):1079-1084.

Kaplan, G.A., T.E. Seeman, R.D. Cohen, L.P. Knudsen, and J. Guralnik
    1987   Mortality among the elderly in the Alameda County study: Behavioral and demographic
            risk factors. *American Journal of Public Health* 77:307-312.
Kaplan, N.M.
    1994   Ethnic aspects of hypertension. *Lancet* 344:450-452.
Keil, J.E., S.E. Sutherland, R.G. Knapp, and H.A. Tyroler
    1992   Does equal socioeconomic status in black and white men mean equal risk of mortality?
            American Journal of Public Health 82:1133-1136.
Kellie, S.E., and J.A. Brody
    1990   Sex-specific and race-specific hip fracture rates. *American Journal of Public Health*
            80(3):326-328.
Kington, R., and J.P. Smith
    In   Socioeconomic status and racial and ethnic differences press in functional status associ-
    press   ated with chronic diseases. *American Journal of Public Health.*
Krieger, N.
    1990   Social class and the black/white crossover in the age-specific incidence of breast cancer:
            A study linking census-derived data to population-based registry records. *American Jour-
            nal of Epidemiology* 131:804-814.
Krieger, N., D.L. Rowley, A.A. Herman, B. Avery, and M.T. Phillips
    1993   Racism, sexism, and social class: Implications for studies of health, disease, and well-
            being. *American Journal of Preventive Medicine* 9:82-122.
Kuczmarski, R.J., K.M. Flegal, S.M. Campbell, and C.L. Johnson
    1994   Increasing prevalence of overweight among U.S. adults. *Journal of the American Medi-
            cal Association* 272:205-211.
LaViest, T.A.
    1994   Beyond dummy variables and sample selection: What health services researchers ought to
            know about race as a variable. *Health Services Research* 29:1-16.
Lewontin, R.C.
    1972   The apportionment of human diversity. *Evolutionary Biology* 6:381-398.
Liberatos, P., B.G. Link, and J.L. Kelsey
    1988   The measurement of social class in epidemiology. *Epidemiology Reviews* 10:87-121.
Macken, C. L.
    1986   A profile of functionally impaired elderly persons living in the community. *Health Care
            Financing Review* 7:33-49.
Manton, K.G., C.H. Patrick, and K.W. Johnson
    1987   Health differentials between blacks and whites: Recent trends in mortality and morbidity.
            Milbank Quarterly 65:129-199.
Massey, D., and N. Denton
    1989   Hypersegregation in U.S. metropolitan areas: Black and Hispanic segregation along five
            dimensions. *Demography* 26(3):373-441.
Menchik, P.L.
    1993   Economic status as a determinant of mortality among black and white and older men:
            Does poverty kill? *Population Studies* 47:427-436.
Mermelstein, R., B. Miller, T. Prohaska, V. Benson, and J.F. Van Nostrand
    1993   Measures of health. *Vital Health Statistics* 3(27):9-21.
Mor, V., J. Murphy, and S. Masterson-Allen
    1989   Risk of functional decline among well-elders. *Journal of Clinical Epidemiology* 42:895-
            904.
Mutchler, J.E., and J.A. Burr
    1991   Racial differences in health and care service utilization in later life: The effect of socio-
            economic status. *Journal of Health and Social Behavior* 32:342-356.

Muurinen, J.M., and J. Le Grand
  1985   The economic analysis of inequalities in health. *Social Science and Medicine* 20:1029-1035.
Osborne, N.G., and M.D. Feit
  1992   The use of race in medical research. *Journal of the American Medical Association* 267(2):275-279.
Otten, M.W., S.M. Teutsch, D.F. Williamson, and J.S. Marks
  1990   The effect of known risk factors on the excess mortality of black adults in the United States. *Journal of the American Medical Association* 263:845-850.
Preston, S.E., and P. Taubman.
  1994   Socioeconomic differences in adult mortality and health status. In *Demography of Aging*, L.G. Martin and S.H. Preston, eds. Washington, DC: National Academy Press.
Rogers, R.G.
  1992   Living and dying in the U.S.A: Sociodemographic determinants of death among blacks and whites. *Demography* 29:287-303.
Rosenzweig, M.R., and T.P. Schultz
  1983   Estimating a household production function: Heterogeneity, the demand for health inputs, and their effects on birth weight. *Journal of Political Economy* 91(5):723-746.
Satariano, W.A.
  1986   Race, socioeconomic status and health: A study of age differences in a depressed area. *American Journal of Preventive Medicine* 2:1-5.
Schoenberg, B.S., D.W. Anderson, and A.R. Haerer
  1986   Racial differentials in the prevalence of stroke. *Archives of Neurology* 43:565-568.
Selden, T.M.
  1993   Uncertainty and health care spending by the poor: The health capital model revisited. *Journal of Health Economics* 12:109-115.
Serjeant, G.R.
  1985   *Sickle Cell Disease.* New York: Oxford University Press.
Smith, J.P.
  1984   Race and human capital. *American Economic Review* 74(4):685-698.
  1994   Hispanics and the American dream. Unpublished manuscript. Santa Monica, CA: RAND.
  1995   Racial and ethnic differences in wealth using the Health and Retirement Study. *Journal of Human Resources* 30:S158-S183.
  In   Wealth inequality among older Americans. *Journal of Gerontology.*
  press
Smith, J.P., and R. Kington
  1996   Demographic and Economic Correlates of Health in Old Age. Santa Monica, CA: RAND, DRU-1316-NIA.
Sobal, J., and A.J. Stunkard
  1989   Socioeconomic status and obesity: A review of the literature. *Psychology Bulletin* 105:260-275.
Sommer, A., J.M. Tielsch, J. Katz, H.A. Quigley, J.D. Gottsch, J.C. Javitt, J.F. Martone, R.M. Royall, K.A. Witt, and S. Ezrine
  1991   Racial differences in the cause-specific prevalence of blindness in East Baltimore. *New England Journal of Medicine* 325:1412-1417.
Sorlie, P., E. Rogot, R. Anderson, N.J. Johnson, and E. Backlund
  1992   Black-white mortality differences by family income. *Lancet* 340:346-350.
Strawbridge, W.J., G.A. Kaplan, T. Camacho, and R.D. Cohen
  1992   The dynamics of disability and functional change in an elderly cohort: Results from the Alameda County study. *Journal of the American Geriatric Society* 40:799-806.

U.S. Department of Health and Human Services
  1990   *Healthy People 2000: National Health Promotion and Disease Prevention Objectives.*
          Washington, DC: U.S. Department of Health and Human Services.
Wagstaff, A.
  1986   The demand for health: Theory and applications. *Journal of Epidemiology and Commu-
          nity Health* 40:1-11.
Waitzman, N.J., and K.R. Smith
  1994   The effects of occupational class transitions on hypertension: Racial disparities among
          working-age men. *American Journal of Public Health* 84:945-950.
Williams, D.R.
  1994   The concept of race in *Health Services Research*: 1966 to 1990. *Health Services Re-
          search* 29(3):261-274.
Williams, D.R., R. Lavizzo-Mourey, and R.C. Warren
  1984   The concept of race and health and status in America. Paper from the CDC-ATSDR
          Workshop on the use of Race and Ethnicity in Public Health Surveillance. *Public Health
          Reports* 109(1):26-41.
Zick, C.D., and K.R. Smith
  1991   Marital transitions, poverty, and gender differences in mortality. *Journal of Marriage
          and the Family* 53:327-336.

5

How Health Behaviors and the Social Environment Contribute to Health Differences Between Black and White Older Americans

Lisa F. Berkman and Jewel M. Mullen

INTRODUCTION

Since data have been collected in the United States on racial differences in health status, blacks have been found to be at increased risk for almost every poor health outcome from most causes of morbidity to mortality and disability. Such inequalities in health are documented for men and women from birth to old age. Even crossovers in very old age in which blacks have been shown to have a survival advantage are now viewed with renewed skepticism (see Elo and Preston, and Manton and Stallard, in this volume). Furthermore, while health status has improved over the last decades for all Americans, the gains have been greater for whites than for blacks, producing an even larger health disparity for blacks in the last decade or two. For instance, during the last 30 years, life expectancy at age 65 increased 2.4 years for white males and only 1.5 years for black males. The corresponding increases for women are 3.1 years for white women and 2.5 years for black women (U.S. Department of Health and Human Services, 1993).

The reasons offered to account for these disparities range from genetic and selection factors to environmental exposures and differential access to medical care. Rather than explore this multitude of possibilities, this paper explores the extent to which health-damaging and health-promoting behaviors explain black-white differences in health status. In addition, we have taken the perspective that while behaviors are de facto performed by individuals, individual behaviors occur in a social context. They are heavily influenced by the larger social structure. For instance, laws regulating the consumption and taxation of alcohol and cigarettes lead directly to altered patterns of consumption. Most behaviors, in fact, vary across social strata. In this paper we are specifically interested in the extent to which there are differences in the distribution of health behaviors or social networks between blacks and whites in the United States and whether this differential distribution is related to underlying differences in socioeconomic status.

The paper is divided into several sections. First we review the evidence on the distribution of health-damaging and health-promoting behaviors among blacks and whites. We take a rather broad perspective on such behaviors, reviewing those that are traditionally called risk behaviors, such as cigarette and alcohol consumption, as well as health-promoting activities, such as physical exercise and maintaining social community ties.

In the second section we examine the distribution of health-damaging and health-promoting behaviors in a large study of older men and women, the New Haven Established Populations for the Epidemiologic Study of the Elderly (EPESE). In that section, we examine both traditional health behaviors and cardiovascular risk factors as well as social conditions related to social networks and socioeconomic status.

THE ROLE OF ATTITUDES AND SOCIAL CONTEXT IN BEHAVIORS THAT DAMAGE OR PROMOTE HEALTH AMONG BLACKS AND WHITES

Comparisons of the health practices of black and white older men and women should not be made without the following considerations:

1. It is now becoming evident that knowledge and information are not the only determinants of behavior. A corollary is that a particular behavior does not necessarily reflect lack of information. People who are aware that exercise helps reduce the risk of heart disease may nonetheless maintain a sedentary lifestyle (Oldridge, 1982). Many cigarette smokers, aware of the association between coronary artery disease or lung cancer and tobacco, continue to smoke (Rigotti et al., 1994). Data about racial differences in knowledge of particular health risks must be considered in the context of other factors that influence the ability or desire to act on that knowledge. Poverty, poor access to medical care, perceived powerlessness and frustration, peer pressure, and differential access to alcohol, tobacco, and food all can impede the adoption of health-enhancing practices (Braithwaite and Lythcott, 1989; Blendon et al., 1989; Rogers, 1992).

2. Even when knowledge and information are adequate, other factors on the health care side of the equation may lead to behavior that is associated with poor health outcomes. Both race and social position have been shown to correlate with the quality and type of screening and therapeutic recommendations that health care providers give their patients (Burstin et al., 1992; American Medical Association Council on Ethical and Judicial Affairs, 1990). Analyzing data from the 1988-1990 Behavioral Risk Factor Surveillance System, Giles et al. (1993) showed that adults consulting a physician for preventive care were less likely to

be screened for hypercholesterolemia if they were black or had not completed high school than if they were white or more educated. Black adults who needed treatment for elevated blood cholesterol were also less likely to be treated. That difference persisted after adjustment for socioeconomic status. In a meta-analysis of studies on behavior of health care providers, Hall et al. (1988) found that social class correlated positively with the information the provider gave the patient: patients of higher social position received superior care, and whites received better care than blacks. Hall et al. found that health care providers were also more likely to engage in "positive talk" with their white patients. That communication style, characterized by reassurance, approbation, and encouragement, correlated positively with patient adherence to treatment.

3. A related phenomenon is that a person's health practices partially reflect the attitudes of his or her health care provider. A clinician's appraisal of a patient's ability to modify health-affecting behavior may cause the clinician to lower his or her expectations for favorable outcomes (Hall et al., 1988). This practice does not necessarily reflect client-centered care. Rather, it may create a self-fulfilling prophecy: with lowered expectations, a health care provider may make less effort to promote health-enhancing behaviors and thereby help to perpetuate the clients' health-damaging behavior. This relationship between provider attitudes and patient practices has been evident in clinical settings, particularly when practitioners have been unsuccessful in helping their patients lose weight, stop smoking, or control their blood sugar. Discouraged by such failure, clinicians can become more accepting of the adverse behaviors of other patients, particularly those from the same racial, social, or ethnic group.

In this section we examine the influence of (and interaction between) race and socioeconomic status on the following attitudes, behaviors, and social environments of black and white older men and women: (1) perceived health and health behavior; (2) diet, smoking, alcohol consumption, and physical exercise; (3) prevalence and control of diabetes and hypertension; and (4) social networks and support. We selected these risk factors because of the recognition that their effects on many chronic diseases, especially cardiovascular and cerebrovascular disease, are interrelated.

Self-Appraisal of Health and Health Behavior

Many investigators suggest that it is important to study preventive health practices of older adults in order to elucidate the behavioral determinants of successful aging (Lubben et al., 1989b; Stults, 1984; Rowe, 1987; Kane, 1985). Others explore racial differences in health practices in an attempt to understand why blacks experience excess morbidity and mortality (Rogers, 1992; Mutchler and Burr, 1991; Duelberg, 1992). Comparisons of health-protective attitudes and behaviors among blacks and whites are also made for the purpose of explaining the possible crossover of their mortality rates (Ford et al., 1990). In a study of the interaction between the extent to which adults worry about heart disease, Ransford (1986) found that at all educational levels, blacks reported greater concern about heart disease. Surprisingly, those concerns translated into more health-protective behavior (exercise, changed dietary habits, or smoking cessation) only among blacks who had less than a high school education. In a survey examining the relationship between socioeconomic characteristics and health beliefs, Weissfeld et al. (1990) found that blacks and those of lower socioeconomic status (measured by a composite of education and income level) placed a higher value on healthful habits than others. After adjustment for race, the association between perceived health threats and socioeconomic status diminished. Ford et al. (1990) reported the results of a cohort study that demonstrated that blacks over age 74 considered themselves less healthy (including mentally) than did whites. A survey by Mutchler and Burr (1991) demonstrated a similar disparity in self-appraisal of health that persisted after adjustment for socioeconomic status. Lubben et al. (1989a) found a similarity between the health practices of black and white Medicaid recipients in California over age 65. Whites were more likely to maintain their desired body weight, but there were no significant racial differences in smoking, exercising, alcohol intake, or maintenance of social networks.

Thus, these studies would suggest, albeit not conclusively, that blacks, especially older blacks, are concerned about chronic disease, appraise their health status as worse than whites, and place an equal or higher value on health-protective behaviors. These findings reinforce the theory that behavior change does not rest on knowledge and awareness alone.

Health Behaviors

Diet and Exercise

The behavioral aspects of obesity have an impact on the difference in disease patterns between blacks and whites. Obesity is associated with hypertension, non-insulin-dependent diabetes mellitus, and osteoarthritis (Pi-Sunyer, 1993), all of which are more prevalent among blacks (National Center for Health Statistics, 1990). It is now believed that weight loss and maintenance are probably best achieved through a combination of dietary control and increased physical activity (DiPietro et al., 1993). For this reason, we will discuss issues related to diet and exercise together.

As many as 60 percent of black women are overweight (Kumanyika, 1987). The higher prevalence of obesity in older black women is related to their higher baseline body mass index in middle age (Williamson et al., 1991) and to their being less likely to lose weight during those years (Kahn et al., 1991). That black women express a positive attitude about their weight more often than white women is a behavioral element that is felt to influence the potential success of dietary interventions designed for them. Although studies about weight perceptions have generally been done in younger populations (Kumanyika et al., 1993; Rucker and Cash, 1991), Stevens et al. (1994) found that elderly black women also have a greater acceptance of being overweight than their white counterparts. Socioeconomic status was not included in that analysis. In a study of dietary patterns of centenarians and adults who were in their sixties and eighties, Johnson et al. (1992) found that three times as many blacks as whites reported a desire to eat more nutritiously. In that study, blacks also reported larger fluctuations in their adult weight. Again, we see that blacks maintain a desire to eat more nutritiously although they tend to be more overweight.

Comparisons of activity levels in elderly racial groups have more often included examination of the effects of socioeconomic status than have studies of dietary patterns (Folsom et al., 1990; Sheridan et al., 1993; Kaplan et al., 1987). Numerous studies have shown that blacks exercise less than whites and engage is less leisure time physical activity (Burke et al., 1992; Washburn et al., 1992; Heath and Smith, 1994): 19 percent of black versus 29.9 percent of white women over age 65 exercise or play sports regularly. The comparative proportions of black and white men who so exercise is 25.1 percent to 36.3 percent. In the cohort above 65 years old, 38.4 percent of black versus 44.9 percent of white women walk for exercise, while for men the rates are 42.6 percent and 52.4 percent, respectively. Folsom et al. (1990) reported data from the Minnesota Heart Survey that demonstrated that the largest difference in leisure time physical activity between blacks and whites occurred in those with a high school education or less. Using data from the National Health Interview Survey (NHIS) and adjusting for education and income, Duelberg showed that these racial differences in exercise patterns could not be entirely explained by socioeconomic status. In a study of how education level and race were associated with risk factors for coronary artery disease among younger men and women, Sheridan et al. (1993) found that lack of regular exercise was more common in blacks, even after adjustment for education. Kaplan et al. (1987) reported that decreased physical activity was a mortality risk factor independent of socioeconomic position in Alameda County elders.

Cigarette Smoking

The prevalence of cigarette smoking among older Americans is complex and is related to cohort effects and different norms among men and women. Population-based estimates provide valuable information about smoking patterns in all blacks and whites, as well as in elderly subgroups. Some general observations are that (1) overall, whites are heavier smokers than blacks; (2) black men smoke more and black women smoke less than their white counterparts; and (3) smoking rates are higher and cessation rates are lower in persons with less education (Centers for Disease Control [CDC] 1994).

In the 1991 NHIS (CDC, 1994), the prevalence of smoking was higher in blacks than whites (29.1% vs. 25.5%), although a higher percentage of blacks reported having never smoked (56.2% vs. 48.9%). Also in that survey, 50 percent of respondents over age 65 had never smoked, compared with 67 percent in 1965. This decrease in the percentage of elderly abstainers was not consistent among all gender and racial subgroups. Whereas abstention rates increased among elderly men, they decreased in women. Moreover, between 1965 and 1991, the net increase in the percentage of those who had never smoked was twice as high for older blacks as for whites (10.4% vs. 5.1%). Despite these trends, smoking rates are higher for elderly black men than for their white counterparts. In women, the rates are higher in whites than in blacks. These differences are illustrated by NHIS data (National Center for Health Statistics, 1993), which show that in 1987, 30 percent of elderly black men were smokers, compared with 16 percent of white men. Whereas 13.9 percent of older white women in that survey smoked, only 11.7 percent of black women did. Although the racial differences in the percentage of smokers among both genders was a bit lower in the 1990 NHIS (National Center for Health Statistics, 1993), the overall trends were identical.

Smaller studies have also described the epidemiology of smoking in older adults. Sheridan et al. (1993) performed a cross-sectional analysis of cardiovascular risk factors in urban South Carolina residents. In his sample, the prevalence of smoking in elderly black and white men and women was very similar to that found in the population-based studies. Other investigators have described similar differences in the tobacco use of black and white elders. For example, in a study of hypertensives, Svetkey et al. (1993) found mean lifetime cigarette consumption higher in whites than blacks. Among Medi-Cal recipients in the study by Lubben et al. (1989b), blacks were 1.66 times less likely to have ever smoked than whites. Finally, Aronow and Kronson (1991) demonstrated a higher smoking rate (9% vs. 7%) in African Americans in their analysis of coronary risk factors in the elderly. Additional research is needed to identify possible correlates (including social class) of tobacco use for older blacks and whites. Smoking cessation confers health benefits on the elderly who have already developed smoking-related cardiovascular or pulmonary disease (CDC, 1990). If low social class explains a large share of the described black-white differences in smoking behavior, strategies to promote quitting should be directed toward a subset of elders of low socioeconomic position, rather than toward those in either racial category.

Alcohol Use

Most studies of alcohol consumption show either no differences by race or increased consumption among white men and women. In the 1990 NHIS (National Center for Health Statistics, 1993), whites displayed a higher overall prevalence of alcohol consumption than did blacks; a similar comparison was also evident in the cohort aged 65 and older: 9 percent of white men and 3.4 percent of white women reported drinking an ounce or more of ethanol in the 2 weeks prior to their interview, compared with 1.9 percent and 0.4 percent of black men and women, respectively. Although the research by Lubben et al. (1989b) on the health of poor elderly adults in California did not find a racial difference in alcohol patterns, a cross-sectional investigation by Molgaard et al. (1990) did. In that study of San Diego County adults age 45 and older, the overall prevalence of drinking was higher in whites than in blacks (79% vs. 50%). For adults 65 and older, drinking rates were also higher in whites (74% vs. 49%). However, those percentages represent only the self-reported prevalence of drinking after age 40. Therefore, direct inferences about current age-specific drinking patterns could not be made.

Health Practices of Elderly Diabetics and Hypertensives

Exercise, dietary control, and adherence to therapy all influence morbidity associated with hypertension and diabetes. Exercise enhances weight reduction with resultant improvement in glucose tolerance in diabetics (Ruderman et al., 1990). However, control of high blood sugars alone does not attenuate diabetics' risk for coronary artery disease. Management of co-morbid conditions such as hypercholesterolemia, hypertension, and cigarette smoking is an essential aspect of diabetic care. Although diabetes is twice as prevalent in older black Americans than in whites (National Center for Health Statistics, 1990), as previously noted, African Americans are less likely to engage in a level of physical activity that might help modulate this condition. This behavioral tendency was demonstrated by Spangler and Konen (1993), who conducted a survey of type I and type II diabetics and found that white diabetics were more likely not only to engage in high levels of exercise, but also to be former smokers. Cowie et al. (1993), evaluating participants in the National Health and Nutrition Survey (NHANES) II, showed that racial differences in the risk for non-insulin-dependent diabetes could not be explained by differences in social status but were strongly correlated with obesity. In a descriptive study of the health behaviors of a small sample of elderly black diabetics in San Francisco, Reid (1992) found that older patients relied more on traditional (rather than folk) medical care than a similar group of younger people. In that study, elders with multiple co-morbid conditions took better care of themselves and adhered more to treatment.

Exercise also has beneficial effects on blood pressure control. Like studies of diabetics, examinations of the health practices of elderly hypertensives often focus on behavioral determinants of obesity (diet, exercise) and salt intake (Svetkey et al., 1993; Spangler and Konen, 1993). Svetkey's study of hypertensive EPESE participants in North Carolina demonstrated that elderly black hypertensives actually had lower salt intake than whites. Lower salt consumption was inversely associated with hypertension risk. In that study, adjustment for socioeconomic status reduced the association between hypertension and race, but did not eliminate it. Having a low-sodium diet was also characteristic of the blacks in Johnson's report on the nutritional habits of centenarians. The authors in both studies hypothesized that black patients, aware of their disproportionate risk of high blood pressure, listen more to messages to moderate their salt intake. Another indicator of such adherence can be found in data from the National Center for Health Statistics (1993), which reveal that a slightly higher percentage of elderly black women and men with high blood pressure also reported that they were taking antihypertensive medications. Sheridan et al. (1993) reported the results of a cross-sectional survey that explored the association between ethnicity and educational level with several behavioral risks for cardiovascular disease in adults between the ages of 20 and 64. Black respondents were less likely than whites to know their own blood pressure or cholesterol level or to accurately indicate what the desirable levels of these risk factors were. These racial differences persisted after adjustment for educational attainment. Since this study did not examine the prevalence of diseases that increase the risk of cardiovascular disease, data about hypertensives and what proportion of them adhered to therapy were not reported. Age-specific data on that topic might clarify whether the observed health practices of elders have been consistent throughout their adult lives and whether the differences in health behaviors between blacks and whites increase or decrease with age. Including social position in such analyses would help illuminate how much it influences those differences.

Health promotion initiatives based on most of the findings presented in this paper would usually reflect secondary or tertiary prevention efforts given the high prevalence of chronic disease in older age groups. How much impact the initiation of cardiovascular risk reduction efforts for these age groups will ultimately have on their mortality will become clearer as prospective studies exploring this issue are done. Most work of this kind has been in younger adults. However, additional studies on the effect that race and socioeconomic status have on health practices of the elderly not only are important for understanding the determinants of successful aging but also can provide insight into the assumption that improvement in education and income level in blacks may be associated with the adoption of more health-enhancing practices and, ultimately, improved morbidity and mortality. If health differences persist in the context of blacks' and whites' having congruent behaviors and seemingly greater economic equality, there is more reason both to examine the influence of racism on overall health and to explicate the role that genetic predisposition plays in certain diseases such as diabetes and hypertension.

Social Networks and Social Support

There is a large body of evidence documenting the role of social networks and social support in influencing survival and life expectancy (Berkman, 1995, House et al., 1988). Among the elderly, social relationships, especially those that are explicitly defined as supportive, are important not only in reducing mortality risk but also in delaying institutionalization and in maintaining functional independence. Studies to date suggest that the important components of network structure or support are the size of networks, the availability of support, and its perceived adequacy. Furthermore, it seems to be more important that the individual identify someone or some group or organization as fulfilling a specific role than that a specific type of person (i.e., kin, non-kin) fill a role. This suggests that older men and women have a number of options that will be equally "protective" in providing supportive relationships. In other words, one doesn't have to be married to experience decreased mortality risk if other intimate ties are available. Most studies indicate that it is only in the absence of any close ties that risks become elevated.

While the major aim of this section is to explore differences in network structure and social support among older black and white men and women, it is important to recognize that social networks assume forms that reflect the broad structure of society and an individual's position in that social structure (Craven and Wellman, 1973; Tilly, 1972; Bultena, 1969). Socioeconomic status, level of urbanization, and geographic and occupational mobility are all associated with network structure. For instance, in the Alameda County study (Berkman and Breslow, 1983), analysis of individual components of the Social Network Index indicated that people of lower socioeconomic status were less likely to be married and to be affiliated with church and voluntary organizations than others. Only with respect to close friends and relatives do lower class men and women compare favorably. Several ethnographers have documented the relative extensiveness of the working class person's contacts with friends and extended family and have described it as a major resource in the face of other considerable challenges and stresses (Stack, 1974; Liebow, 1967). Thus, it is important to review the evidence that black-white differences in networks and support may be related to social and economic conditions, which may vary between ethnic groups. Only in some studies have the social and economic conditions been thoroughly discussed.

The Alameda County study, conducted in the mid-1960s and 1970s, suggests that there are very small differences between blacks and whites in the percentage of men and women who appear to be isolated on the Social Network Index, a composite index of marital status, contact with friends and relatives, and church and group membership (Berkman and Breslow, 1983). Among men, 38 percent of blacks and 32 percent of whites score in the top two categories of isolation, and 46 percent of black women compared with 44 percent of white women score in the same range. Of more interest are variations within subcategories of the index.

In this area, blacks were less likely to be married or to report membership in voluntary organizations than whites but they were more likely to belong to church groups and to have more contacts with friends and relatives. The strong role of the church in the life of black Americans and the importance of the extended family and three-generation networks have been extensively noted in many studies, most of which are qualitative ethnographic studies (George, 1988; Taylor and Chatters, 1986).

In one of the most thorough and insightful reviews of social networks and support among older black Americans, Taylor (1988) provides both a theoretical overview of a model of family support relationships and a review of non-kin sources of support. The reader is referred to this paper for a more extensive review of the literature than is provided here. Among the more notable studies in this newer wave of research on black Americans is the National Survey of Black Americans. This survey studied a nationally representative cross-sectional sample of the adult black population living in the continental United States that was based on the 1970 census. The study resulted in 2,107 interviews with a response rate of 69 percent. Among a subsample ($n = 581$) of older blacks, 67 percent of respondents said that their families were very close in their feelings for one another, and only 8 percent stated that their families were either not too close or not close at all (Chatters et al., 1985, 1986). Of helper networks, 56 percent were composed exclusively of immediate family and another 33 percent were composed of immediate family and others. Neither family income nor education was associated with network composition. There were, however, regional variations, with southern blacks having larger helper networks than those in other regions of the United States. Since most studies have been based in communities rather than on national samples, it will be important to consider whether regional variations may account for differences in network structure and support between black and whites.

Finally, there is a consistent body of evidence indicating that older blacks are less likely to live alone than older whites. While older blacks are less likely to be married, they are more likely to live in extended households with children and grandchildren. Three-generation households or households whose members do not belong to a nuclear family may have particular advantages for old people, especially those with limited economic resources or functional limitations. When families live as units that share resources and tasks, the individuals in those families may experience benefits that they would not obtain alone or in small nuclear families. At the same time, multigenerational households, if they are bound together only for financial or logistic reasons, may place strains on older people that have not been well identified (George, 1988).

As is suggested by George, there are more similarities in the maintenance of social relationships in late life between blacks and whites than there are differences. The major similarities between blacks and whites are that (1) black and white elders maintain frequent contact with families, especially their children, and (2) both black and white women tend to have more extensive contacts with family members than do men. Both blacks and whites have a similar hierarchy by which support is provided to older members of the family. This principle of hierarchy developed by Cantor (1979, 1983) suggests that spouses are the first choice of source of support, followed by children (especially daughters) if spouses are unavailable. More distant relatives are the source of support if members of a nuclear family are unavailable. George reviews multiple studies indicating that this hierarchy applies to both racial groups.

On the other hand, most studies indicate that older blacks both receive and provide more social support than do older whites.

RACIAL AND SOCIOECONOMIC DIFFERENCES IN HEALTH AND SOCIAL BEHAVIORS: FINDINGS FROM THE NEW HAVEN EPESE

In this section we examine differences in health and social behaviors among older black and white men and women. Data are analyzed from the New Haven EPESE program, which is based on a probability sample of 2,806 noninstitutionalized men and women living in New Haven, Connecticut, in 1982. Details of the sampling frame have been reported elsewhere (Berkman et al., 1986). This study has the advantage of including (1) a very heterogeneous sample in terms of race, socioeconomic status, and health status and (2) a broad array of health behaviors and social conditions. Since it is a community sample of older men and women in an urban area of the Northeast, the associations found in this cohort may not be generalizable to other areas of the United States. In fact, our earlier review suggested that there may be substantial geographic variations in patterns of behaviors and social conditions.

Briefly, the sampling frame included samples drawn from three housing strata reflecting the most common types of housing for those aged 65 years and older: (1) public elderly housing, which is age and income restricted; (2) private elderly housing, which is age restricted; and (3) private community houses and apartments. In public housing, all eligible persons were interviewed, whereas women were subsampled in both the private and the community strata. The overall response rate was 82 percent.

Table 5-1 shows the distribution of a broad range of risk factors, including both standard risk factors such as smoking, alcohol consumption, and prevalence of chronic diseases (e.g., diabetes and hypertension) and aspects of social networks and support. Neither blacks nor whites have a consistently greater prevalence of high-risk behaviors. For instance, older black men and women are less likely to have ever smoked cigarettes than are whites, but among people who have ever smoked, whites are significantly more likely than blacks to have quit smoking. Though data are not shown for cohort effects for both blacks and whites, younger old men and women (i.e., those in their sixties) are more likely to be current smokers than are older generations.

TABLE 5-1   Percentage of Blacks and Whites With Various High-Risk
Health and Social Behaviors by Gender: New Haven EPESE (N = 2,806),
1982, Weighted Percentages

	Men		Women	
High-Risk Characteristic	Blacks (%)	Whites (%)	Blacks (%)	Whites (%)
Health Practices:				
Cigarette smoking				
Current	25	21	14	18[a]
Past	35	45	16	20
Any alcohol consumption	50	67	21	49[b]
Chronic Conditions:				
Body mass index ≥ 28%	24	26	48	28[b]
Hypertensive	39	38	68	47[b]
Diabetic	15	12	20	12
Social Networks and Support:				
Social ties of 0 to 1 (0-4 scale)	27	26	29	36
Not married	48	31[b]	79	70
Low contact with friends, relatives	37	32	33	32
No group membership	60	59	44	60[b]
No church membership	41	54[c]	33	47[b]
No sources of instrumental support	29	31	20	22
No sources of emotional support	36	31	28	26

[a]$p \geq .05$.
[b]$p \geq .001$.
[c]$p \geq .01$.

Black and white men show no differences in body weight. Substantial differences in weight are observed, however, between black and white women.
Almost 50 percent of black women fall into the upper tercile of body mass
assessed by the Quetelet Index compared with 28 percent of white women
($p \geq .01$).

With regard to alcohol consumption, the New Haven data are consistent with
many other reports indicating that older blacks are less likely to consume alcohol
than are whites. Among black women, only 21 percent report any alcohol consumption compared with 49 percent of white women and 50 percent and 67
percent of black and white men, respectively. This lower prevalence of alcohol
consumption and, to a lesser extent, cigarette consumption among black Americans, especially women, in part reflects the strong cultural value placed on absti-
nence in that older generation. Since norms regarding these behaviors have
changed over time, we may expect to see substantially different patterns of use
among new cohorts of Americans as they enter older ages.

As discussed in the earlier section, blacks tend to have higher levels of chronic conditions that lead to greatly increased mortality risks. In the New Haven EPESE study, the prevalence of diabetes and hypertension among black and white men is similar, but black women have a higher prevalence than all other groups. The prevalence of self-reports of physician-diagnosed hypertension is 68 percent among black women compared with 47 percent among white women ($p \geq .001$). The prevalence of diabetes is also higher in black women compared with white women (20% vs. 12%), although this difference is not statistically significant.

A very balanced picture comes into view when we examine the distribution of aspects of social network and support. First we examine a summary measure of social ties composed of four components: marital status, contacts with friends and relatives, church membership, and group membership. Contacts with friends and relatives is a summary measure of the number of close friends and relatives the respondent identified. Group membership is assessed by an affirmative response to participation in any groups (e.g., voluntary, public service, self-help, community, or work related). The percentage of people who scored zero on this summary scale, indicating social isolation, is very similar across racial and gender groups. There are no statistically significant differences among these groups. When each component of the measure is examined individually, a different picture emerges. For instance, both white men and women are more likely to be married than their black counterparts ($p \geq .001$). Black men and women, on the other hand, are more likely than their white counterparts to belong to a church group. Almost 60 percent of black men belong to a church versus 46 percent of white men ($p \geq .01$). The respective percentages for women are 67 percent versus 53 percent ($p \geq .001$). Contact with friends and relatives is very similar among all groups. Only among women are racial differences in group involvement in voluntary activities revealed, with black women being less likely to report voluntary group membership than white women ($p \geq .001$) or men of either race.

We now turn to an examination of differences between older blacks and whites in the availability of social support. We report here on two domains. The availability of instrumental support is assessed by a response of yes to the question, "When you need some extra help, can you count on anyone to help you with daily tasks like grocery shopping, house cleaning, cooking, telephoning, giving you a ride?" The availability of emotional support is assessed by a response of yes to the question, "Can you count on anyone to provide you with emotional support (talking over problems or helping you make a difficult decision)?" There are no differences in the degree to which blacks and whites report the availability of emotional and instrumental support though, in general, men are less likely than women to report having support. Overall, these data indicate that there are not substantial differences in the extent to which blacks and whites maintain social ties and obtain social support. While there are differences in the degree to which blacks and whites engage in specific relationships, overall differences balance out. Since most data have indicated that it is overall levels of social ties or emotional support that are critical to well-being rather than absolute levels on any single one domain or type of relationship, it is unlikely that the extent to which blacks and whites maintain social networks accounts for differences in health status between older blacks and whites.

The above percentages do not take into consideration the possibility that differences between races may be the result of underlying differences between blacks and whites in socioeconomic status. Indeed, many recent reports have suggested that race per se does not reflect a meaningful biological grouping but rather a social grouping defined by social and economic circumstances. To the extent that differences between blacks and whites reflect underlying differences in socioeconomic status or position, we would expect that controlling statistically for socioeconomic status would diminish differences between blacks and whites in health and social behaviors.

Table 5-2 shows the results of individual multiple logistic models in which we examined the odds that black men and women would maintain a specific behavior or have a specific condition compared with whites. For each behavior, we conducted two analyses: one in which we controlled for age and a second in which we controlled for age and education, the strongest indicator we have of socioeconomic status in this study. In all analyses, we used the Professional Software for Survey Data Analysis (SUDAAN) (SAS Inc., Cary, N.C.) to adjust for possible design effects of the stratified sampling design that was used to construct the New Haven EPESE cohort. In 1982, we designed the cohort by stratifying on type of housing and we oversampled men. The SUDAAN software computes sampling variances for parameter estimates using the Taylor series approximation method. It is important to use design-based variance estimates with these data (Freeman et al., 1992).

Table 5-2 reveals that some differences between blacks and whites in the prevalence of health-promoting and health-damaging behaviors reflect underlying distributions of age and, more importantly, socioeconomic status. For instance, while the odds of being a current or past smoker are less for blacks than for whites, once we adjust for covariates, especially education, these differences become nonsignificant. On the other hand, even adjustment for age and education does not reduce differences in alcohol consumption. Black women are about a third as likely to drink alcohol as white women, and black men are half as likely to drink as white men. When we control for age and especially for education the odds of being hypertensive or diabetic are reduced, while for black women the odds of being overweight remain substantial.

The availability of social networks and social support patterns are consistent with earlier bivariate analyses. While there are no significant differences in the level of social ties when we look at the summary measure, there are differences in the specific domains even after adjustment for age and educational level. Specifically, black men and women are about twice as likely to be unmarried as whites.

TABLE 5-2   Odds Ratios (ORs) for High-Risk Health and Social Behaviors for Black and White Older Men and Women (Results of Weighted Multiple Logistic Regressions, New Haven EPESE Baseline, 1982, Data)

High-Risk Characteristic	Black Versus White Men		Black Versus White Women	
	OR	95% CI	OR	95% CI
Cigarette smoking				
Age adjusted	0.72	0.42, 1.25	0.58	0.39, 0.88
Age and education adjusted	0.62	0.35, 1.09	0.71	0.45, 1.11
Alcohol consumption				
Age adjusted	0.48	0.38, 0.61	0.27	0.18, 0.40
Age and education adjusted	0.53	0.41, 0.70	0.32	0.22, 0.47
Hypertensive				
Age adjusted	1.02	0.75, 1.40	2.34	1.52, 3.60
Age and education adjusted	1.08	0.79, 1.48	2.18	1.39, 3.42
Diabetic				
Age adjusted	1.30	0.83, 2.04	1.70	0.91, 3.18
Age and education adjusted	1.08	0.69, 1.70	1.57	0.82, 3.00
Body mass index ≥ 28%				
Age adjusted	0.85	0.55, 1.31	2.22	1.60, 311
Age and education adjusted	0.68	0.42, 1.08	1.80	1.27, 2.57
Social ties of 0-1 (0-4 scale)				
Age adjusted	1.11	0.76, 1.60	0.80	0.48, 1.34
Age and education adjusted	0.82	0.50, 1.34	0.71	0.43, 1.19
Unmarried				
Age adjusted	2.29	1.58, 3.33	2.03	1.46, 2.84
Age and education adjusted	1.92	1.27, 2.89	1.93	1.33, 2.81
Low contact with friends and relatives				
Age adjusted	1.34	1.04, 1.72	1.09	0.82, 1.47
Age and education adjusted	1.28	1.02, 1.62	0.99	0.72, 1.36
No group membership				
Age adjusted	1.08	0.79, 1.48	0.54	0.36, 0.80
Age and education adjusted	0.75	0.55, 1.02	0.36	0.24, 0.56
No church membership				
Age adjusted	0.61	0.43, 0.86	0.58	0.42, 0.79
Age and education adjusted	0.59	0.41, 0.85	0.62	0.45, 0.85

Continued on following page

TABLE 5-2   Continued

High-Risk Characteristic	Black Versus White Men		Black Versus White Women	
	OR	95% CI	OR	95% CI
No instrumental support				
Age adjusted	0.91	0.68, 1.26	0.86	0.65, 1.13
Age and education adjusted	1.14	0.79, 1.65	0.98	0.73, 1.32
Emotional support				
Age adjusted	1.23	0.80, 1.90	1.14	0.76, 1.72
Age and education adjusted	1.36	0.85, 2.18	1.08	0.70, 1.67

Note: The odds ratios presented here reflect the odds of being in the high-risk category for each condition. Thus, odds ratios over 1 indicate that black men or women have higher odds of belonging in a high-risk category (e.g., reporting diabetes or being unmarried) than whites of the same sex, whereas odds ratios of less than 1 indicate that black men or women are less likely to be in a high-risk category (e.g., consume alcohol or be current smokers).

For instance, the odds ratios (ORs) for black men are 2.29 with 95 percent confidence intervals (CIs) not overlapping 1 (CI = 1.58, 3.33).

Black men are also somewhat less likely than white men to have few contacts with friends and relatives (OR = 1.28; 95% CI = 1.02, 1.62). After adjusting for age and education, however, blacks—both men and women—are much more likely to belong to church than are whites.

These multivariate analyses indicate that black-white differences in most health behaviors are only slightly reduced by controlling for education. Greater reductions were seen for the risks associated with a history of hypertension or diabetes when we controlled for education. Thus, part of the explanation for increased rates of these important causes of morbidity and mortality among black women may be their lower socioeconomic status.

CONCLUSIONS

In this paper we have examined differences between black and white older men and women in a broad array of health-promoting and health-damaging behaviors. Overall, we find inconsistent patterns, with blacks' having a higher prevalence of some behaviors and chronic conditions and a lower prevalence of other conditions. With regard to social networks and support, while there are differences in the degree to which older black Americans maintain some type of ties when compared with whites, there are no overall differences in summary measures of social ties or social support. Finally, when the level of education is introduced as a control for socioeconomic status, differences between blacks and whites are occasionally reduced, but the strongest associations remain significant.

Our results suggest that the mortality disadvantage experienced by older black Americans is unlikely to be the sole result of their high-risk practices or behaviors. In addition, differences in the extent to which blacks and whites maintain close and effective social ties are minimal. Other conditions more closely linked to social class and environmental exposures, as well as stressful experiences related to discrimination, are worthy of serious investigation.

REFERENCES

American Medical Association Council on Ethical and Judicial Affairs
   1990   Black-white disparities in health care. *Journal of the American Medical Association* 263(17):2344-2346.
Aronow, W.S., and I. Kronson
   1991   Prevalence of coronary risk factors in blacks and whites. *Journal of the American Geriatric Society* 39:567-570.
Berkman, L.F.
   1995   The role of social relations in health promotion. *Psychosomatic Medicine* 57(3):245-254.
Berkman, L.F., C.S. Berkman, S. Kasl, D.H. Freeman Jr., L. Leo, A.M. Ostfeld, J. Cornoni-Huntley, and J.A. Brody
   1986   Depressive symptoms in relation to physical health and functioning in the elderly. *American Journal of Epidemiology* 124:372-388.
Berkman, L.F., and L. Breslow
   1983   *Health and Ways of Living: The Alameda County Study.* New York: Oxford University Press.
Blendon, R.J., L.H. Aiken, H.E. Freeman, and C.R. Corey
   1989   Access to medical care for black and white Americans. A matter of continuing concern. *Journal of the American Medical Association* 261(2):278-281.
Braithwaite, R.L., and N. Lythcott
   1989   Community empowerment as a strategy for health promotion for black and other minority populations. *Journal of the American Medical Association* 261(2):282-283.
Bultena, G.L.
   1969   Rural-urban differences in the familial interaction of the aged. *Rural Sociology* 34(1):5-15.
Burke, G.L., P.J. Savage, T.A. Manolio, J.M. Sprafka, L.E. Wagenknecht, S. Sidney, L.L. Perkins, K. Liu, and D.R. Jacobs
   1992   Correlates of obesity in young black and white women: The CARDIA study. *American Journal of Public Health* 82(12):1621-1625.
Burstin, H.R., S.R. Lipsitz, and T.A. Brennan
   1992   Socioeconomic status and risk for substandard medical care. *Journal of the American Medical Association* 268(17):2383-2387.
Cantor, M.H.
   1979   The informal support system of New York's inner city elderly: Is ethnicity a factor? Pp. 153-174 in *Ethnicity and Aging: Theory, Research and Policy*, D.E. Gelfand and A.J. Kutzik, eds. New York: Springer.
   1983   Strain among caregivers: A study of experience in the United States. *Gerontologist* 23:597-604.
Centers for Disease Control
   1990   The surgeon general's 1990 report on the health benefits of smoking cessation. *Morbidity and Mortality Weekly Report* 39:RR12.

    1994   Surveillance for selected tobacco use behaviors—United States, 1900-1994. *Morbidity and Mortality Weekly Report CDC Surveillance Summaries* 43:3.

Chatters, L.M., R.J. Taylor, and J.S. Jackson
    1985   Size and composition of the informal helper networks of elderly blacks. *Journal of Gerontology* 40(5):605-614.
    1986   Aged blacks' choices for an informal helper network. *Journal of Gerontology* 41(1):94-100.

Cowie, C.C., M.I. Harris, R.E. Silverman, E.W. Johnson, and K.F. Rust
    1993   Effect of multiple risk factors on differences between blacks and whites in the prevalence of non-insulin dependent diabetes mellitus in the United States. *American Journal of Epidemiology* 137(7):719-732.

Craven, S., and B. Wellman
    1973   The network city. *Sociological Enquiry* 43:57-88.

DiPietro, L., D.F. Williamson, C.J. Caspersen, and E. Eaker
    1993   The descriptive epidemiology of selected physical activities and body weight among adults trying to lose weight: The Behavioral Risk Factor Surveillance System survey, 1989. *International Journal of Obesity* 17:69-76.

Duelberg, S.I.
    1992   Preventive health behavior among black and white women in urban and rural areas. *Social Science and Medicine* 34(2):191-198.

Folsom, A.R., T.C. Cook, J.M. Sprafka, G.L. Burke, S.W. Norstead, and D.R. Jacobs
    1990   Differences in leisure time physical activity levels between blacks and whites in population-based samples: The Minnesota Heart Survey. *Journal of Behavioral Medicine* 14(1):1-9.

Ford, A.B., M.R. Haug, P.K. Jones, A.W. Roy, and S.J. Folmar
    1990   Race-related differences among elderly urban residents: A cohort study, 1975-1984. *Journal of Gerontology: Social Sciences* 45(4):163-171.

Freeman, D.H., M.M. Livingston, P.J. Leaf, and L.F. Berkman
    1992   Sampling strategies for studying older populations. Pp. 46-59 in *The Epidemiologic Study of the Elderly*, R. Wallace and R. Woolson, eds. New York: Oxford University Press.

George, L.K.
    1988   Social participation in later life: Black-white differences. Pp. 99-126 in *The Black American Elderly: Research on Physical and Psychosocial Health*, J.S. Jackson, ed. New York: Springer.

Giles, W.H., R.F. Anda, D.H. Jones, M.K. Serdula, R.K. Merritt, and F. DeStefano
    1993   Recent trends in identification and treatment of high blood cholesterol by physicians: Progress and missed opportunities. *Journal of the American Medical Association* 269(9):1133-1138.

Hall, J.A., D.L. Roter, and N.R. Katz
    1988   Meta-analysis of correlates of provider behavior in medical encounters. *Medical Care* 26(7):657-675.

Heath, G.W., and J.D. Smith
    1994   Physical activity patterns among adults in Georgia: Results from the 1990 Behavioral Risk Factor Surveillance System. *Southern Medical Journal* 87(4):435-439.

House, J.S., K.R. Landis, and D. Umberson
    1988   Social relationships and health. *Science* 241(4865):540-545.

Johnson, M.A., M.A. Brown, L.W. Poon, P. Martin, and G.M. Clayton
    1992   Nutritional patterns of centenarians. *International Journal of Aging and Human Development* 34(1):57-76.

Kahn, H.S., D.F. Williamson, and J.A. Stevens
    1991   Race and weight change in U.S. women: The roles of socioeconomic and marital status. *American Journal of Public Health* 81(3):319-323.

Kane, R.L.
    1985   Prevention and the elderly: Risk factors. *Health Services Research* 19:945-1006.
Kaplan, G.A., Seeman, T.E., R.D. Cohen, L.P. Knudsen, and J. Guralnik
    1987   Mortality among the elderly in the Alameda County Study: Behavioral and demographic
            risk factors. *American Journal of Public Health* 77(3):307-312.
Kumanyika, S.
    1987   Obesity in black women. *Epidemiologic Reviews* 9:31-50.
Kumanyika, S., J. Wilson, and M. Guilford-Davenport
    1993   Weight-related attitudes and behaviors of black women. *Journal of the American Dietetic
            Association* 93:416-422.
Liebow, E.
    1967   *Tally's Corner: A Study of Negro Streetcorner Men.* Boston: Little, Brown.
Lubben, J.E., P.G. Weiler, and I. Chi
    1989a   Gender and ethnic differences in the health practices of the elderly poor. *Journal of
            Clinical Epidemiology* 42(8):725-733.
    1989b   Health practices of the elderly poor. *American Journal of Public Health* 79(6):731-734.
Molgaard, C.A., C.M. Nakamura, E.P. Stanford, K.M. Peddecord, and D.J. Morton
    1990   Prevalence of alcohol consumption among older persons. *Journal of Community Health*
            15(4):239-251.
Mutchler, J.E., and J.A. Burr
    1991   Racial differences and health care utilization in later life: The effect of socioeconomic
            status. *Journal of Health and Social Behavior* 32:342-356.
National Center for Health Statistics
    1990   *Current Estimates from the National Health Interview Survey, 1989.* Hyattsville, MD:
            Public Health Service.
    1991   *Health, United States, 1990.* Hyattsville, MD: Public Health Service.
    1993   *Health Promotion and Disease Prevention, United States, 1990.* Hyattsville, MD: Public
            Health Service.
Oldridge, N.B.
    1982   Compliance and exercise in primary and secondary prevention of coronary heart disease:
            A review. *Preventative Medicine* 11:56-70.
Pi-Sunyer, F.X.
    1993   Medical hazards of obesity. *Annals of Internal Medicine* 119(7):655-660.
Ransford, H.E.
    1986   Race, heart disease, worry and health protective behavior. *Social Science and Medicine*
            2(12):1355-1362.
Reid, B.V.
    1992   It's like you're down on a bed of affliction: Aging and diabetes among black Americans.
            Social Science and Medicine 34(12):1317-1323.
Rigotti, N.A., K.M. McKool, and S. Shiffman
    1994   Predictors of smoking cessation after coronary artery bypass graft surgery: Results of a
            randomized trial with 5-year follow-up. *Annals of Internal Medicine* 120(4):287-293.
Rogers, R.P.
    1992   Living and dying in the U.S.A.: Sociodemographic determinants of death among blacks
            and whites. *Demography* 29(2):287-303.
Rowe, J.W.
    1987   Human aging: Usual and successful. *Science* 237:143-149.
Rucker, C., and T. Cash
    1991   Body images, body size perceptions, and eating behaviors among African American and
            white college women. *International Journal of Eating Disorders* 12:291-299.

Ruderman, N., A.Z. Apelian, and S.H. Schneider
    1990   Exercise in therapy and prevention of type II diabetes. *Diabetes Care* 13(11):1163-1168.
Sheridan, D.P., C.A. Hornung, E.P. McCutcheon, and F.C. Wheeler
    1993   Demographic and educational differences in smoking in a tobacco growing state. *American Journal of Preventive Medicine* 9(3):155-159.
Spangler, J.G., and J.C. Konen
    1993   Predicting exercise and smoking behavior in diabetic and hypertensive patients. *Archives of Family Medicine* 2(Feb.):149-155.
Stack, C.B.
    1974   *All Our Kin.* New York: Harper and Row.
Stevens, J., S.K. Kumanyika, and J.E. Keil
    1994   Attitudes toward body size and dieting: Differences between elderly black and white women. *American Journal of Public Health* 84(8):322-325.
Stults, B.M.
    1984   Preventive health care and the elderly. *Western Journal of American Medicine* 141:832-845.
Svetkey, L.P., L.K. George, B.M. Burchett, P.A. Morgan, and D.G. Blazer
    1993   Black/white differences in hypertension in the elderly: An epidemiologic analysis in central North Carolina. *American Journal of Epidemiology* 137(1):64-73.
Taylor, R.J.
    1988   Aging and supportive relationships. Pp. 259-281 in *The Black American Elderly: Research on Physical and Psychosocial Health*, J.S. Jackson, ed. New York: Springer.
Taylor, R.J., and L.M. Chatters
    1986   Church-based informal support among elderly blacks. *The Gerontologist* 26:637-642.
Tilly, C.
    1972   An interactional scheme for analysis of communities, cities, and urbanization. Unpublished manuscript, Department of Sociology, University of Michigan, Ann Arbor.
U.S. Department of Health and Human Services
    1993   Chartbook on Health Data on Older Americans: United States, 1992. *Vital and Health Statistics* 3:29.
Washburn, R.A., G. Kline, D.T. Lackland, and F.C. Wheeler
    1992   Leisure time physical activity: Are there black/white differences? *Preventative Medicine* 21(1):127-135.
Weissfeld, J.L., J.P. Kirscht, and B.M. Brock
    1990   Health beliefs in a population: The Michigan blood pressure survey. *Health Education Quarterly* 17(2):141-155.
Williamson, D.F., H.S. Kahn, and T. Byers
    1991   The 10-y incidence of obesity and major weight gain in black and white U.S. women aged 30-55 y. *American Journal of Clinical Nutrition* 53(suppl.):1515-1518.

6

Black-White Differences in the Use of Medical Care by the Elderly: A Contemporary Analysis

José J. Escarce and Frank W. Puffer

INTRODUCTION

Reduced access to medical care among black Americans, as compared with whites, has concerned researchers and policy makers for many years. Although racial differences in access to care are important at all stages of the life cycle, such differences are especially significant when they occur among the elderly. Older persons bear a high burden of chronic disease and may be particularly vulnerable to the deleterious effects of impaired access to care. Elderly blacks have poorer health status and higher mortality rates than elderly whites (Manton et al., 1987; Gibson 1994), and the difference in life expectancy between blacks and whites who reach age 65 is increasing (Manton et al., 1987).

Socioeconomic and racial differences in the elderly's use of medical care were sizable prior to the enactment of the Medicare program in 1965. For instance, in 1964, white elders had 20 percent higher rates of physician visits than black elders (Davis et al., 1981; Long and Settle, 1984), and whites were nearly twice as likely as blacks to be hospitalized (Long and Settle, 1984). By providing insurance coverage for hospital and physician services to the elderly, the Medicare program substantially improved access to medical care among previously underserved populations. Racial differences in physician visit rates largely disappeared by the late 1970s (Davis et al., 1981; Long and Settle, 1984). Indeed, some studies suggest that older blacks currently see physicians more often than older whites (Kleinman et al., 1981; Wan, 1982; Wolinsky et al., 1989; Furner, 1993). Results for inpatient hospital utilization are mixed; the most recent studies find a higher probability of hospitalization and more hospital nights among blacks (Wolinsky et al., 1989), and earlier studies report persistently higher use of hospitals by whites (Wan, 1982; Long and Settle, 1984). Nonetheless, all studies agree that racial differences in hospital utilization have narrowed markedly during the past three decades.

Two caveats are important in interpreting these encouraging trends. First, studies comparing rates of physician visits and hospitalization for black and white elders either have not adjusted for racial differences in health status (Davis et al., 1981; Wolinsky et al., 1989) or have used limited measures of physical health in the adjustment (Kleinman et al. 1981; Wan, 1982; Long and Settle, 1984; Furner, 1993). However, black-white differences in the health status of the elderly encompass multiple and varied dimensions of health. Older blacks not only have higher mortality rates than older whites; they also have higher rates of many common and frequently disabling chronic conditions, such as hypertension, diabetes, stroke, circulatory disease, end-stage kidney disease, arthritis and other musculoskeletal impairments, open-angle glaucoma, and certain cancers (Manton et al., 1987; Haywood, 1990; Anderson and Felson, 1988; Polednak, 1989; Leske and Rosenthal, 1979; Byrne et al., 1994). Not unexpectedly, blacks suffer from much more disability and functional impairment than whites (Manton et al., 1987). Black elders also have higher rates of mental and nervous disorders than whites (Manton et al., 1987; Polednak, 1989). Adjusting for racial differences in health status, therefore, requires more comprehensive health status measures than are generally employed. Failure to take a comprehensive approach may result in overlooking persistent and clinically important racial differences in medical care utilization.

Second, most of the studies focus on racial differences in the quantity of medical care received by older persons (e.g., numbers of physician visits and hospital nights) and do not address differences in the type or quality of care. Recent research has documented racial disparities in important qualitative aspects of medical care utilization. For instance, whereas white elders are more likely than black elders to obtain their regular ambulatory care from private physicians, blacks are more likely than whites to use neighborhood health centers, hospital outpatient departments, or emergency rooms (Wan, 1982; Kotranski et al., 1987). These practice settings are characterized by long waiting times, less satisfactory patient-physician relationships, and less continuity of care than private physicians' offices (Petchers and Milligan, 1988; Dutton, 1985).

In addition, elderly blacks are less likely than elderly whites to receive a wide array of specialized or high-technology medical services, including coronary angiography, angioplasty, and bypass surgery; carotid angiography and endarterectomy; cataract extraction; glaucoma surgery; hip and knee replacement; kidney transplantation; and magnetic resonance imaging (Wenneker and Epstein, 1989; Ford et al., 1989; Escarce et al., 1993; Ayanian et al., 1993; Kjellstrand, 1988; Javitt et al., 1991; Held et al., 1988; Oddone et al., 1993). Compared with white elders, hospitalized black elders receive worse processes of care, have more medical instability at discharge, and are less likely to receive follow-up physician care (Kahn et al., 1994; Moy and Hogan, 1993). Blacks also receive less appropriate cancer care than whites (McWhorter and Mayer, 1987; Diehr et al., 1989; Mayer and McWhorter, 1989). Perhaps not surprisingly, blacks are less satisfied than whites with many aspects of their care (Blendon et al., 1989).

In this study, we examine the current status of black-white differences in the use of medical care among elderly Americans. We focus mainly on racial differences in the quantity of medical care, although some of our analyses address qualitative aspects of care. Our study goes beyond most previous research on the elderly in two ways. First, in addition to physician visits and inpatient hospital utilization, we examine racial differences in total medical care expenditures, which serve as a rough index of the total amount of medical care received.

Second, using multivariate methods, we assess the independent effect of race on utilization from two alternative perspectives. Under a "demand-based" perspective, we adjust for all other available variables that may influence the *demand* for medical care, including demographic and socioeconomic characteristics, health status, and attitudes and beliefs about the efficacy of care. The demand-based analyses, therefore, address whether black and white elders of similar socioeconomic status and in similar health use the same quantity of medical care. Under a "need-based" perspective, we adjust for variables that affect individuals' *need* for medical care, conceptualized as health status, but exclude most demographic and socioeconomic characteristics. Thus, the need-based analyses address whether black and white elders in similar health have the same medical care utilization irrespective of socioeconomic factors. By comparing the results of the two analyses, we assess whether the current allocation of medical care services between older blacks and whites mainly reflects observed racial differences in medical need or continues to be substantially influenced by socioeconomic variables. The measures of health status used in the study are multidimensional and comprehensive.

DATA AND METHODS

Data and Study Sample

The source of data for this study is the Household Survey component of the 1987 National Medical Expenditure Survey conducted by the Agency for Health Care Policy and Research. The sample for the Household Survey was a stratified multistage area probability sample of about 35,000 individuals in 14,000 households, and excludes residents of nursing or personal care homes or facilities for the mentally retarded. Several population groups of particular policy interest, including blacks and the elderly, were oversampled (Cohen et al., 1991).

Each family in the Household Survey received a core interview four times over a period of 16 months to obtain information about each family member's health, use of medical care, medical care expenditures, and insurance coverage in 1987 (Edwards and Berlin, 1989). In addition, detailed information about health status and access to medical care was gathered from special supplementary questionnaires that were administered once during the year. This study uses data from the core interviews, the health status supplement, and the access supplement.

The Household Survey included 5,725 individuals who were 65 years or older in 1987. Of these, 5,573 individuals were white (n = 4,828) or black (n = 745) and substantially completed the core interviews. These individuals constitute the sample used in the descriptive analyses of utilization and demographic and socioeconomic characteristics (see below), which thus are representative of noninstitutionalized white and black elderly individuals in the United States (institutionalized elders are excluded owing to the design of the Household Survey). In addition, 4,957 individuals (4,324 whites and 633 blacks) also provided a basic set of responses to the health status supplement. These individuals constitute the sample used in the descriptive analyses of health status and attitudes. Finally, 4,288 (3,815 whites and 473 blacks) of the individuals who responded to the health status supplement answered all the questions needed to construct the complete set of variables for the multivariate analyses.

Elders in the complete sample of 5,573 differed from those who responded to the health status supplement and provided enough answers for inclusion in the multivariate analyses. Specifically, elders in the complete sample were older (mean age, 74.0 vs. 73.6), less healthy (mean disability days, 25.3 vs. 23.0), more likely to be black (13% vs. 11%), and more likely not have completed grade school (19% vs. 16%). Elders in the complete sample also had higher mean total medical care expenditures ($4,397 vs. $3,924) and hospital nights (2.91 vs. 2.34), although their mean number of contacts with physicians was slightly lower (6.6 vs. 6.7). Since the health status supplement was largely self-administered, nonrespondents were more likely than respondents to be cognitively impaired. Therefore, the descriptive analyses of health status and attitudes and the multivariate analyses are representative of white and black noninstitutionalized elders who do not suffer from severe cognitive impairment.

Variables

In this study, we make use of variables measuring utilization of medical care, demographic and socioeconomic characteristics, health status, and attitudes and beliefs about the efficacy of medical care.

Utilization of Medical Care

We examine three main quantitative measures of medical care utilization during 1987: total medical care expenditures, physician visits, and inpatient hospital nights. Total medical care expenditures are defined as the sum of all expenditures for medical care, irrespective of source of payment, including facility and professional fees and expenditures on pharmaceuticals and medical equipment. Physician visits are defined as face-to-face contacts with physicians in physicians' offices, group practices, or clinics; neighborhood or family health centers; free-standing surgical centers; hospital outpatient departments; emergency rooms; or patients' homes. Inpatient hospital nights are defined as nights in acute care hospitals, excluding long-term care facilities. Expenditures, physician visits, and hospital nights have frequently been used in studies of access to or demand for medical care (Blendon et al., 1989; Manning et al., 1981, 1982, 1987; Wolinsky et al., 1989; Stoller, 1982; Evashwick et al., 1984; Wan 1982).

In addition, we examine telephone contacts with physicians and contacts with nonphysician providers, with the latter defined as face-to-face contacts in any setting with nonphysician medical care providers such as chiropractors, optometrists, podiatrists, audiologists, physician assistants, nurse practitioners, physical or occupational therapists, social workers, or home health aides.

Finally, we examine several qualitative measures of utilization, including the site or setting of physician visits; whether individuals have a usual source of care; the type of usual source, if any; whether individuals usually see a particular physician at their usual source of care; and the specialty of this physician, if any.

Demographic and Socioeconomic Characteristics

The key demographic variable in the study is race, categorized as white or black according to individuals' self-identification. Additional demographic and socioeconomic characteristics used in the analyses are age, sex, employment status, educational attainment, family income, marital status, family size, insurance coverage, and location of residence. Age is categorized as 65 to 69, 70 to 74, 75 to 79, 80 to 84, or 85 and older. Educational attainment is categorized as no high school, some high school, high school graduate, or college graduate. Family income is categorized as poor, near poor (100% to 125% of poverty), low income (125% to 200%), middle income (200% to 400%), or high income (> 400%). Marital status is categorized as married; widowed more than 1 year; divorced or separated more than 1 year; widowed, divorced, or separated within the past year; or never married. Insurance coverage is categorized as Medicare only (this category also includes a small number of patients with only private insurance or Medicaid), Medicare plus Medicaid (or other public program), Medicare plus private supplementary insurance, or uninsured. Location of residence is categorized as a large metropolitan area (one of the 19 largest Metropolitan Statistical Areas), a small metropolitan area (any other Metropolitan Statistical Area), or a nonmetropolitan area. A substantial body of literature confirms the association of these variables with utilization of medical care (Blendon et al., 1989; Manning et al., 1982; Wolinsky et al., 1989; Dor and Holahan, 1990; Arling, 1985; Stoller, 1982; Evashwick et al., 1984).

Health Status

Assessing the independent effect of race on the utilization of medical care requires comprehensive adjustment for differences in health status. The World Health Organization (1948) defines health as "a state of complete physical, mental, and social well-being and not merely the absence of disease or infirmity." This definition implies that comprehensive measures of health status are multidimensional, with distinct physical, mental, and social components (Manning et al., 1982). Further, whenever possible, the range of measured values for each component should extend beyond the absence of illness to include the degree to which positive states of health are enjoyed.

Studies of access to or demand for medical care that use multivariate analyses have found that health status is the most important determinant of medical care utilization (Manning et al., 1982; Evashwick et al., 1984; Wolinsky et al., 1989; Wan, 1982; Arling, 1985). However, most such studies of the elderly have used limited measures of health status. In this study, we adopt the framework developed by Manning et al. (1982), in which measures of health status include a measure of general health in addition to measures of physical, mental, and social health. This approach has been found to substantially enhance the explanatory power of regression models for the use of medical care (Manning et al., 1982; Arling, 1985).

The measure of general health status used in the study was individuals' self-rating of their current health as excellent, good, fair, or poor. Four variables were used to measure physical health: (1) a count of limitations on functional status, which assesses limits in physical activities such as walking, running, and lifting (range, 0 to 7); (2) a count of chronic conditions, which assesses the burden of chronic diseases such as diabetes, emphysema, heart disease, and arthritis (0 to 11); (3) a count of acute symptoms experienced during the preceding 30 days, such as weight loss, fatigue, abdominal pain, or shortness of breath (0 to 9); and (4) the number of disability days during the study year, defined as days in which illness or injury caused the individual to stay in bed more than half the day or otherwise cut down on usual activities. In addition, we determined whether individuals were current smokers. Although this is not a direct measure of physical health, smoking has multiple harmful effects on physical health.

Mental health was measured with two variables: (1) degree of emotional instability, measured by summing the scores on three ordinal items that assess manifestations of depression and anxiety (range, 3 to 18), and (2) degree of positive emotional states, measured by summing the scores on two items that assess feelings of calmness and happiness (2 to 12). The measure of social health was the sum of four ordinal items that assess participation in voluntary organizations (e.g., church, clubs, lodges) and the frequency of social interactions with family and friends (4 to 28).

Attitudes and Beliefs

Assessing the independent effect of race on the utilization of medical care also requires adjusting for differences in attitudes and beliefs regarding the efficacy of medical care. An important component of these beliefs is individuals' perceived "health locus of control," a construct from social learning theory that refers to whether health and health outcomes are under individuals' personal control, the control of medical care providers, or chance (Rotter, 1966; Lau and Ware, 1981; Marshall et al., 1990). In this study, beliefs regarding health locus of control were measured with two variables: (1) degree of belief in the efficacy of self-care for health problems, measured by summing the scores on three ordinal items that assess attitudes toward the relative benefits of self-care versus physician care (range, 3 to 15), and (2) degree of belief in luck as an important factor in health outcomes (1 to 5). Prior studies have found such variables to be associated with the utilization of medical care (Manning et al., 1982; Stoller, 1982).

Statistical Analysis

We conducted bivariate analyses to examine differences between black and white elders with regard to quantitative and qualitative measures of medical care utilization, demographic and socioeconomic characteristics, health status, and attitudes and beliefs. Quantitative utilization measures were adjusted for age and sex by using direct standardization (Kleinbaum et al., 1982). Statistical significance was assessed through the use of t tests for continuous variables and chi-square tests for proportions.

To determine the independent effect of race on medical care utilization, we conducted multivariate regression analyses with total medical care expenditures, physician visits, and inpatient hospital nights as dependent variables. Our primary analyses employed a demand-based perspective. In these analyses, the explanatory variables included all demographic and socioeconomic characteristics and measures of health status and attitudes and beliefs described in the preceding section. Employment status may influence the demand for medical care through its effect on the cost of care in terms of time spent. Education is expected to influence the demand for care because better educated individuals may be more efficient producers of health (Grossman, 1972). Marital status and family size can affect the demand for care because family members may encourage older persons to seek care for symptoms that otherwise would be ignored or, alternatively, may serve as substitutes for formal medical care. Insurance coverage is expected to influence the demand for care through its effect on the out-of-pocket price of care. Metropolitan versus nonmetropolitan residence may be a proxy for certain nonmonetary costs of care (e.g., travel time). Measures of health status are expected to influence the demand for care because they reflect individuals' stock of health capital (Grossman, 1972). Finally, attitudes and beliefs are expected to affect the demand for care because they shape individuals' preferences. The explanatory variables used in our demand-based analyses are similar to those used in other studies of the demand for medical care (Manning et al., 1981, 1982; Wedig, 1988).

In addition, we performed secondary analyses employing a need-based perspective. These analyses included as explanatory variables only age, sex, and the measures of health status and attitudes and beliefs; other demographic and socioeconomic characteristics were excluded.

Multivariate analyses were based on the two-part model of medical care utilization (Manning et al., 1981, 1987; Duan et al., 1982). The first part of the two-part model is an equation for whether or not an individual has non-zero medical care expenditures (or physician visits or hospital nights) during the year and is estimated by using logistic regression. This equation, which separates users of medical care from nonusers, assesses the factors that influence the decision to spend on care. From a statistical viewpoint, it also deals with the fact that an appreciable proportion of the population does not use any medical care during a year. The second part of the two-part model is an equation for the logarithm of medical care expenditures (or physician visits or hospital nights) conditional on non-zero expenditures and is estimated by using ordinary least squares. This equation assesses the factors that affect the level of use among those who use care. The logarithmic transformation of the dependent variable deals with the marked skewness of the distribution of medical care expenditures and use, and results in more robust and efficient estimates (Manning et al., 1981, 1987; Duan et al., 1982). Standard errors were obtained by using White's (1980) heteroskedasticity-consistent covariance matrix estimator.

All analyses were weighted with weights that reflect both the sample design of the Household Survey and complete and partial survey nonresponse (Cohen et al., 1991). A p value of .10 or less was chosen as the criterion for statistical significance.

RESULTS

Bivariate Analyses

Elderly whites constituted 91.3 percent of the weighted study sample and elderly blacks constituted 8.7 percent. Table 6-1 compares the demographic and socioeconomic characteristics of elderly whites and blacks. Whites and blacks were similar in age and sex distribution and had similar rates of labor force participation. However, whites had more education and higher incomes than blacks and were more likely than blacks to be married, although blacks lived in larger families. Insurance coverage differed substantially for white and black elders. Specifically, blacks were much more likely than whites to have Medicare only—that is, without either public or private supplementary coverage—and to

TABLE 6-1   Demographic and Socioeconomic Characteristics

Variable	Whites	Blacks
Age category (%)		
65-69	33.6	36.3
70-74	26.5	25.3
75-79	20.1	18.6
80-84	11.3	11.6
≥85	8.5	8.2
Sex (%)		
Male	41.4	40.2
Female	58.6	59.8
Employment status (%)		
Employed	10.4	11.4
Unemployed	89.6	88.6
Educational attainment (%)[a]		
No high school	14.2	45.6
Some high school	32.7	30.9
High school graduate	43.2	21.0
College graduate	10.0	2.6
Income category (%)		
Poor	9.8	33.6
Near poor	7.4	12.0
Low income	20.4	22.4
Middle income	36.1	25.0
High income	26.3	7.0
Marital status (%)[a]		
Married	54.8	42.1
Widowed > 1 year	32.7	41.4
Divorced or separated > 1 year	5.6	10.6
Widowed or divorced < 1 year	2.3	1.9
Never married	4.5	4.0
Family size (mean)[a]	1.86	2.25
Insurance coverage (%)[a]		
Medicare only	11.4	26.7
Medicare plus Medicaid	7.6	31.9
Medicare plus private	83.4	44.7
Uninsured	0.6	2.2
Location of residence (%)[a]		
Large metropolitan area	24.4	34.5
Small metropolitan area	48.0	39.1
Nonmetropolitan area	27.6	26.4

[a]$p < .01$ for test of difference between whites and blacks for numbers in this category.
Notes: The weighted sample consisted of 5,088 whites and 485 blacks; the sample was weighted to reflect the sample design and complete and partial nonresponse. Percentages for insurance coverage add to more than 100 because some individuals had both Medicaid and private supplementary insurance in addition to Medicare.

have Medicaid or other public coverage in addition to Medicare. In contrast, whites were much more likely than blacks to have private supplementary insurance in addition to Medicare. Blacks were more likely than whites to live in large metropolitan areas, but the proportion of individuals residing in nonmetropolitan areas was similar for both races.

As Table 6-2 shows, older whites perceived themselves to be in much better general health than older blacks. For instance, 9.3 percent of elderly whites assessed their current health as excellent, whereas only 5.5 percent of elderly blacks did so. Conversely, 11.0 percent of whites assessed their current health as poor, compared with 16.4 percent of blacks. White elders also had more favorable indicators of physical, mental, and social health than black elders. Compared with blacks, whites had fewer functional status limitations, chronic condi-

TABLE 6-2 Health Status and Attitudes and Beliefs

Variable	Whites	Blacks
Health Status		
General health (%)[a]		
Excellent	9.3	5.5
Good	44.4	31.7
Fair	35.3	46.4
Poor	11.0	16.4
Physical health (mean)		
Functional status limitations[a]	2.88	3.81
Chronic conditions[b]	2.32	2.45
Acute symptoms in preceding 30 days[a]	1.50	1.73
Disability days[a]	22.89	32.49
Mental health (mean)		
Emotional instability[a]	6.18	6.93
Positive emotional states[a]	8.39	8.04
Social health (mean)		
Social activities[c]	15.03	14.56
Current smoker (%)		
Yes	14.9	16.7
No	85.1	83.3
Attitudes and beliefs		
Health locus of control (mean)		
Efficacy of self-care	7.56	7.43
Luck as a factor in health[a]	1.94	2.16

[a] $p < .01$ for test of difference between whites and blacks for numbers in this category.
[b] $p < .10$ for test of difference between whites and blacks for numbers in this category.
[c] $p < .05$ for test of difference between whites and blacks for numbers in this category.

tions, acute symptoms during the preceding 30 days, and disability days. Whites also had lower degrees of emotional instability and higher degrees of positive emotional states, and were more involved in social activities. Similar proportions of white and black elders were current smokers.

Elderly whites and blacks were similar in their beliefs regarding the efficacy of self-care (vs. physician care) for health problems, but blacks had stronger beliefs than whites regarding the importance of luck as a factor in health outcomes.

Descriptive analyses of quantitative measures of utilization uncovered interesting patterns, as Table 6-3 shows. Mean total medical care expenditures for white and black elders were not statistically significantly different. However, this finding masks racial differences in the probability of spending on medical care and in the level of use among those who use care. Thus, whereas whites were more likely than blacks to have non-zero expenditures ($p < .01$), among individuals who spent on care blacks had higher mean expenditures than whites ($p < .10$). The findings for physician visits were similar to those for total medical care expenditures. Specifically, although elderly whites and blacks had similar rates of physician visits, whites were more likely than blacks to have at least one

TABLE 6-3   Medical Care Utilization

Variable	Whites	Blacks
Total medical care expenditures		
Mean, all individuals	$4,236	$4,764
Percentage of individuals		
with non-zero expenditures	94.6[a]	88.2[a]
Mean, individuals with		
non-zero expenditures	$4,477[b]	$5,401[b]
Hospital nights		
Mean, all individuals	2.74	3.33
Percentage of individuals		
with non-zero nights	20.3	21.4
Mean, individuals with		
non-zero nights	13.49	15.54
Physician visits		
Mean, all individuals	6.64	6.41
Percentage of individuals		
with non-zero visits	87.9[a]	81.9[a]
Mean, individuals with		
non-zero visits	7.55	7.83

[a]$p < .01$ for test of difference between whites and blacks.
[b]$p < .10$ for test of difference between whites and blacks.
Note: Adjusted for age and sex using direct standardization.

visit ($p < .01$). By contrast, measures of inpatient hospital use did not differ between whites and blacks.

Older whites averaged more telephone contacts with physicians than older blacks (whites, 0.23; blacks, 0.10; $p < .01$), but blacks had more face-to-face contacts with nonphysician providers of medical care than whites (blacks, 12.38; whites, 8.46; $p < .05$).

An important question pertains to the burden of out-of-pocket expenditures for medical care. Mean out-of-pocket expenditures were $944 for white elders compared with $522 for black elders ($p < .01$), indicating a higher absolute burden for whites. However, the relative burden, measured as the proportion of family income (adjusted for family size) devoted to the older individual's out-of-pocket expenditures, was similar in the two races (whites, 5.2%; blacks, 5.1%; $p > .10$).

The results presented above and in Table 6-3 indicate that racial differences in quantitative measures of medical care utilization were relatively small. Analyses of qualitative aspects of utilization, on the other hand, tell a different story. For example, as Table 6-4 shows, elderly blacks saw physicians in hospital outpatient departments at more than twice the rate of elderly whites, and they saw physicians in emergency rooms nearly one and one-half times as often. Overall, 25.9 percent of physician visits by black elders took place in hospital outpatient departments or emergency rooms, compared with 13.4 percent of physician visits by white elders. Conversely, whites saw physicians in physicians' offices, group practices, or clinics or in neighborhood or family health centers at a higher rate than blacks.

Analyses of elders' usual source of medical care were consistent with these findings. Thus, whereas elderly blacks were only slightly less likely than elderly whites to have a usual source of care (blacks, 87.7%; whites, 91.0%; $p < .05$), among individuals with a usual source, blacks were much more likely than whites to report a hospital outpatient department, emergency room, or neighborhood or

TABLE 6-4   Mean Physician Visits, by Site

Site	Whites	Blacks
Physician office, group practice, or clinic or neighborhood or family health center[a]	5.65[b]	4.67[b]
Hospital outpatient department	0.63[b]	1.30[b]
Emergency room	0.26[b]	0.36[b]
Home	0.10	0.07

[a]The data did not allow us to distinguish physicians' offices or group practices from neighborhood or family health centers.

[b]$p < .01$ for test of difference between whites and blacks.

TABLE 6-5   Percentage Distribution of Usual Source of Care, by Type[a]

Type[b]	Whites	Blacks
Physician office, group practice, or clinic	92.0	77.4
Neighborhood or family health center	1.7	6.1
Hospital outpatient department	3.8	11.9
Emergency room	0.4	1.8
Other[c]	2.2	2.8

[a]Includes only individuals with a usual source of care.
[b]$p < .01$ for test of difference between whites and blacks.
[c]Includes company clinics, walk-in centers, patients' homes, and miscellaneous other sites.

family health center as their usual source as Table 6-5 shows. Whites were more likely than blacks to report a physician's office, group practice, or clinic as their usual source of care.

Not surprisingly, 94.6 percent of whites with a usual source of care had a regular physician at their usual source, compared with 87.3 percent of blacks ($p < .01$). Whites also were more likely than blacks to report having a specialist (vs. a general practitioner) as their regular physician (whites, 36.5%; blacks, 28.5%; $p < .01$). Without further information, however, it is difficult to say whether greater use of specialists is associated with higher quality of care.

Multivariate Analyses

We used multivariate regression to assess the independent effect of race on quantitative measures of medical care utilization. Our primary analyses, which employed a demand-based perspective, adjusted for demographic and socioeconomic characteristics, health status, and attitudes and beliefs regarding medical care. Table 6-6 reports the results of logistic regression models for the first part of two-part models for medical care expenditures, physician visits, and hospital nights. When adjustment was made for other demand factors, elderly blacks were less likely than elderly whites to spend on medical care ($p < .10$). However, the racial difference in adjusted probabilities of spending on care (whites, 94.3%; blacks, 91.7%) was smaller than the difference in unadjusted probabilities (shown in Table 6-3). Race did not have a statistically significant independent effect on the probability of having at least one physician visit or on the probability of being hospitalized.

Other demographic and socioeconomic variables generally had expected effects on the decision to spend on medical care and on the likelihood of having at least one physician visit (Table 6-6). Thus, older age, female sex, higher income,

TABLE 6-6   Regression Results on Whether a Person Has Non-zero Expenditures (or Physician Visits or Hospital Nights) During the Year: Part I of a Two-Part Model Using a Demand-Based Perspective[a]

Variable[b]	Non-zero Medical Care Expenditures	Non-zero Physician Visits	Non-zero Hospital Nights
Demographic and socioeconomic characteristics			
Black	−0.419[c]	−0.178	−0.077
	(1.73)	(0.89)	(0.42)
Age 70-74	0.246	0.146	−0.033
	(1.20)	(1.03)	(0.27)
Age 75-79	0.511[d]	0.385[d]	0.237[c]
	(2.12)	(2.32)	(1.85)
Age 80-84	0.327	0.362[c]	0.211
	(1.06)	(1.68)	(1.40)
Age ≥ 85	0.955[d]	0.776[e]	0.194
	(2.13)	(2.83)	(1.04)
Female	0.450[e]	0.302[d]	−0.481[e]
	(2.62)	(2.54)	(4.60)
Employed	0.155	0.028	0.147
	(0.64)	(0.18)	(0.91)
Some high school	0.160	−0.159	0.160
	(0.67)	(0.89)	(1.14)
High school graduate	0.327	0.099	0.296[d]
	(1.31)	(0.55)	(2.08)
College graduate	1.081[d]	0.298	0.204
	(2.43)	(1.18)	(1.00)
Near poor	0.162	0.623[d]	0.341[c]
	(0.47)	(2.37)	(1.74)
Low income	0.338	0.573[e]	0.319[c]
	(1.12)	(2.63)	(1.87)
Middle income	0.657[d]	0.716[e]	0.184
	(2.17)	(3.33)	(1.09)
High income	0.999[e]	0.971[e]	0.250
	(2.89)	(4.06)	(1.31)
Widowed > 1 year	−0.772[e]	−0.388[d]	0.114
	(3.38)	(2.47)	(0.83)
Divorced > 1 year	−1.249[e]	−0.390	0.089
	(3.67)	(1.42)	(0.42)
Separated > 1 year	−0.774	−0.602	0.193
	(1.23)	(1.30)	(0.49)
Widowed or divorced < 1 year	−1.061[d]	−0.655[d]	−0.321
	(2.53)	(2.05)	(1.05)
Never married	−0.622[c]	−0.491[d]	0.353
	(1.66)	(1.96)	(1.49)
Family size[f]	−2.275[e]	−1.617[e]	0.010
	(4.92)	(4.72)	(0.03)
Medicare plus Medicaid	0.379	0.536[d]	0.258
	(1.30)	(2.26)	(1.59)
Medicare plus private	0.723[e]	0.571[e]	0.214
	(3.65)	(4.05)	(1.63)
Uninsured	0.444	−0.121	−0.106
	(0.47)	(0.23)	(0.13)

TABLE 6-6   Continued

Variable[b]	Non-zero Medical Care Expenditures	Non-zero Physician Visits	Non-zero Hospital Nights
Small metropolitan area	0.277	−0.061	0.049
	(1.42)	(0.46)	(0.45)
Nonmetropolitan area	0.240	−0.052	0.139
	(1.09)	(0.34)	(1.12)
Health status			
Good general health	−0.310	0.144	−0.104
	(1.28)	(0.89)	(0.49)
Fair general health	−0.038	0.283	0.070
	(0.12)	(1.31)	(0.30)
Poor general health	0.389	0.176	0.069
	(0.54)	(0.48)	(0.26)
Functional limitations[g]	1.142[e]	0.573[d]	0.721[e]
	(3.32)	(2.45)	(3.51)
Chronic conditions	0.510[e]	0.395[e]	0.109[e]
	6.73	8.58	3.69
Acute symptoms[g]	0.533	0.246	−0.289
	(1.25)	(0.90)	(1.40)
Disability days[f]	1.041[e]	0.910[e]	0.936[e]
	(4.83)	(8.45)	(16.43)
Emotional instability	−0.098[d]	−0.022	−0.016
	(2.16)	(0.70)	(0.72)
Positive emotional states	−0.037	−0.033	−0.057[c]
	(0.69)	(0.86)	(1.93)
Social activities	0.051[e]	0.037[e]	−0.029[e]
	(2.74)	(2.89)	(2.84)
Current smoker	−0.470[d]	−0.284[d]	−0.170
	(2.35)	(1.99)	(1.36)
Attitudes and beliefs			
Efficacy of self-care	−0.151[e]	−0.134[e]	−0.082[e]
	(5.01)	(6.88)	(5.13)
Luck as a factor in health	−0.041	−0.062	0.094[d]
	(0.51)	(1.23)	(2.31)
Intercept	1.952[d]	0.809	−1.940[d]
	(2.36)	(1.27)	(3.85)
Log likelihood	−651.14	−1,221.78	−1,692.30
N	4,288	4,288	4,288

[a]The equation for the first part of the model is estimated using logistic regression; t ratios are in parentheses.

[b]The omitted category for age is 65 to 69; for educational level, no high school; for income category, poor; for marital status, married; for insurance coverage, Medicare only; for location of residence, large metropolitan area; and for general health, excellent.

[c]$p < .10$.

[d]$p < .05$.

[e]$p < .01$.

[f]In the regressions, the variable was replaced by its natural logarithm to reduce the effect of skewness.

[g]In the regressions, the variable was replaced by the natural logarithm of 1 plus the variable to reduce the effect of skewness.

and having private supplementary insurance in addition to Medicare were associated with a higher probability of having non-zero medical care expenditures and physician visits, while a larger family and being widowed or divorced were associated with a lower probability. By contrast, most demographic and socioeconomic characteristics did not have a statistically significant influence on the probability of being hospitalized.

The findings for measures of health status and attitudes shown in Table 6-6 are noteworthy. Worse physical health (i.e., more functional limitations, chronic conditions, and disability days) was generally associated with a higher probability of having non-zero medical care expenditures, physician visits, and hospital nights, whereas worse mental and social health (i.e., emotional instability and low involvement in social activities) were associated with a lower probability of non-zero expenditures but a higher probability of being hospitalized. Interestingly, the impact of individuals' self-rating of their current health as excellent, good, fair, or poor did not achieve statistical significance in any of the logistic regression models; this suggests that the influence of general health status on the use of medical care was fully captured by the measures of physical, mental, and social health. A stronger belief in the efficacy of self-care for health problems was associated with a lower probability of non-zero expenditures, physician visits, and hospital nights.

Table 6-7 reports the results of linear models for the second part of two-part models for medical care expenditures, physician visits, and hospital nights. In these equations, the sample is restricted to those who have non-zero utilization and the dependent variable is the logarithm of the level of utilization. Race did not have a statistically significant independent effect on the level of medical care expenditures among users of medical care, the number of physician visits among individuals who saw a physician, or the number of hospital nights among elders who were hospitalized.

Among those who spent on medical care, higher educational attainment, higher income, and having private supplementary insurance or Medicaid in addition to Medicare were associated with higher medical care expenditures, whereas female sex, a larger family, and living in a nonmetropolitan area were associated with lower expenditures. The findings were similar for the number of physician visits among elders who saw a physician, although nonmetropolitan residence was not associated with fewer visits. Demographic and socioeconomic characteristics had little impact on the number of hospital nights among elders who were hospitalized, with the notable exception that living in a small metropolitan area or a nonmetropolitan area was associated with fewer nights.

Turning to the findings for health status and attitudes and beliefs, we note that individuals' self-rating of their current health as poor was associated with higher medical care expenditures and more physician visits, whereas worse physical health was generally associated with higher expenditures, more physician visits, and more hospital nights. Worse mental health, as manifested by a higher degree of emotional instability, was associated with more hospital nights. A stronger belief in the efficacy of self-care for health problems was associated with lower medical care expenditures and fewer physician visits and hospital nights.

We also conducted secondary analyses, employing a need-based perspective, which adjusted only for age, sex, health status, and attitudes and beliefs. Table 6-8 reports the estimated coefficients of the black race indicator variable in these analyses and compares them with the estimated coefficients from the demand-based analyses (shown in Tables 6-6 and 6-7).

Race had statistically significant and important independent effects on medical care expenditures and physician visits in the need-based analyses. As shown in Table 6-8, elderly whites were more likely than elderly blacks to spend on medical care after adjustment for the other explanatory variables, and the racial difference in adjusted probabilities of spending on care (whites, 94.9%; blacks, 85.0%) was larger than the difference in unadjusted probabilities (shown in Table 6-3). Moreover, among individuals who spent on care, adjusted medical care expenditures were 11.5 percent higher for whites than for blacks. Similarly, white elders were more likely than black elders to see a physician, and the racial difference in adjusted probabilities of having at least one physician visit (whites, 88.2%; blacks, 77.8%) was nearly twice as large as the difference in unadjusted probabilities (shown in Table 6-3). Among individuals who saw a physician, whites made 4.4 percent more physician visits than blacks. Race did not have a statistically significant impact on the utilization of inpatient hospital care.

Finally, because the effect of race on the utilization of medical care may differ among population subgroups, we repeated our demand-based and need-based analyses after including interaction terms between race and sex, race and income, and race and self-rated health in the regression models. The only statistically significant interactions in these analyses were between race and self-rated health in the equations for the number of hospital nights among elders who were hospitalized. Specifically, hospitalized older blacks who reported excellent health spent fewer nights in the hospital than their white counterparts, whereas there were no differences in the level of hospital use between hospitalized older blacks and whites who reported good, fair, or poor health. Owing to small cell sizes, however, the lack of significant interactions should be interpreted with caution.

DISCUSSION

This study indicates that racial differences in the quantity of medical care received by elderly persons in the United States have largely disappeared. In particular, bivariate analyses found that in 1987, white and black elders had similar mean annual total medical care expenditures, physician visits, and inpa-

TABLE 6-7   Regression Results on Expenditures (or Physician Visits or
Hospital Nights) on Non-zero Use During the Year: Part II of a Two-Part
Model Using a Demand-Based Perspective[a]

Variable[b]	Level of Medical Care Expenditures	Number of Physician Visits	Number of Hospital Nights
Demographic and socioeconomic characteristics			
Black	−0.032	0.001	0.068
	(0.80)	(0.03)	(1.22)
Age 70-74	−0.016	0.004	0.077[c]
	(0.65)	(0.25)	(1.78)
Age 75-79	0.031	0.021	0.036
	(1.09)	(1.17)	(0.78)
Age 80-84	0.067[c]	0.001	0.124[d]
	(1.78)	(0.05)	(2.36)
Age ≥ 85	−0.001	−0.047	0.113
	(0.01)	(1.60)	(1.53)
Female	−0.079[e]	−0.028[c]	−0.051
	(3.39)	(1.94)	(1.44)
Employed	−0.003	−0.007	−0.011
	(0.08)	(0.33)	(0.18)
Some high school	0.052	0.008	0.063
	(1.50)	(0.39)	(1.30)
High school graduate	0.148[e]	0.044[d]	0.081[c]
	(4.22)	(2.08)	(1.70)
College graduate	0.200[e]	0.055[c]	0.014
	(4.41)	(1.77)	(0.21)
Near poor	0.124[d]	−0.013	0.073
	(2.41)	(0.42)	(1.08)
Low income	0.118[e]	0.013	0.009
	(2.87)	(0.51)	(0.15)
Middle income	0.118[e]	0.021	0.049
	(2.84)	(0.84)	(0.75)
High income	0.180[e]	0.056[d]	0.035
	(4.15)	(2.10)	(0.54)
Widowed > 1 year	−0.0002	−0.017	0.058
	(0.01)	(0.86)	(1.24)
Divorced > 1 year	0.084	0.024	0.069
	(1.52)	(0.84)	(0.82)
Separated > 1 year	−0.057	−0.135[d]	−0.068
	(0.54)	(2.02)	(0.40)
Widowed or divorced < 1 year	−0.017	−0.041	0.104
	(0.26)	(0.98)	(1.02)
Never married	−0.010	−0.001	0.121
	(0.16)	(0.04)	(1.47)
Family size[f]	−0.189[d]	−0.111[d]	0.025
	(2.48)	(2.43)	(0.23)
Medicare plus Medicaid	0.171[e]	0.040[c]	−0.028
	(4.23)	(1.77)	(0.49)
Medicare plus private	0.077[d]	0.044[d]	0.052
	(2.38)	(2.30)	(1.14)
Uninsured	−0.240	−0.069	0.504[e]
	(0.75)	(0.62)	(4.75)

TABLE 6-7   Continued

Variable[b]	Level of Medical Care Expenditures	Number of Physician Visits	Number of Hospital Nights
Small metropolitan area	−0.041	−0.014	−0.089[d]
	(1.58)	(0.89)	(2.12)
Nonmetropolitan area	−0.094[e]	−0.016	−0.164[e]
	(3.22)	(0.93)	(3.61)
Health status			
Good general health	0.035	0.035	−0.074
	(0.90)	(1.42)	(0.87)
Fair general health	0.086[c]	0.053[c]	−0.058
	(1.86)	(1.88)	(0.61)
Poor general health	0.146[d]	0.094[d]	0.030
	(2.36)	(2.52)	(0.27)
Functional limitations[g]	0.260[e]	0.117[e]	0.145[c]
	(5.54)	(4.11)	(1.82)
Chronic conditions	0.060[e]	0.038[e]	−0.014
	(8.49)	(8.43)	(1.36)
Acute symptoms[g]	−0.027	0.056[c]	−0.0001
	(0.56)	(1.87)	(0.001)
Disability days[f]	0.297[e]	0.129[e]	0.114[e]
	(19.99)	(14.43)	(5.66)
Emotional instability	0.007	0.001	0.019[d]
	(1.29)	(0.42)	(2.28)
Positive emotional states	−0.005	−0.001	0.007
	(0.80)	(0.34)	(0.57)
Social activities	−0.002	0.003[c]	−0.002
	(0.79)	(1.83)	(0.69)
Current smoker	−0.090[e]	−0.056[e]	0.056
	(3.00)	(2.90)	(1.09)
Attitudes and beliefs			
Efficacy of self-care	−0.024[e]	−0.014[e]	−0.018[e]
	(6.80)	(6.32)	(2.89)
Luck as a factor in health	0.002	0.005	0.029[c]
	(0.23)	(0.75)	(1.95)
Intercept	2.579[e]	0.438[e]	0.530[d]
	(21.21)	(5.95)	(2.47)
R^2	0.30	0.22	0.18
N	4,055	3,782	792

[a]The logarithmic equation for the second part of the model is estimated using ordinary least squares regression; t ratios are in parentheses.

[b]The omitted category for age is 65 to 69; for educational level, no high school; for income category, poor; for marital status, married; for insurance coverage, Medicare only; for location of residence, large metropolitan area; and for general health, excellent.

[c]$p < .10$.

[d]$p < .05$.

[e]$p < .01$.

[f]In the regressions, the variable was replaced by its natural logarithm to reduce the effect of skewness.

[g]In the regressions, the variable was replaced by the natural logarithm of 1 plus the variable to reduce the effect of skewness.

tient hospital nights, although whites were slightly more likely than blacks to spend on medical care and to see a physician during the year. These data generally agree with other recent studies of medical care utilization by the elderly (Kleinman et al., 1981; Wolinsky et al., 1989; Wan, 1982; Long and Settle, 1984; Furner, 1993).

Interpreting descriptive findings, however, requires careful consideration of differences between older whites and blacks in demographic and socioeconomic characteristics, health status, and attitudes and beliefs regarding medical care. Consistent with prior research (Manton et al., 1987; Polednak, 1989), we found that elderly blacks fared worse than elderly whites on multiple and varied indicators of health status, including individuals' self-rating of their current health as well as measures of physical, mental, and social health. Worse health would be expected to lead to higher use of medical care among blacks. On the other hand, compared with black elders, white elders had more education, higher incomes, and much higher rates of private insurance coverage to supplement Medicare, all of which could result in higher utilization among whites.

We assessed the independent effect of race on the utilization of medical care using multivariate regression analysis. Our primary analyses employed a demand-based perspective that adjusted for all available variables that may influence the demand for care. The explanatory variables in these analyses thus included a full complement of demographic and socioeconomic characteristics, comprehensive measures of health status, and measures of attitudes and beliefs about the efficacy of medical care. These analyses found that race generally did not have statistically significant independent effects on medical care expenditures, physician visits, or hospital nights. The only exception was that black elders were slightly less likely than white elders to spend on medical care after adjustment for other demand factors, but the racial disparity in the adjusted probabilities of non-zero expenditures was very small.

The finding that race has little independent influence on the demand for medical care among the elderly, however, does not necessarily imply that the current allocation of medical care services between older whites and older blacks is socially desirable. Researchers on the equity of access to and delivery of medical care have long maintained that an equitable and desirable allocation of medical care services occurs when these services are distributed among individuals according to their "need" for care, which is usually conceptualized as health status (Aday and Andersen, 1981; Andersen and Newman, 1973; Aday, 1975; Culyer et al., 1992; van Doorslaer and Wagstaff, 1992). Policy makers in many other industrialized countries also accept this view (van Doorslaer and Wagstaff, 1992). But allocation of services according to the demand for care may fall short of this criterion. In particular, features of the medical care delivery system may result in individuals of high socioeconomic status receiving more services than their lower socioeconomic status counterparts.

To address this issue, we performed additional multivariate analyses em-

TABLE 6-8 Medical Care Expenditures, Physician Visits, and Hospital
Nights: Coefficients of Black Race in Multivariate Regression Analyses
Employing Need-Based and Demand-Based Perspectives[a]

	Part of model[b]	
Utilization Measure and Perspective	Part I	Part II
Total medical care expenditures		
Need-based perspective	-1.227^c	-0.109^c
	(5.59)	(3.09)
Demand-based perspective[e]	-0.419^d	-0.032
	(1.73)	(0.80)
Physician visits		
Need-based perspective	-0.704^c	-0.044^d
	(3.87)	(1.93)
Demand-based perspective[e]	-0.178	0.001
	(0.89)	(0.03)
Hospital nights		
Need-based perspective	-0.182	0.016
	(1.07)	(0.31)
Demand-based perspective[e]	-0.077	0.068
	(0.42)	(1.22)

[a]Parentheses contain *t* ratios.

[b]Part I of the model is an equation for whether an individual has non-zero expenditures (or
physician visits, or hospital nights) and is estimated with logistic regression. Part II of the model is
an equation for the logarithm of expenditures (or physician visits, or hospital nights) and is estimated
with an ordinary least squares regression. The demand-based findings of the model are presented in
detail in Tables 6-6 and 6-7.

[c] $p < .10$.

[d] $p < .01$.

[e] From Tables 6-6 and 6-7.

ploying a need-based perspective. The explanatory variables in these analyses
included only age, sex, and the measures of health status and attitudes and beliefs; educational attainment, income, insurance coverage, and indicators of family structure were excluded. Thus, the need-based analyses addressed the question of whether older whites and blacks of similar health status have the same
medical care utilization irrespective of socioeconomic factors.

The results of the need-based analyses differed strikingly from the findings
of the demand-based analyses. Specifically, the need-based analyses revealed
that, with adjustment made for the other explanatory variables, elderly blacks
were considerably less likely than elderly whites to spend on medical care or to
see physicians. Moreover, among users of medical care, black elders had lower
adjusted medical care expenditures than white elders, and among individuals
who saw a physician, blacks had fewer physician visits than whites. These
findings indicate that elderly blacks, as compared with whites, received less

medical care and saw physicians less often than would be expected given their health status.

Why are white and black older persons in equal need of medical care treated differently? Comparison of our demand-based and need-based analyses suggests that a large portion of the racial discrepancy in the use of medical care found in the need-based analyses is due to racial differences in socioeconomic variables. Socioeconomic status may influence the allocation of medical care among elderly Americans through several mechanisms.

Socioeconomic status is positively associated with elders' likelihood of having private insurance to supplement Medicare (Rice and McCall, 1985; Nelson et al., 1989). Private supplementary coverage may influence patient behavior by reducing the out-of-pocket price of care and may influence provider behavior through more generous reimbursement. Other financial and nonfinancial barriers to care may also differ across socioeconomic groups. For instance, individuals of low socioeconomic status are more likely than those of high socioeconomic status to travel long distances to receive care, rely on public transportation, and reside in areas where medical care providers—especially private physicians—are scarce (LeGrand, 1982; Aday, 1975; Dutton, 1985; Ernst and Yett, 1985). High socioeconomic status may also be associated with increased ability to navigate successfully within the complex health care delivery system in the United States.

A potential objection to our analyses is that socioeconomic status, not race, is the important factor and that, consequently, our need-based analyses are misleading. However, there are at least three reasons why it is meaningful to ask whether the allocation of medical care services between elderly blacks and whites corresponds to observed racial differences in need. First, socioeconomic status and race are inextricably linked in American society, and race directly affects educational and economic opportunities through societal mechanisms such as stratification, segregation, and discrimination (Wallace, 1990). Second, it is likely that a portion of the racial disparity in medical care utilization observed in the need-based analyses is due to race per se rather than to socioeconomic status (Wallace, 1990). Physicians may tend to avoid areas with large minority populations when establishing private practices (Ernst and Yett, 1985). Some observers believe that patient race may also have a direct influence on clinical decision making by physicians (Eisenberg, 1979; Maynard et al., 1986; Yergan et al., 1987; Escarce et al., 1993). Third, racial inequalities in the use of medical care have long interested both researchers and policy makers. Our comparison of demand-based and need-based analyses makes a novel contribution to the literature on this topic.

Another potential objection to our analyses is that they overlook the full richness and complexity of the relationships among race, socioeconomic status, and health status. A comprehensive model of these relationships, for instance, would explicitly acknowledge the impact of race on socioeconomic opportunities as well as the effects of socioeconomic factors on health and vice versa (Feinstein, 1993; Williams et al., 1994). Such a comprehensive model is best formulated and empirically tested using a life-cycle perspective, however, and is beyond the scope of our study and our cross-sectional data. Rather, our study focuses on the more modest goal of assessing the influence of race on medical care utilization, with health status and socioeconomic status being taken as given.

Our study also is limited by imperfect measurement of health status, since it is unlikely that even our comprehensive approach captured all of the relevant racial differences in health. But if omitted health status variables are correlated with socioeconomic characteristics, then the difference between our demand-based and need-based analyses may be partly explained by omitted variable bias.

To conclude, our study indicates that the evidence that the Medicare program has substantially improved access to medical care for older blacks in the United States is subject to strong qualification. Simple descriptive analyses comparing whites and blacks and multivariate analyses employing a demand-based perspective suggest that racial differences in elders' use of medical care are small. On the other hand, multivariate analyses employing a need-based perspective reveal that elderly blacks and whites in similar health do not receive the same amount of medical care. In particular, blacks spend substantially less on care than would be expected given their health status. Our findings are consistent with those of van Doorslaer and Wagstaff (1992), who performed an international comparison of equity in the delivery of medical care among industrialized nations. Their study, which also conceptualized equity as equal treatment for persons with equal medical need, found that the United States was characterized by inequity, with elderly persons of higher socioeconomic status being favored.

The findings of our study have two implications. First, the poorer health status of elderly blacks, as compared with whites, may be partially related to inadequate medical care. Older blacks do not receive the quantity of care that would be expected based on their medical need. There are also qualitative differences in care between black and whites. Although the contribution of racial differences in medical care utilization to differences in health may be small relative to the contribution of other influences, such as socioeconomic factors, elimination of the disparity in the use of care would be a positive step.

Second, additional policies to efface the relationship between socioeconomic status and the use of medical care in the United States may be helpful. Potential policies include extension of insurance coverage to low-income elderly individuals, incentives or programs to locate private physicians in undeserved areas, and development of clinical practice guidelines to mitigate the undue influence of patient race (or other demographic factors) on clinical decision making by physicians. Two recent policies that may have salutary effects on the use of care by older blacks with Medicare insurance are the extension of public supplementary coverage to a higher proportion of the low-income elderly, which is expected to decrease out-of-pocket payments for this group, and the implementation of the resource-based Medicare fee schedule (Health Care Financing Administration, 1991), which is likely to reduce the difference in physician reimbursement between Medicare patients with private and with public supplementary coverage. We must acknowledge, however, that health policy has only limited ability to reverse the effects of societal mechanisms and structures that constrain black Americans' economic opportunities and adversely affect their health.

REFERENCES

Aday, L.A.
    1975   Economic and noneconomic barriers to the use of needed medical services. *Medical Care* 13:447-456.
Aday, L.A., and R.M. Andersen
    1981   Equity of access to medical care: A conceptual and empirical overview. *Medical Care* 19(suppl.):4-27.
Andersen, R., and J.F. Newman
    1973   Societal and individual determinants of medical care utilization in the United States. *Milbank Memorial Fund Quarterly* 51:95-124.
Anderson, J.J., and D.T. Felson
    1988   Factors associated with osteoarthritis of the knee in the first National Health and Nutrition Examination Survey (HANES I). *American Journal of Epidemiology* 128:179-189.
Arling, G.
    1985   Interaction effects in a multivariate model of physician visits by older people. *Medical Care* 23:361-371.
Ayanian, J.Z., S. Udvarhelyi, C.A. Gatsonis, C.L. Pashos, and A.M. Epstein
    1993   Racial differences in the use of revascularization procedures after coronary angiography. *Journal of the American Medical Association* 269:2642-2646.
Blendon, R.J., L.H. Aiken, H.E. Freeman, and C.R. Corey
    1989   Access to medical care for black and white Americans: A matter of continuing concern. *Journal of the American Medical Association* 261:278-281.
Byrne, C., J. Nedelman, and R.G. Luke
    1994   Race, socioeconomic status, and the development of end-stage renal disease. *American Journal of Kidney Diseases* 23:16-22.
Cohen, S.B., R. DiGaetano, and J. Waksberg
    1991   *Sample Design of the 1987 Household Survey.* National Medical Expenditure Survey Methods 3, Agency for Health Care Policy and Research. AHCPR publication 91-0037. Rockville, MD: Public Health Service.
Culyer, A.J., E. van Doorslaer, and A. Wagstaff
    1992   Comment: Utilization as a measure of equity. *Journal of Health Economics* 11:43-98.
Davis, K., M. Gold, and D. Makuc
    1981   Access to health care for the poor: Does the gap remain? *Annual Review of Public Health* 1:159-182.
Diehr, P., J. Yergan, J. Chu, P. Feigl, G. Glaefke, R. Moe, M. Bergner, and J. Rodenbaugh
    1989   Treatment modality differences for black and white breast-cancer patients treated in community hospitals. *Medical Care* 27:942-958.
Dor, A., and J. Holahan
    1990   Urban-rural differences in Medicare physician expenditures. *Inquiry* 27:307-318.
Duan, N., W.G. Manning, C.N. Morris, and J.P. Newhouse
    1982   *A Comparison of Alternative Models for the Demand for Medical Care.* R-2754-HHS. Santa Monica, CA: RAND Corporation.
Dutton, D.
    1985   Financial, organizational and professional factors affecting health care utilization. *Social Science and Medicine* 20:721-735.

Edwards, W.S., and M. Berlin
  1989   *Questionnaires and Data Collection Methods for the Household Survey and the Survey of American Indians and Alaska Natives.* National Medical Expenditure Survey Methods 3, National Center for Health Services Research and Health Care Technology Assessment. DHHS publication 89-3450. Rockville, MD: Public Health Service.

Eisenberg, J.M.
  1979   Sociologic influences on decision making by clinicians. *Annals of Internal Medicine* 90:957-964.

Ernst, R.L., and D.E. Yett
  1985   Econometric and statistical studies of the geographic distribution of physicians. Pp. 179-226 in *Physician Location and Specialty Choice*, R.L. Ernst and D.E. Yett, eds. Ann Arbor, MI: Health Administration Press.

Escarce, J.J., K.R. Epstein, D.C. Colby, and J.S. Schwartz
  1993   Racial differences in the elderly's use of medical procedures and diagnostic tests. *American Journal of Public Health* 83:948-954.

Evashwick, C., G. Rowe, P. Diehr, and L. Branch
  1984   Factors explaining the use of health care services by the elderly. *Health Services Research* 19:357-382.

Feinstein, J.S.
  1993   The relationship between socioeconomic status and health: A review of the literature. *Milbank Quarterly* 71:279-322.

Ford, E., R. Cooper, A. Castaner, B. Simmons, and M. Mar
  1989   Coronary arteriography and coronary bypass surgery among whites and other racial groups relative to hospital-based incidence rates for coronary artery disease: Findings from the NHDS. *American Journal of Public Health* 79:437-440.

Furner, S.E.
  1993   Chartbook on health data on older Americans: United States, 1992. Health care use and its cost. *Vital and Health Statistics* 3(29):21-36.

Gibson, R.C.
  1994   The age-by-race gap in health and mortality in the older population: A social science research agenda. *Gerontologist* 34:454-462.

Grossman, M.
  1972   On the concept of health capital and the demand for health. *Journal of Political Economy* 80:223-255.

Haywood, L.J.
  1990   Hypertension in minority populations. *American Journal of Medicine* 88(suppl. 3B):17S-20S.

Health Care Financing Administration, U.S. Department of Health and Human Services
  1991   Medicare program: Fee schedule for physicians' services: Final rule. *Federal Register* 56:59502-59811, November 25.

Held, P.J., M.V. Pauly, R.R. Bovbjerg, J. Newmann, and O. Salvatierra
  1988   Access to kidney transplantation: Has the United States eliminated income and racial differences? *Archives of Internal Medicine* 148:2594-2600.

Javitt, J.C., A.M. McBean, G.A. Nicholson, J.D. Babish, J.L., Warren, and H. Krakauer
  1991   Undertreatment of glaucoma among black Americans. *New England Journal of Medicine* 325:1418-1422.

Kahn, K.L., M.L. Pearson, E.R. Harrison, K.A. Desmond, W.H. Rogers, L.V. Rubenstein, R.H. Brook, and E.B. Keeler
  1994   Health care for black and poor hospitalized Medicare patients. *Journal of the American Medical Association* 271:1169-1174.

Kjellstrand, C.M.
  1988   Age, sex, and race inequality in renal transplantation. *Archives of Internal Medicine* 148:1305-1309.
Kleinbaum, D.G., L.L. Kupper, and H. Morgenstern
  1982   Epidemiologic Research: Principles and Quantitative Methods. New York: Van Nostrand Reinhold.
Kleinman, J.C., M. Gold, and D. Makuc
  1981   Use of ambulatory medical care by the poor: Another look at equity. *Medical Care* 19:1011-1029.
Kotranski, L., J. Bolick, and J. Halbert
  1987   Neighborhood variations in the use of city-supported primary health care services by an elderly population. *Journal of Community Health* 12:231-245.
Lau, R.R., and J.E. Ware
  1981   Refinements in the measurement of health-specific locus-of-control beliefs. *Medical Care* 19:1147-1157.
LeGrand, J.
  1982   *The Strategy of Equality: Redistribution and the Social Services.* London, England: Allen and Unwin.
Leske, M.C., and J. Rosenthal
  1979   Epidemiologic aspects of open-angle glaucoma. *American Journal of Epidemiology* 109:250-272.
Long, S.H., and R.F. Settle
  1984   Medicare and the disadvantaged elderly: Objectives and outcomes. *Milbank Quarterly* 62:609-656.
Manning, W.G., C.N. Morris, J.P. Newhouse, L.L. Orr, N. Duan, E.B. Keller, A. Leibowitz, K.H. Marquis, M.S. Marquis, and C.E. Phelps
  1981   A two-part model of the demand for medical care: Preliminary results from the Health Insurance Study. Pp. 103-123 in *Health, Economics, and Health Economics*, J. van der Gaag and M. Perlman, eds. Amsterdam, Netherlands: North Holland.
Manning, W.G., J.P. Newhouse, N. Duan, E.B. Keeler, A. Leibowitz, and M.S. Marquis
  1987   Health insurance and the demand for medical care: Evidence from a randomized experiment. *American Economic Review* 77:251-278.
Manning, W.G., J.P. Newhouse, and J.E. Ware
  1982   The status of health in demand estimation: Or, beyond excellent, good, fair, and poor. Pp. 143-184 in *Economic Aspects of Health*, V.R. Fuchs, ed. Chicago: University of Chicago Press.
Manton, K.G., C.H. Patrick, and K.W. Johnson
  1987   Health differentials between blacks and whites: Recent trends in mortality and morbidity. *Milbank Quarterly* 65(suppl. 1):129-199.
Marshall, G.N., B.E. Collins, and V.C. Crooks
  1990   A comparison of two multidimensional health locus of control instruments. *Journal of Personality Assessment* 54:181-190.
Mayer, W.J., and W.P. McWhorter
  1989   Black/white differences in non-treatment of bladder cancer patients and implications for survival. *American Journal of Public Health* 79:772-774.
Maynard, C., L.D. Fisher, E.R. Passamani, and T. Pullum
  1986   Blacks in the Coronary Artery Surgery Study (CASS): Race and clinical decision making. *American Journal of Public Health* 76:1446-1448.
McWhorter, W.P., and W.J. Mayer
  1987   Black/white differences in type of initial breast cancer treatment and implications for survival. *American Journal of Public Health* 77:1515-1517.

Moy, E., and C. Hogan
  1993   Access to needed follow-up services: Variations among different Medicare populations. *Archives of Internal Medicine* 153:1815-1823.
Nelson, L., A. Ciemnecki, N. Carlton, and K. Longwell
  1989   *Assignment and the Participating Physician Program: An Analysis of Beneficiary Aware-ness, Understanding, and Experience.* Background paper 89-1. Washington, DC: Physi-cian Payment Review Commission.
Oddone, E.Z., R.D. Horner, M.E. Monger, and D.B. Matchar
  1993   Racial variations in the rates of carotid angiography and endarterectomy in patients with stroke and transient ischemic attack. *Archives of Internal Medicine* 153:2781-2786.
Petchers, M.K., and S.E. Milligan
  1988   Access to health care in a black urban elderly population. *Gerontologist* 28:213-217.
Polednak, A.P., ed.
  1989   *Racial and Ethnic Differences in Disease.* New York: Oxford University Press.
Rice, T., and N. McCall
  1985   The extent of ownership and the characteristics of Medicare supplemental policies. *In-quiry* 22:188-200.
Rotter, J.B.
  1966   Generalized expectancies for internal versus external control of reinforcement. *Psycho-logical Monographs* 80:1-28.
Stoller, E.P.
  1982   Patterns of physician utilization by the elderly: A multivariate analysis. *Medical Care* 20:1080-1089.
van Doorslaer, E., and A. Wagstaff
  1992   Equity in the delivery of health care: Some international comparisons. *Journal of Health Economics* 11:389-411.
Wallace, S.P.
  1990   The political economy of health care for elderly blacks. *International Journal of Health Services* 20:665-680.
Wan, T.T.H.
  1982   Use of health services by the elderly in low-income communities. *Milbank Quarterly* 60:82-107.
Wedig, G.J.
  1988   Health status and the demand for health. *Journal of Health Economics* 7:151-163.
Wenneker, M.B., and A.M. Epstein
  1989   Racial inequalities in the use of procedures for patients with ischemic heart disease in Massachusetts. *Journal of the American Medical Association* 261:253-257.
White, H.
  1980   A heteroskedasticity consistent covariance matrix and a direct test for heteroskedasticity. *Econometrica* 48:817-838.
Williams, D.R., R. Lavizzo-Mourey, and R.C. Warren
  1994   The concept of race and health status in America. *Public Health Reports* 109:26-41.
Wolinsky, F.D., B.E. Aguirre, L-J. Fann, V.M. Keith, C.J. Arnold, J.C. Niederhauer, and K. Dietrich
  1989   Ethnic differences in the demand for physician and hospital utilization among older adults in major American cities: Conspicuous evidence of considerable inequalities. *Milbank Quarterly* 67:412-449.
World Health Organization
  1948   Constitution. *Basic Documents.* Geneva, Switzerland: World Health Organization.
Yergan, J., A.B. Flood, J.P. LoGerfo, and P. Diehr
  1987   Relationship between patient race and the intensity of hospital services. *Medical Care* 25:592-603.

7

Are Genetic Factors Involved in Racial and Ethnic Differences in Late-Life Health?

James V. Neel

INTRODUCTION

In the United States, when we think about racial or ethnic differences in late-life health (and the possible genetic bases for these differences), our thoughts tend to center on the comparison of blacks and whites, and because there is so much more information on these two groups than any others, this presentation concentrates on some possible differences between them. First, I briefly discuss two well-understood disease entities of early onset that are almost entirely restricted to blacks and use these diseases as a point of departure for the possible health implications of racial and ethnic differences in allele frequencies with respect to single-locus polymorphisms. (An allele is any one of two or more different genes that may occupy the same position on a specific chromosome.) I then turn to more complex situations and consider two diseases that result from an interaction between a complex genetic substrate and an equally complex environment. Both of these diseases are characterized by black-white differences in morbidity and mortality. Finally, I briefly discuss the prospects for improving our understanding of whether there really are any genetic differences between blacks and whites with respect to susceptibility to the major diseases of late (as contrasted to early) life.

At the outset, I would like to acknowledge the debt this paper owes the comprehensive treatment entitled *Genetic Variation and Disorders in Peoples of African Origin* by Bowman and Murray (1990). Documentation of statements not otherwise referenced will as a rule be found there. However, I of course assume full responsibility for my interpretive statements.

TWO SIMPLE MONOGENIC DISORDERS DIFFERING IN FREQUENCY IN BLACKS AND WHITES

The two very well-known diseases of blacks that are the point of departure for this presentation are sickle cell anemia and the hemolytic anemia of glucose-6-phosphate dehydrogenase (G-6-PD) deficiency. At first blush, because these diseases typically have their onset in early life, they seem very out of place in a discussion of racial and ethnic differences in late-life diseases. However, they illustrate some of the genetic nuances that enter into a discussion of late-life disease susceptibilities.

Sickle cell anemia is a severe, chronic anemia, usually terminating fatally in early life, that results from homozygosity for a nucleotide substitution at the 17th position in the first intron of the gene coding for the beta chain of hemoglobin, located on chromosome 11. In the United States, about 1.8 in 1,000 black live-born children will develop the disease. Heterozygosity for the allele, designated as β^S, results in the sickle cell trait and is not associated with anemia. Eight percent to nine percent of all American blacks are trait carriers. In black Africans, the frequency of trait carriers varies: it is as high as 35 percent to 50 percent in several tribes of Uganda and Tanzania and is as low as 1 percent to 2 percent in several of the Liberian tribes, with corresponding differences in the incidence of sickle cell anemia. Serjeant's monograph (1985; see also Bowman and Murray, 1990; Honig and Adams, 1986; Livingstone, 1967, 1983) presents an excellent review of the disease and its precise distribution.

As soon as the genetic basis for sickle cell anemia and the sickle cell trait became apparent (Neel, 1947, 1949; Pauling et al., 1949), geneticists confronted a great paradox. Most recessively inherited, serious, essentially lethal disorders—and technically sickle cell anemia is recessively inherited—are quite rare, with an incidence of on the order of 1 in 100,000. Examples are such diverse diseases as Werdnig-Hoffman disease, mucopolysaccharidosis IV (Morquio's syndrome), branched chain ketoaciduria (maple syrup urine disease), and mucolipidosis II (I-cell disease), diseases so uncommon that only medical specialists recognize them. Noting that the sickle cell gene originated in a tropical ecosystem in which malaria, especially *Plasmodium falciparum* malaria, was a major cause of morbidity and mortality, Allison (1954) suggested that the relatively high frequency of the sickle cell gene was due to the fact that the sickling phenomenon conferred protection against the disease. This followed an earlier suggestion by Haldane (1949) that another hematological disorder, thalassemia major (a severe chronic anemia usually fatal in childhood), known at that time to be relatively common in parts of Italy, owed its incidence to the fact that people heterozygous for a thalassemia gene (those with thalassemia minor) were resistant to malaria. There followed a period of intense research activity concerning the validity of the hypothesis. Three distinct lines of evidence now suggest it is correct (details in Bowman and Murray, 1990; Livingstone, 1967, 1983):

1. There is a strong positive correlation between the frequency of the hemoglobin S allele in a given geographic area and the present (or past) prevalence of infection with falciparum malaria.

2. The morbidity and mortality associated with infections with falciparum malaria are less in persons with the sickle cell trait than in persons without the trait.

3. Although the findings are not without controversy, a number of studies suggest that the red blood corpuscles of persons with the sickle cell trait provide a suboptimal environment for the growth of the parasite *P. falciparum*.

Conversely, on the basis of samples collected in Africa, our group was unable to find evidence for the high mutation rate required if such a high rate was the mechanism maintaining the frequency of the hemoglobin S allele (Vanderpitte et al., 1955).

Thus, in a malarial environment, heterozygosity for the hemoglobin S allele confers protection against *P. falciparum*, and means increased survival and reproduction of these heterozygotes. This improved survival of the heterozygote offsets the loss of hemoglobin S alleles when they are in the homozygous state. It is a successful genetic adaptation, but it carries a rather high price tag.

The G-6-PD deficiency trait came to medical attention in a somewhat unusual fashion. Following World War II, there was a major effort to develop better antimalarial drugs, especially those effective against *P. falciparum* malaria. Much of this investigation involved synthesizing and clinically testing compounds of the 8-aminoquinoline family; the clinical investigations took place largely at the University of Chicago under the direction of A. Alving and associates. In field trials, it became apparent that two early antimalarial compounds (pamaquine and primaquine) induced a transitory hemolytic anemia in some blacks, but more rarely in whites. A long series of investigations demonstrated that the anemia was the result of an inherited defect in the gene encoding for the enzyme G-6-PD, located on the sex chromosome. With respect to G-6-PD deficiency, hemizygous males (with one X chromosome) were either positive or negative, but females could be positive/positive, positive/negative, or negative/negative. In females, only the third genotype is affected, and since this requires the presence of two defective alleles (rather than one, as in males), G-6-PD deficiency is much less common in females than in males.

Extensive genetic studies that included biochemical characterization of the deficient enzyme revealed that the molecular basis of the G-6-PD deficiency was rather different from that of the sickling trait. Whereas a single very specific mutation of the beta globin locus produces the sickling trait, with respect to the G-6-PD protein, many different mutations affect the amount in which the enzyme occurs and the efficiency of its action. G-6-PD deficiency is now known to be the cause of the transient hemolytic anemia that some people experience after eating the fava bean and is sometimes associated with a congenital nonspherocytic hemolytic anemia. The deficiency may precipitate anemia in some individuals with viral infections, such as viral hepatitis. In deficient individuals, in addition to the 8-aminoquinolines, an impressive list of other drugs may cause a hemolytic anemia.

By now, population surveys for the frequency of the G-6-PD deficiency are almost as numerous as surveys for the frequency of the sickle cell trait. More than 300 different G-6-PD variants have been identified, and at least 100 of these are relatively common in the males of the populations in which they occur. The higher frequencies are encountered in peoples living in tropical or near-tropical environments. Thus, in addition to African blacks (in whom the frequency of deficient males may vary from zero to 32%, according to tribal affiliation), the frequency of G-6-PD deficient males is as high as 36 percent in some communities of Sephardic Jews, up to 48 percent in areas of Sardinia, 20 percent in some Iranian groups, 15 percent in the Khmer of Cambodia, and 13 percent in the Punjabis of India. The frequency in male African Americans is some 14 percent.

The high frequency of G-6-PD deficient males in these various populations raises the same questions as the high frequency of the hemoglobin S allele, and a similar explanation, the relative resistance of allele carriers to malaria, has been put forth. The evidence in favor of this explanation is similar to the types of evidence adduced earlier to explain the frequency of the hemoglobin S allele, although in general not as convincing. Again, a trait, G-6-PD deficiency, that under certain conditions appears to be deleterious has been carried to a relatively high frequency because it confers a benefit in a specific situation.

The frequency of the allele of the beta globin chain of hemoglobin associated with the sickling phenomenon, and the deficiency alleles of the G-6-PD locus, are examples of genetic polymorphisms. A genetic locus is said to be polymorphic if one or more variant alleles are known for that locus and at least one of the variant alleles has a frequency of 1 percent. This is an arbitrary definition—there is no magic, logical dividing line at 1 percent—but the definition is operationally useful. The genetic loci encoding for the ABO and Rh blood groups are other well-known examples of polymorphic systems. Genetic polymorphisms are in theory of three principal types. First, there are transient polymorphisms that result when an established allele is in the process of being replaced by an allele that confers a selective advantage. Second, there are genetic polymorphisms that result when a new mutation of no particular selective value by chance "drifts" upward in its frequency, to the point where it is polymorphic. Such polymorphisms are most often encountered in small, isolated populations. Third, there are balanced polymorphisms, maintained by the operation of opposing selective forces.

The sickling alleles and the G-6-PD deficiency alleles are representatives of balanced polymorphisms. Homozygosity for the hemoglobin S allele is usually inconsistent with reproduction because the homozygotes usually die in childhood. Homozygosity for a G-6-PD deficiency allele (or hemizygosity in the case of a male) by no means confers the handicap of sickle cell anemia but must still be regarded as impairing the fitness of the homozygote. But in both cases, the alleles have a positive side, conferring resistance to malaria, and the frequency of the allele in a population is determined by a balance between positive and negative selective forces.

What possible light do these two genetic systems throw on disease susceptibilities in late life? Very simply, in an environment where *P. falciparum* malaria is epidemic—and malaria is making a comeback—people with the sickle cell trait or with G-6-PD deficiency trait should at any age level enjoy superior health through a "natural" resistance to the disease. On the other hand, the drug sensitivities of the male with the G-6-PD deficiency persist throughout life and may first become manifest with the increased medication of senior citizens. But these two diseases illustrate an additional point: as the environment alters, a genetic trait that once conferred a selective advantage may lose its advantage.

For the record, I should make it clear that the possession of certain unusual alleles in relatively high frequency is by no means unique to blacks. I think of the Tay-Sachs alleles in Ashkenazic Jews, cystic fibrosis alleles in white populations of North European extraction, and beta-thalassemia alleles in whites of the eastern Mediterranean basin. The beta-thalassemia alleles in heterozygotes probably confer protection against *P. falciparum* malaria, but the reason for the relatively high frequency of the other two sets of alleles is unknown.

DIFFERENCES IN ALLELE FREQUENCY FOR GENETIC POLYMORPHISMS IN BLACKS AND WHITES

Not until genetics took on strong biochemical overtones, in the 1950s and 1960s, was it appreciated how common genetic polymorphisms were. The technique of electrophoresis, combined with enzyme activity stains, revealed that roughly half the proteins studied could have genetic polymorphisms. With the advent of DNA genetics in the 1970s and 1980s, especially the use of so-called restriction site enzymes to define restriction fragment length polymorphisms (the now well-known RFLPs), it became apparent that polymorphisms were very common at the DNA level; we have recently estimated that humans are polymorphic at something like 3×10^6 nucleotide sites (Bittles and Neel, 1994).

Geneticists have been overtaken by an avalanche of genetic variations, and defining their functional significance is a core problem of contemporary population genetics. How much of this variation is flotsam and jetsam, noise in an imperfect genetic system (i.e., neutral polymorphisms), and how much is of biological significance, representing balanced polymorphisms such as the sickle cell and G-6-PD systems, or polymorphisms in which one allele is in the course of being substituted for another through biological selection? On theoretical grounds (Kimura, 1983) and from the results of studies on the outcome of consanguineous marriages (Bittles and Neel, 1994; Neel, 1993), we can argue that much of this variation has no effect on survival and reproduction, but the examples of the sickle cell trait and G-6-PD deficiency—not to mention evolutionary theory—force us to assume that some of the variation has functional significance that we must strive to understand. Most of the readers of this paper will be surprised to learn how poorly sorted out the polymorphisms are in this regard.

Perhaps the best current example of human polymorphic loci associated with disease susceptibilities is the major histocompatibility complex, a set of genetic loci that are responsible for the near immunological uniqueness of each human being (except identical twins). The best known of the loci in this complex code for the *h*uman *l*eukocyte *a*ntigens are termed HLA loci; the four best defined of the loci are designated HLA-A, HLA-B, HLA-C, and HLA-D, with HLA-D a series of sub-loci. Each of these loci is highly polymorphic; at last count, the number of established alleles at each locus varied from 18 to 60 for the A, B, and C loci and from 4 to 58 for the 6 D sub-loci, and the number is still growing. The various possible combinations of these alleles in each individual (plus other inherited antigenic differences not discussed in this paper) create an almost astronomical number of immunological genotypes and phenotypes (references in Ayala et al., 1994; see also Tsugi et al., 1992).

It is now well established that certain HLA alleles confer susceptibility to specific diseases of middle or late life. Many of these diseases are autoimmune disorders, so called because they appear to occur when a person's immune system elaborates specific antibodies that react with that person's own tissues. The precise basis for these disease associations remains under active debate: Is it the specific HLA allele that confers the susceptibility or a gene closely linked to the HLA allele? In fact, the associations undoubtedly result from a mixture of both mechanisms. Be this as it may, some of the more striking disease associations established in whites are shown in Table 7-1.

It is noteworthy that blacks are not represented in these studies. It is not clear whether the diseases in question are much less common in blacks than in whites or whether the necessary studies simply have not been carried out. Note that there are significant and even striking differences between blacks and whites in the frequency of some of the alleles of the HLA system, including alleles A2, A3, and B27, which are associated with several diseases in whites, as Table 7-2 shows (see also Tsugi et al., 1992). Most of these HLA-associated diseases are rare, but collectively, they represent a considerable medical burden.

Of special interest in the present context is the recently demonstrated protection against *P. falciparum* malaria in West Africans conferred by an HLA-B-group haplotype, HLA-Bw53, and a D-group haplotype, DRB1*1302-DQB1*0501 (Hill et al., 1991, 1992). These haplotypes, relatively common in West Africa, are rare in other racial groups. The protection to the individual is not as great as that conferred by heterozygosity for the sickle cell allele, but since these alleles have a higher frequency in West Africa than the sickle cell allele, the protection to the population as a whole appears to be somewhat greater than that afforded by hemoglobin S heterozygosity. Here would seem to be a clear ex-

TABLE 7-1 Some Associations Between HLA Type and Specific Diseases

Disease	Group	HLA type	Antigen Frequency		Relative risk[a]	P value	Number of Studies[b]
			Patients	Control Subjects			
Joint Disease							
Ankylosing spondylitis	White	B27	89.8	8.0	87.8	1.0×10^{-10}	17
	Japanese	B27	66.7	0.0	305.7	1.0×10^{-10}	1
	Haida Indians	B27	100.0	50	34.4	1.7×10^{-9}	1
	Bella Coola Indians	B27	100.0	20.2	20.2	1.9×10^{-2}	1
	Pima Indians	B27	36.0	18.0	2.6	1.0×10^{-3}	1
Reiter's disease	White	B27	78.2	8.4	35.9	1.0×10^{-10}	8
Yersinia arthritis	White	B27	79.4	9.4	24.3	1.0×10^{-10}	2
Salmonella arthritis	White	B27	66.7	8.6	17.6	3.6×10^{-10}	2
Psoriatic arthritis	White	B13	19.8	5.5	4.8	9.6×10^{-10}	5
Central joints		B27	40.2	8.7	8.6	1.0×10^{-4}	5
		Bw17	11.6	5.5	2.5	4.6×10^{-3}	5
		Bw38	22.7	2.9	9.1	5.6×10^{-6}	5
Peripheral joints	White	B13	9.9	5.5	2.3	9.5×10^{-3}	5
		B27	15.5	8.7	2.5	3.5×10^{-4}	5
		Bw17	24.8	5.5	5.8	1.0×10^{-10}	5
		Bw38	12.6	2.9	4.5	$3.2 \times :0^{-4}$	5
Juvenile rheumatoid arthritis	White	B27	26.4	8.5	4.7	1.0×10^{-10}	7
Rheumatoid arthritis	White	Dw4	42.2	15.7	3.0	1.0×10^{-5}	2
	White	Cw3	30.0	17.0	2.7	1.0×10^{-2}	1

Disease of the Endocrine Glands

Thyroid disease							
Graves' disease	White	B8	36.7	21.7	2.13	1.0×10^{-6}	6
		Dw3	50.0	21.7	4.0	1.0×10^{-4}	3
	Japanese	Bw35	56.8	20.5	4.97	1.0×10^{-5}	1
deQuervain's thyroiditis	White	Bw35	76.9	12.5	22.2	1.0×10^{-10}	2
Adrenal disease							
Addison's disease	White	B8	50.0	22.7	3.9	7.3×10^{-6}	2
		Dw3	70.0	21.7	10.5	1.0×10^{-3}	1
Pancreatic disease							
Diabetes	White	B8	36.7	21.8	2.1	1.0×10^{-10}	8
Juvenile onset diabetes		Bw15	22.8	14.9	2.1	1.0×10^{-10}	8

Gastrointestinal Tract Disease

Chronic active hepatitis	White	A1	41.6	28.4	1.8	6.4×10^{-5}	5
		B8	44.2	20.3	3.0	1.0×10^{-10}	5
		Dw3	60.0	21.7	7.2	1.0×10^{-3}	2
Celiac disease (gluten enteropathy)	White	A1	63.7	29.5	4.2	1.0×10^{-10}	7
		B8	71.2	23.1	8.8	1.0×10^{-10}	9
		Dw3	98.0	15.0	278	1.0×10^{-5}	1
Hemochromatosis	White	A3	78.4	27.0	9.5	2.1×10^{-11}	2
		B14	25.5	3.4	9.23	5.3×10^{-5}	1
Ulcerative colitis	Japanese	B5	80.0	30.8	9.3	1.0×10^{-3}	1
Pernicious anemia	White	B7	35.8	22.1	2.2	1.2×10^{-4}	3

Continued on following page

TABLE 7-1 Continued

Disease	Group	HLA type	Antigen Frequency Patients	Antigen Frequency Control Subjects	Relative risk[a]	P value	Number of Studies[b]
Skin Disease							
Psoriasis	White	B13	19.7	4.5	4.65	1.0×10^{-10}	6
		Bw17	26.2	7.8	4.7	1.0×10^{-10}	6
		Bw37	7.7	1.4	5.4	1.0×10^{-10}	3
Dermatitis herpetiformis	White	A1	69.0	30.1	4.4	1.0×10^{-10}	5
		B8	77.0	24.7	9.2	1.0×10^{-10}	6
Pemphigus vulgaris	White	A10	39.3	12.7	3.1	1.2×10^{-4}	3
Herpes labialis	White	A1	55.6	25.1	3.7	1.3×10^{-6}	1
		B8	33.3	16.8	2.5	3.5×10^{-4}	1
Eye Disease							
Anterior uveitis	White	B27	56.8	7.7	15.4	1.0×10^{-4}	2
Vogt-Koyanagi-Harada disease	Japanese	B22J	42.9	13.2	4.5	2.0×10^{-2}	1
Malignant Disease							
Hodgkin's disease	White	A1	31.1	39	1.4	1.0×10^{-6}	17
		B5	10.6	16	1.6	1.0×10^{-6}	17
		B8	23.7	29	1.3	1.0×10^{-4}	17
		Bw18	7.1	13	1.9	1.0×10^{-6}	17
Acute lymphatic leukemia	White	A2	60.0	53.6	1.3	1.0×10^{-2}	10
		B8	29.0	23.7	1.3	1.0×10^{-2}	10
		Bw18	29.0	25.2	1.3	1.0×10^{-2}	10
Nasopharyngeal cancer	Chinese	Sia2	44.0	21.0	1.9	1.0×10^{-3}	1

[a]The relative risk is the ratio of the proportion of diseased individuals among carriers of a specific genetic trait to the proportion of diseased individuals among people who do not carry that trait.

[b]The relative risk figures are derived from the combined data set.

SOURCE: Adapted from Vogel and Motulsky, 1979.

TABLE 7-2   A Comparison of Three Ethnic Groups with Respect to the
Frequency of Certain HLA Types

	HLA-A Frequency				HLA-B Frequency		
Gene Locus	European Whites ($n = 228$)	African Blacks ($n = 102$)	Japanese ($n = 195$)	Gene Locus	European Whites ($n = 228$)	African Blacks ($n = 102$)	Japanese ($n = 195$)
A1	0.16	0.04	0.01	B5	0.06	0.03	0.21
A2	0.27	0.09	0.25	B7	0.10	0.07	0.07
A3	0.13	0.06	0.007	B8	0.09	0.07	0.002
A23	0.02	0.11	—	B12	0.17	0.13	0.07
A24	0.09	0.02	0.37	B13	0.03	0.02	0.008
A25	0.02	0.04	—	B14	0.02	0.04	0.005
A26	0.04	0.05	0.13	B18	0.06	0.02	—
A11	0.05	—	0.07	B27	0.05	—	0.003
A28	0.04	0.09	—	B15	0.05	0.03	0.09
Aw29	0.06	0.06	0.002	Bw38	0.02	—	0.02
Aw30	0.04	0.22	0.005	Bw39	0.04	0.02	0.05
Aw31	0.02	0.04	0.87	B17	0.06	0.16	0.006
Aw32	0.03	0.02	0.005	Bw21	0.02	0.02	0.02
Aw33	0.007	0.01	0.02	Bw22	0.04	—	0.07
Aw43	—	0.04	—	Bw35	0.10	0.07	0.09
Blank	0.02	0.11	0.04	B37	0.01	—	0.008
				B40	0.08	0.02	0.22
				Bw41	—	0.02	—
				Bw42	—	0.12	—
				Blank	0.04	0.18	0.08

	HLA-C Frequency				HLA-DR Frequency		
Gene Locus	European Whites ($n = 321$)	African Blacks ($n = 101$)	Japanese ($n = 203$)	Gene Locus	European Whites ($n = 334$)	African Blacks ($n = 77$)	Japanese ($n = 164$)
Cw1	0.05	—	0.11	DRw1	0.06	—	0.05
Cw2	0.05	0.11	0.01	DRw2	0.11	0.09	0.17
Cw3	0.09	0.06	0.16	DRw3	0.09	0.12	—
Cw4	0.13	0.14	0.04	DRw4	0.08	0.04	0.14
Cw5	0.08	0.01	0.01	DRw5	0.15	0.07	0.05
Cw6	0.13	0.18	0.02	DRw6	0.09	0.10	0.07
Blank	0.47	0.50	0.53	DRw7	0.16	0.07	—
				W1A8	0.06	0.07	0.07
				Blank	0.21	0.45	0.45

SOURCE: Bowman and Murray, 1990: Table 5.3.   Original data from Conference Workshop on Histocompatibility Testing (1978: Table 6.1-6.4). Reprinted by permission of Munksgaard International Publishers.

ample of an ethnic difference in susceptibility to a disease as great as the sickle cell example. Other possible genetic protective mechanisms against malaria in blacks have been recently reviewed by Miller (1994, 1995). It is clear that in meeting the serious challenge to survival that malaria poses, the process of natural selection has drawn on multiple, diverse genetic mechanisms to blunt the effects of the disease.

A possible polymorphism-disease association of whites that is currently receiving a great deal of attention is the highly significant correlation between Alzheimer's disease and possession of the ε 4 allele of the apolipoprotein E (Apo E) system (Chartier-Harlin et al., 1994; Corder et al., 1993; Noguchi et al., 1993; Payami et al., 1993; Poirier et al., 1993; Saunders et al., 1993; Strittmatter et al., 1993). Eight abstracts from the fall 1994 meeting of the American Society of Human Genetics confirmed this association (Crawford et al., 1994; Houlden and Rossor, 1994; Jarvik et al., 1994; Kamboh et al., 1994; Martinez et al., 1994; Okuizumi et al., 1994; Poduslo and Schwankhaus, 1994; Sahota et al., 1994). For whites, this is now one of the most firmly established marker-disease associations in genetic medicine. Linkage studies have already suggested that there are at least three genetic loci where the presence of an abnormal allele may result in a condition that meets the criteria of Alzheimer's disease (e.g., Corder et al., 1993; Goldin and Gershon, 1993; Pericak-Vance et al., 1993); heterogeneity is also suggested by segregation analysis (Rao et al., 1994). It will be very important to determine whether the three types of Alzheimer's disease that these loci define all exhibit the Apo E ε 4 association. If the association is with only one of these three loci, then the high statistical correlation that has been observed would require a very strong association with that one locus.

The ε 4 allele occurs about twice as frequently in U.S. blacks (0.26) as in U.S. whites (0.13) (summary in Gerdes et al., 1992). The data on black-white differences in the frequency of Alzheimer's disease are scanty but favor a lower incidence of Alzheimer's in blacks (de la Monte et al., 1989; Molgaard et al., 1990; Schoenberg et al., 1985). The limited data on an Apo E ε 4 allele association with Alzheimer's in blacks are contradictory; Mayeux et al. (1993) find no relationship but Sahota et al. (1994) find a strong association. Further studies on this association will be as important as further studies on the associations of HLA alleles with disease in blacks, since cross-racial studies of both of these disease associations will reveal much about the specificity of the association.

Most of the human genetic polymorphisms have been discovered in white populations, and studies of the comparative frequency of the variant alleles in whites and blacks are often limited. However, in a majority of instances where proper population surveys have been done, there are statistically significant differences between the allele frequencies of the polymorphisms in the two racial groups. In some instances, these differences are very striking. For instance, the frequency of the R_0 (cDe) allele of the Rh system, associated with Rh hemolytic disease, is relatively very high in black Africans and African Americans (0.50 to

0.90), whereas in most white populations, the frequency is in the neighborhood of 0.03. With respect to the Duffy blood group systems, the Fy^a allele has a frequency of 0.421 in whites and 0.053 in blacks, whereas the Fy allele, whose presence has been associated with a resistance to *P. vivax* malaria (Miller et al., 1975, 1976), has a frequency of 0.825 in West Africans but only 0.030 in whites. There are numerous other differences in allele frequencies where no health effect has yet related to the allele. Finally, there are a few further polymorphisms that, like the sickle cell polymorphism, have thus far been encountered only in blacks or whites (the rare exceptions are explicable by racial admixture). An example of a polymorphism unique to blacks is the PGM_2^2 allele of the phosphoglucomutase-2 enzyme system, which in blacks has a frequency of 3 percent to 4 percent but is absent in whites.

It is axiomatic that if an allele-disease association is established for one racial or ethnic group, it cannot be automatically assumed to prevail in a different group. Even for the strongest allele-disease associations, only a minority of the carriers of the allele develop the disease. Realization of the potential disease relationship undoubtedly depends on both modifying genetic factors and environmental variables. Thus, although the difference between blacks and whites in the frequency of the HLA alleles, or the alleles of the Apo E system, raises the possibility of racial and ethnic differences in the frequency of the diseases associated with these alleles, it remains for detailed studies to determine whether that possibility is realized. Indeed, the possible role of racial and ethnic differences in late-life diseases related to differences in allele frequencies with respect to known polymorphism is still poorly understood.

SOME GENETICALLY COMPLEX, ENVIRONMENTALLY INFLUENCED DISORDERS DIFFERING IN FREQUENCY IN BLACKS AND WHITES

This section considers the possible role of genetic factors in two diseases that differ in frequency in blacks and whites, namely, diabetes mellitus of the non-insulin-dependent type and essential hypertension, that is, hypertension that is not a consequence of renal or other disease. These two diseases have been arbitrarily selected from among the many diseases of late-life onset, but they raise questions about genetic differences in blacks and whites in susceptibility to these diseases that also arise for many other disorders of late-life onset.

Two facts about these diseases are very important to anyone considering their genetic basis. First, unlike the traits considered thus far, both the ability to metabolize glucose and the level of the systolic and diastolic blood pressure are continuously distributed variables. Under these conditions, the definition of disease is arbitrary. By convention, the physician makes the diagnosis of essential hypertension when the resting systolic blood pressure exceeds 160 mm Hg and the diastolic, 95 mm Hg (some would make the diagnosis at a pressure of

140/90). The justification is the belief that when these or higher levels are sustained over a prolonged period of time, there are departures from health, however that be defined. Likewise, the definition of diabetes mellitus is reached when the fasting plasma glucose exceeds 140 mg/dl or when the plasma glucose exceeds 200 mg/dl 2 hours after the ingestion of a standard (75 grams) load of glucose. Again, this is based on the belief that at this level of impairment of glucose metabolism, there are departures from health. It is customary to distinguish between two principal types of diabetes: (1) diabetes of relatively early life and sudden onset, in the medical management of which insulin is necessary from the outset, and (2) diabetes of relatively late life and gradual onset, in the medical management of which insulin is not necessary until late in the disease if at all. The former is termed insulin-dependent diabetes mellitus, the latter non-insulin-dependent diabetes mellitus. In this brief presentation, we consider only the second type of diabetes.

That there are differences between blacks and whites in the frequency and severity of these two diseases is well established (Anderson and McManus, 1996; see also Roseman, 1985). However, there are some tricky aspects to these racial comparisons. The National Health and Nutrition Examination Survey (NHANES) of 1979-1982 revealed that for all ages, the rate of diagnosed diabetes per 1,000 people was 32 for blacks and 24 for whites. The vast majority of these diagnoses were of non-insulin-dependent diabetes mellitus (insulin-dependent diabetes mellitus seems less common in blacks). However, I remind you that the inability to metabolize glucose is a continuously distributed trait. The NHANES during 1979-1981 administered oral glucose tolerance tests to a large sample of blacks and whites in whom diabetes had not been diagnosed. For all ages (20 to 74 years) and both sexes, the prevalence of undiagnosed diabetes mellitus was 80/1,000 in whites and 123/1,000 in blacks, but the prevalence of impaired glucose tolerance (which may be regarded as a way station to non-insulin-dependent diabetes mellitus) was 95/1,000 in whites and 34/1,000 in blacks. For all three categories combined—the diagnosed, those with undiagnosed diabetes, and those with impaired glucose tolerance—the prevalence was 189/1,000 in blacks and 199/1,000 in whites. One could argue from this finding that the magnitude of the predisposed group was about the same in blacks and in whites but that a larger fraction of blacks have realized that predisposition, as the disease is now defined.

The second salient point about these two diseases is that they are of very gradual onset. In the children of parents with non-insulin-dependent diabetes mellitus, there are statistically significant departures from normal glucose metabolism in the third decade, even though the degree of impairment that justifies the (arbitrary) diagnosis of non-insulin-dependent diabetes mellitus is not usually reached until the fifth or sixth decade (cf. Neel et al., 1965). Likewise, in retrospect, individuals with borderline hypertension (average age 31.4 years) exhibited, in comparison with control subjects, small but significant elevations during childhood and immediately after puberty (Julius et al., 1990).

The argument over the degree to which these ethnic differences in non-insulin-dependent diabetes are environmentally triggered versus the degree to which they are based on specific genes that differ in frequency in the two ethnic groups—like the polymorphisms previously discussed—goes back to the recognition of the racial and ethnic differences. Since there is no agreement as to the basic defect or defects in either of the two diseases, the argument has been relatively uninhibited by troublesome facts. One salient point is clear: both of these diseases are diseases of modern civilization, however civilization be defined. Hypertension is very uncommon in tribal populations adhering to traditional lifestyles (reviewed in Page, 1978). For instance, we encountered no hypertensives in quite unacculturated Xavante and Yanomama Amerindians (Neel et al., 1964; Oliver et al., 1975). Numerous studies on native Africans document the increase in blood pressure that occurs with the transition from a relatively unacculturated rural setting to urban life, with hypertension then apparently as prevalent as in U.S. blacks (reviewed in Kaufman and Barkey, 1993; see especially Scotch, 1963). The "triggers" that have been invoked to explain this increase range from a greater salt intake to a complex of socioeconomic factors that create stress. Since tribal life is by no means without its stresses, one must be careful not to use the term *stress* loosely. Non-insulin-dependent diabetes mellitus is likewise less prevalent in rural African blacks than in urban African blacks, but in both groups it is well below the prevalence in U.S. blacks (reviewed in Roseman, 1985).

With reference to the genetics of hypertension, numerous studies have established its familial nature (reviewed in Burke and Motulsky, 1990; Ward, 1990). Although most of these studies involve whites, the disease is no less familial in blacks (Rotini et al., 1994). However, the correlation between adult siblings usually varies from 0.2 to 0.3 for both systolic and diastolic pressures, and for parents and offspring, the variation is the same or somewhat lower (reviewed in Burke and Motulsky, 1990). For monozygous twins, the correlations were 0.55 for systolic pressure and 0.58 for diastolic, whereas for dizygous twins, the corresponding figures were 0.25 and 0.27. These are, of course, significant but well below those expected of a continuously distributed trait that is completely determined genetically. Thus, while these data certainly establish the familial nature of hypertension, I have to remind you of the old truism that all that is familial is not genetic, a stricture especially appropriate for a disease such as hypertension (cf. especially Cooper and Rotini, 1994).

With reference to the genetics of non-insulin-dependent diabetes mellitus, the disease has long been recognized as strongly familial, and various modes of inheritance have been suggested. Many of the problems recognized 30 years ago in attempts to elucidate its genetic basis (reviewed in Neel, 1962; Neel et al., 1965) persist today (Leslie, 1993). In one representative study, the risks for siblings and children of a person with the disease were placed at 38 percent and 33 percent, respectively (Köbberling and Tillil, 1982), and these are minimal estimates because additional cases will develop subsequent to the study. Concordance in monozygotic twins, given the detection of the disease in a parent or sibling, is greater than 90 percent (Barnett et al., 1981). Although in several studies only about 10 percent to 30 percent of the children of two diabetic parents were similarly affected (Ganda and Soeldner, 1977; Tattersall and Fajans, 1975), correction for the age of onset brought the anticipated proportion of those affected to 90 percent to 100 percent. Again, one must remember that all that is familial does not necessarily have a genetic basis in the sense of segregating, identifiable alleles.

Although essential hypertension and non-insulin-dependent diabetes mellitus are diseases of later life, they may develop during reproductive life and impose a reproductive handicap in their various manifestations. The genes for susceptibility appear to be relatively common and widespread. This pattern raises the same question as was raised by the frequency of the sickle cell trait. Some years ago, I raised the possibility that what we now regard as genes for susceptibility to diabetes mellitus served a useful function prior to civilization but did not become fixed because they were balanced by opposing selective forces. I referred to the diabetic predisposition as a "thrifty genotype," which contributed to our metabolic efficiency in lean times (Neel, 1962, 1976, 1982). Others have pursued a similar hypothesis regarding the predisposition to hypertension (Julius and Jamerson, 1994). As we come to better understand the molecular genetics for these predispositions, it will be of interest to see how this hypothesis plays out.

Investigators accept that diseases as varied in age of onset and course as non-insulin-dependent diabetes mellitus and essential hypertension are genetically heterogeneous. A number of rare subtypes of each, often associated with syndromes, are known, and these are excluded from this general discussion. But the remaining cases are almost surely genetically heterogeneous, and efforts to tease out subtypes continue. The most notable success in recognizing a subtype of non-insulin-dependent diabetes mellitus involves the relatively uncommon maturity onset diabetes of youth, in which impairment of sugar metabolism has an early onset, progresses slowly, and appears to be inherited as a simple dominant trait (Tattersall, 1974). In the 20 years since its recognition, the maturity onset diabetes of youth has been divided into three subtypes, one tightly linked to the genetic markers ADA and D20S16 on chromosome 20q, one due to abnormalities in the glucokinase gene on chromosome 7p, and one with neither of these genetic linkages (reviewed in Fajans et al., 1994). Likewise, there are rare, simply inherited types of hypertension (reviewed in Williams et al., 1994). For example, a rare type of hypertension identified some 20 years ago (New and Peterson, 1967; Sutherland et al., 1966) has been shown to be due to a chimeric 11 beta-hydroxylase/aldosterone synthetase gene located on chromosome 8q (Lifton et al., 1992). Further rare genetic subtypes of both diseases will undoubtedly be defined, but the body of both diseases will remain complexly multifactorial.

Both non-insulin-dependent diabetes mellitus and essential hypertension are often encountered in obese individuals. Since obesity is also accompanied by a decreased life expectancy, it may be defined as a disease, and it too is a disease rare in tribal peoples. As in the case of non-insulin-dependent diabetes mellitus and essential hypertension, the race to identify "obesity susceptibility" genes is on. Because all three of these diseases are relatively common, they might be expected occasionally to occur together by chance. In fact, the frequency of the congruence of truncal/abdominal (android) obesity with non-insulin-dependent diabetes mellitus and hypertension in the same person far exceeds the expectation based on chance (cf. Carmelli et al., 1994; Rice et al., 1994; Sims and Berchtold, 1982). It is increasingly necessary to see these three conditions as a disease complex (e.g., Björntorp, 1992; Landsberg, 1986; Reaven, 1988; Rice et al., 1994) that has emerged with the profound changes in lifestyle that accompany modern civilization, and the genetic studies of the future must deal with this complex, which amounts to the thrifty genotype updated.

As we all know, the disease manifestations of non-insulin-dependent diabetes mellitus and essential hypertension are numerous and varied. These manifestations appear to differ in blacks and whites. For instance, it appears that blacks with non-insulin-dependent diabetes mellitus may have a relatively higher frequency of microvascular disease, retinopathy, renal disease, and peripheral vascular disease than whites (Cowie et al., 1989; Harris et al., 1994; Roseman, 1985). Adjusting these findings for the differences in the duration and severity of the disease in the two groups is difficult; it is not clear whether these differences result from specific organ susceptibilities in blacks or an earlier onset of the disease. Likewise, for hypertension, blacks have a lower risk for coronary artery disease but a higher risk for stroke and renal failures (cf. Burke and Motulsky, 1990). The data on ethnic differences in end-stage renal disease from the U.S. Renal Data System are especially striking, the incidence of blacks with end-stage renal disease averaging three to four times higher than for whites, at all age groups (Lopes et al., 1993, 1994). While the Renal Data System does not include all persons with end-stage renal disease in the United States, underreporting is more probable for blacks than for whites. Again, the question arises as to whether this reflects a greater duration of the disease in blacks.

PROSPECTS FOR A BETTER UNDERSTANDING OF THE BASIS FOR DIFFERENCES IN LATE-LIFE DISEASES

What should by now be clear is that except for a relatively few simply inherited diseases or disease-associated traits, knowledge about the possible genetic basis for the different patterns of adult onset and late-life diseases in blacks and whites is still meager.

I close with a brief comment on the prospects for improving this situation. First, however, a comment on maintaining perspective is in order. Some years ago (Neel, 1981), I pointed out that on the basis of 11 proteins that had been sequenced in humans (presumably from whites) and the chimpanzee, the deduced number of nucleotide substitutions distinguishing the two species was only 6 in the 4,326 nucleotides of the exons coding for these proteins in the two species. There is a 99.85 percent similarity. Now, with the use of genetic-distance techniques, the genetic distance between the major human racial and ethnic groups, based on the "standard" allele for the genes used in the study, can be shown to be only 1/25 to 1/60 of that between the human and the chimpanzee (King and Wilson, 1975). Blacks and whites then are genetically very similar indeed, leading to the expectation of resemblance, not differences, in the great majority of their genetic responses in disease-producing situations.

Most of the major diseases differing in frequency between whites and blacks appear to be diseases of complex etiology, with a multifactorial genetic basis and a strong environmental component in the determination of how this inherited susceptibility is expressed. It is quite likely that there are various allele combinations that create the susceptibility and various environments that facilitate the expression of this genetic susceptibility. The varying patterns of interaction between the gene products and the milieu in which these products function create a complex epigenetic nexus that is difficult to penetrate, especially since the interactions between the components of the epigenetic nexus may be nonlinear. (I use the term *epigenetic* as synonymous with the complex of interactions that may intervene between gene products and their ultimate phenotypic expression.) My personal bias is that at present this epigenetic nexus differs so much between blacks and whites that it is difficult if not impossible to reach any but the simplest inferences concerning racial differences in susceptibility to complex diseases. I find myself in full accord with the pungent documentation of this viewpoint developed by Cooper and Rotini (1994), with particular reference to hypertension.

Although the application of the techniques of molecular biology to genetic studies of non-insulin-dependent diabetes mellitus and essential hypertension will undoubtedly result in significant insights into the genetic component of these two diseases over the next several decades, I suspect that really definitive insights into the differences between blacks and whites that I have discussed must await progress in equalizing the epigenetic factors at work on white and black genotypes, or research designs that take advantage of unusual social circumstances. The usual research designs for epidemiological studies of traits with a strong environmental overlay—paired control subjects matched as closely as possible socioeconomically to the case subjects—do not work well in genetic studies of complex diseases because whereas it is difficult enough to match individuals, it is much more difficult to match families. Yes, there are genetic differences between blacks and whites; yes, there are clear differences in the frequency of some of the severe genetic diseases of childhood. But with reference to the diseases that are the purview of this volume, we still know very little about innate genetic differences in susceptibility, and the prospects for definitive studies are dim until ways are found to deal more adequately with the epigenetic factors influencing interracial and interethnic studies.

REFERENCES

Allison, A.C.
1954   Protection afforded by sickle-cell trait against subtertian malarial infection. *British Medical Journal* 1:290-294.

Anderson, N.B., and C. McManus
1996   *Hypertension in Blacks Across the Life Course: A Biopsychosocial Analysis.* New York: Springer.

Ayala, F.J., A. Escalante, C. O'Huigin, and J. Klein
1994   Molecular genetics of speciation and human origins. *Proceedings of the National Academy of Sciences of the United States of America* 91:6787-6794.

Barnett, A.H., C. Eff, R.D.G. Leslie, and D.A. Pyke
1981   Diabetes in identical twins: A study of 200 pairs. *Diabetologia* 20:87-93.

Bittles, A.H., and J.V. Neel
1994   The costs of human inbreeding and their implications for variation at the DNA level. *Nature Genetics* 8:117-121.

Björntorp, P.
1992   Abdominal obesity and the metabolic syndrome. *Annals of Medicine* 24:465-468.

Bowman, J.E., and R.F. Murray
1990   *Genetic Variation and Disorders in Peoples of African Origin.* Baltimore, MD: Johns Hopkins University Press.

Burke, W., and A.G. Motulsky
1990   Hypertension. Pp. 170-191 in *The Genetic Basis of Common Diseases*, R.A. King, J.I. Rotter, and A.G. Motulsky, eds. New York: Oxford University Press.

Carmelli, D., L.R. Cardon, and R. Fabsitz
1994   Clustering of hypertension, diabetes, and obesity in adult male twins: Same genes or same environment? *American Journal of Human Genetics* 55:566-573.

Chartier-Harlin, M.C., M. Parfitt, S. Legrain, J. Perez-Tur, T. Brousseau, A. Evans, C. Berr, O. Vidal, P. Roques, V. Gourlet, J. Fruchart, A. Delacourte, M. Rossor, and P. Amouyel
1994   Apolipoprotein E, ε4 allele as a major risk factor for sporadic early and late-onset forms of Alzheimer's disease: Analysis of the 19q13.2 chromosomal region. *Human Molecular Genetics* 3:569-574.

Cooper, R., and C. Rotini
1994   Hypertension in populations of West African origin: Is there a genetic predisposition? *Journal of Hypertension* 12:215-227.

Corder, E.H., A.M. Saunders, W.J. Strittmatter, D.E. Schmechel, P.C. Gaskell, G.W. Small, A.D. Roses, J.L. Haines, and M.A. Pericak-Vance
1993   Gene dose of apolipoprotein E type 4 allele and the risk of Alzheimer's disease in late onset families. *Science* 261:921-923.

Cowie, C.C., F.K. Port, R.A. Wolfe, P.J. Savage, P.P. Moll, and V.M. Hawthorne
1989   Disparities in incidence of diabetic end-stage renal disease according to race and type of diabetes. *New England Journal of Medicine* 321:1074-1079.

Crawford, F., C. Bennett, A. Osborne, P. Diaz, J. Hoyne, R. Lopez, P. Roques, R. Duara, M. Rossor, and M. Mullan
1994   The APOE locus advances disease progression in late onset familial Alzheimer's disease but is not causative. *American Journal of Human Genetics* 55(suppl.):149(abstract).

de la Monte, S.M., G.M. Hutchins, and G.W. Moore
   1989   Racial differences in the etiology of dementia and frequency of Alzheimer lesions in the brain. *Journal of the National Medical Association* 81:644-652.
Fajans, S.S., G.I. Bell, D.W. Bowden, J.B. Halter, and K.S. Polonsky
   1994   Maturity-onset diabetes of the young. *Life Sciences* 55:413-422.
Ganda, O.P., and S.S. Soeldner
   1977   Genetic, acquired, and related factors in the etiology of diabetes mellitus. *Archives of Internal Medicine* 137:461-469.
Gerdes, L.U., I.C. Klausen, I. Sihm, and O. Faergeman
   1992   Apolipoprotein E polymorphism in a Danish population compared to findings in 45 other study populations around the world. *Genetic Epidemiology* 9:155-167.
Goldin, L.R., and E.S. Gershon
   1993   Linkage of Alzheimer's disease to chromosome 21 and chromosome 19 markers: Effect of age of onset assumptions. *Genetic Epidemiology* 10:449-454.
Haldane, J.B.S.
   1949   Disease and evolution. *La Ricerca Scientifica* Supplementa 19:68-76.
Harris, E.L., M. Sheldon-Rubio, C.R. Robinson, S. Sherman, and A. Georgopoulos
   1994   Racial differences in risk of developing retinopathy among persons with non-insulin-dependent diabetes (NIDDM). *American Journal of Human Genetics* 55(suppl.):153- (abstract).
Hill, A.V.S., C.E.M. Allsopp, D. Kwiatkowski, N.M. Anstey, P. Twumasi, P.A. Rowe, S. Bennett, D. Brewster, A.J. McMichael, and B.M. Greenwood
   1991   Common West African HLA antigens are associated with protection from severe malaria. *Nature* 352:595-600.
Hill, A.V.S., J. Elvin, A.C. Willis, M. Aidoo, C.E.M. Allsopp, F.M. Gotch, X.M. Gao, M. Takiguchi, B.M. Greenwood, A.R.M. Townsend, A.J. McMichael, and H.C. Whittle
   1992   Molecular analysis of the association of HLA-B53 and resistance to severe malaria. *Nature* 360:434-439.
Honig, G.R., and J.G. Adams
   1986   *Human Hemoglobin Genetics.* New York: Springer Verlag.
Houlden, H., and M. Rossor
   1994   Clustering and age of onset in familial late onset Alzheimer's disease are determined at the apolipoprotein E locus. *American Journal of Human Genetics* 55(suppl.):152(abstract).
Jarvik, G.P., W.A. Kukull, K. Goddard, G.D. Schellenberg, E.B. Laron, and E.M. Wijsman
   1994   Family history and apo E genotype interaction in Alzheimer disease (AD). *American Journal of Human Genetics* 55(suppl.):152(abstract).
Julius, S., and K. Jamerson
   1994   Sympathetics, insulin resistance and coronary risk in hypertension: The "chicken-and-egg" question. *Journal of Hypertension* 12:495-502.
Julius, S., K. Jamerson, A. Mejia, L. Krause, N. Schork, and K. Jones
   1990   The association of borderline hypertension with target organ changes and higher coronary risk. *Journal of the American Medical Association* 264:354-358.
Kamboh, M.I., S.T. DeKosky, and R.E. Ferrell
   1994   Over-representation of the APOE*4 allele in autopsy confirmed early- and late-onset sporadic Alzheimer's disease. *American Journal of Human Genetics* 55(Suppl.):152- (abstract).
Kaufman, J., and N. Barkey
   1993   Hypertension in Africa: An overview of prevalence rates and causal risk factors. *Ethnicity and Disease* 3(suppl.):83-101.
Kimura, M.
   1983   *The Neutral Theory of Molecular Evolution.* Cambridge, England: Cambridge University Press.

King, M.-C., and A.C. Wilson
1975   Evolution at two levels in humans and chimpanzees. *Science* 188:107-116.

Köbberling, J., and H. Tillil
1982   Empirical risk figures for first degree relatives of non-insulin dependent diabetics. Pp. 201-209 in *The Genetics of Diabetes Mellitus*, J. Köbberling and R. Tattersall, eds. London, England: Academic Press.

Landsberg, L.
1986   Diet, obesity, and hypertension: An hypothesis involving insulin, the sympathetic nervous system, and adaptive thermogenesis. *Quarterly Journal of Medicine* 61:1081-1090.

Leslie, R.D.G.
1993   *Causes of Diabetes: Genetic and Environmental Factors.* Chichester, England: John Wiley and Sons.

Lifton, R.P., R.G. Dluhy, M. Powers, G.M. Rich, C. Cook, S. Ulick, and J.M. Lalouel
1992   A chimeric 11β-hydroxylase/aldosterone synthetase gene causes glucocorticoid-remedial aldosteronism and human hypertension. *Nature* 355:262-265.

Livingstone, F.B.
1967   *Abnormal Hemoglobins in Human Populations: A Summary and Interpretation.* Chicago: Aldine.
1983   The malaria hypothesis. Pp. 15-44 in *Distribution and Evolution of Hemoglobin and Globin Loci*, J.E. Bowman, ed. New York: Elsevier.

Lopes, A.A.S., K. Hornbuckle, S.A. James, and F.K. Port
1994   The joint effects of race and age on the risk of end-stage renal disease attributed to hypertension. *American Journal of Kidney Diseases* 24:554-560.

Lopes, A.A.S., F.K. Port, S.A. James, and L. Agodoa
1993   The excess risk of treated end-stage renal disease in blacks in the United States. *Journal of the American Society of Nephrology* 3:1961-1971.

Martinez, M., J. Perez-Tur, C. Campion, F. Clerget-Darpoux, M.C. Chartier-Harlin, and the French Alzheimer Collaborative Group
1994   Increase of the Apo E4 allele frequency in a subgroup of early-onset Alzheimer's patients. *American Journal of Human Genetics* 55(suppl.):157(abstract).

Mayeux, R., Y. Stern, R. Ottman, T.K. Tattemichi, M.-X. Tang, G. Maestre, C. Ngai, B. Tycko, and H. Ginsberg
1993   The apolipoprotein ε4 allele in patients with Alzheimer's disease. *Annals of Neurology* 34:752-754.

Miller, L.H.
1994   Impact of malaria on genetic polymorphism and genetic diseases in Africans and African Americans. *Proceedings of the National Academy of Sciences of the United States of America* 91:2415-2419.
1995   Impact of malaria on genetic polymorphism and genetic diseases in Africans and African Americans. Pp. 99-111 in *Infectious Diseases in an Age of Change*, B. Roizman, ed. Washington, DC: National Academy Press.

Miller, L.H., S.J. Mason, D.F. Clyde, and M.H. McGinniss
1976   The resistance factor to *Plasmodium vivax* in blacks: The Duffy-blood-group genotype, FyFy. *New England Journal of Medicine* 295:302-304.

Miller, L.H., S.J. Mason, J.A. Dvorak, M.H. McGinniss, and I.K. Rothman
1975   Erythrocyte receptors for *Plasmodium knowlesi* malaria: Duffy blood group determinants. *Science* 189:561-563.

Molgaard, C.A., E.P. Stanford, D.J. Morton, L.A. Ryden, K.R. Schubert, and A.L. Golbeck
1990   Epidemiology of head trauma and neurocognitive impairment in a multi-ethnic population. *Neuroepidemiology* 9:233-242.

Neel, J.V.
1947   The clinical detection of the genetic carriers of inherited disease. *Medicine* 26:115-153.
1949   The inheritance of sickle cell anemia. *Science* 110:64-66.
1962   Diabetes mellitus: A "thrifty" genotype rendered detrimental by "progress"? *American Journal of Human Genetics* 14:353-362.
1976   Diabetes mellitus—A geneticist's nightmare. Pp. 1-11 in *The Genetics of Diabetes Mellitus*, W. Creutzfeldt, J. Köbberling, and J.V. Neel, eds. Heidelberg, Germany: Springer-Verlag.
1981   The major ethnic groups: Diversity in the midst of similarity. *American Naturalist* 117:83-87.
1982   The thrifty genotype revisited. Pp. 137-147 in *The Genetics of Diabetes Mellitus*, J. Köbberling and R. Tattersall, eds. Amsterdam, Netherlands: Academic Press.
1993   Human consanguinity effects revisited: Why is the measurable impact of inbreeding so small? Pp. 58-82 in *Genetics of Cellular, Individual, Family, and Population Variability*, C.F. Sing and C.R. Hanis, eds. New York: Oxford University Press.
Neel, J.V., S.S. Fajans, J.W. Conn, and R. Davidson
1965   Diabetes mellitus. Pp. 105-132 in *Genetics and the Epidemiology of Chronic Diseases*, J.V. Neel, M.W. Shaw, and W.J. Schull, eds. Washington, DC: Government Printing Office, Publication No. 1163.
Neel, J.V., F.M. Salzano, P.C. Junqueira, F. Keiter, and D. Maybury-Lewis
1964   Studies on the Xavante Indians of the Brazilian Mato Grosso. *American Journal of Human Genetics* 16:52-140.
New, M.I., and R.E. Peterson
1967   A new form of congenital adrenal hyperplasia. *Journal of Clinical Endocrinology and Metabolism* 27:300-305.
Noguchi, S., K. Murakami, and N. Yamada
1993   Apolipoprotein E genotype and Alzheimer's disease. *Lancet* 342:737.
Okuizumi, K., O. Onodera, S. Naruse, H. Tanaka, H. Kobayashi, H. Takahashi, K. Oyanagi, K. Seki, M. Tanaka, H. Fujigasaki, H. Hirasawa, H. Mizusawa, I. Kanazawa, and S. Tsuji
1994   Apolipoprotein E-ε4 and early-onset Alzheimer's disease. *American Journal of Human Genetics* 55(suppl.):160(abstract).
Oliver, W.J., E.L. Cohen, and J.V. Neel
1975   Blood pressure, sodium intake, and sodium related hormones in the Yanomamo Indians, a "no-salt" culture. *Circulation* 52:146-151.
Page, L.B.
1978   Hypertension and atherosclerosis in primitive and acculturating societies. Pp. 1-12 in *Hypertension Update*, J. C. Hurt, ed. Bloomfield, NJ: Health Learning Systems.
Pauling, L., H.A. Itano, S.J. Singer, and I.C. Wells
1949   Sickle cell anemia, a molecular disease. *Science* 110:543-548.
Payami, H., J. Kaye, L.L. Heston, T.D. Bird, and G.D. Schellenberg
1993   Apolipoprotein E genotype and Alzheimer's disease. *Lancet* 342:738.
Pericak-Vance, M.A., P.H. St. George-Hyslop, P.C. Gaskell Jr., J. Growdon, B.J. Crain, C. Hulette, J.F. Gusella, L. Yamaoka, R.E. Tanzi, A.D. Roses, and J.L. Haines
1993   Linkage analysis in familial Alzheimer disease: Description of the Duke and Boston data sets. *Genetic Epidemiology* 10:361-364.
Poduslo, S.E., and J.D. Schwankhaus
1994   Apolipoprotein E alleles in Alzheimer's and Parkinson's patients. *American Journal of Human Genetics* 55(suppl.):162(abstract).
Poirier, J., J. Davignon, D. Bouthillier, S. Kogan, P. Bertrand, and S. Gauthier
1993   Apolipoprotein E polymorphism and Alzheimer's disease. *Lancet* 342:697-699.

Rao, V.S., C.M. van Duijn, L. Connor-Lacke, L.A. Cupples, J.H. Growdon, and L.A. Farrer
    1994   Multiple etiologies for Alzheimer disease are revealed by segregation analysis. *American Journal of Human Genetics* 55:991-1000.

Reaven, G.M.
    1988   Role of insulin resistance in human disease. *Diabetes* 37:1959-1607.

Rice, T., M. Province, L. Pérusse, C. Bouchard, and D.C. Rao
    1994   Cross-trait familial resemblance for body fat and blood pressure: Familial correlations in the Québec Family Study. *American Journal of Human Genetics* 55:1019-1029.

Roseman, J.N.
    1985   Diabetes in black Americans. Pp. 1-24 in *Diabetes in America*, M.I. Harris and R.F. Hamman, eds. Bethesda, MD: National Institutes of Health, Publication 85-1468.

Rotini, C., R. Cooper, G. Cao, C. Sundarum, and D. McGee
    1994   Familial aggregation of cardiovascular disease in African-American pedigrees. *Genetic Epidemiology* 11:397-407.

Sahota, A., H.C. Hendrie, K.S. Hall, S. Hui, D.K. Lahiri, M. Farlow, A. Brashear, B.O. Osuntokun, and G.D. Schellenberg
    1994   Apolipoprotein E genotypes and Alzheimer's disease in a community-based study of elderly African-Americans. *American Journal of Human Genetics* 55(suppl.):164 (abstract).

Saunders, A., W.J. Strittmatter, D. Schmechel, P.H. St. George-Hyslop, M.A. Pericak-Vance, S.H. Joos, B.L. Rosi, J.F. Gusella, D.R. Crapper-MacLachlan, M.J.Alberts, C. Hulette, B. Crain, D. Goldgaber, and A.D. Roses
    1993   Association of apolipoprotein E allele ε4 with late-onset familial and sporadic Alzheimer's disease. *Neurology* 43:1467-1472.

Schoenberg, B.S., D.W. Anderson, and A.F. Haerer
    1985   Severe dementia: Prevalence and clinical features in a biracial U.S. population. *Archives of Neurology* 42:740-743.

Scotch, N.A.
    1963   Sociocultural factors in the epidemiology of Zulu hypertension. *American Journal of Public Health* 53:1205-1213.

Serjeant, G. R.
    1985   *Sickle Cell Disease*. Oxford, England: Oxford University Press.

Sims, E.A.H., and P. Berchtold
    1982   Obesity and hypertension: Mechanisms and implications for management. *Journal of the American Medical Association* 24:49-52.

Strittmatter, W.J., A.M. Saunders, D. Schmechel, M. Pericak-Vance, J. Enghild, G.S. Salvesen, and A.D. Roses
    1993   Apolipoprotein E: High-avidity binding to β-amyloid and increased frequency of type 4 allele in late-onset familial Alzheimer disease. *Proceedings of the National Academy of Sciences of the United States of America* 90:1977-1981.

Sutherland, D.J., J.L. Ruse, and J.C. Laidlaw
    1966   Hypertension, increased aldosterone secretion and low plasma renin activity relieved by dexamethasone. *Canadian Medical Association Journal* 95:1109-1119.

Tattersall, R.B.
    1974   Mild familial diabetes with dominant inheritance. *Quarterly Journal of Medicine* 43:339-357.

Tattersall, R.B., and S.S. Fajans
    1975   Prevalence of diabetes and glucose intolerance in 199 offspring of thirty-seven conjugal diabetic parents. *Diabetes* 24:452-462.

Tsugi, K., M. Aizawa, and T. Sasasaki
    1992   *HLA '90-'91*. New York: Oxford University Press.

Vanderpitte, J.M., W.W. Zuelzer, J.V. Neel, and J. Colaert
    1955   Evidence concerning the inadequacy of mutation as an explanation of the frequency of
            the sickle cell gene in the Belgian Congo. *Blood* 10:341-350.
Vogel, F., and A.G. Motulsky
    1979   *Human Genetics: Problems and Approaches.* Berlin, Germany: Springer-Verlag.
Ward, R.
    1990   Familial aggregation and genetic epidemiology of blood pressure. Pp. 81-100 in *Hypertension: Pathophysiology, Diagnosis, and Management,* J.H. Laragh and B.M. Brenner, eds. New York: Raven Press.
Williams, R.R., S.C. Hunt, P.N. Hopkins, L.L. Wu, and J.M. Lalouel
    1994   Evidence for single gene contributions to hypertension and lipid disturbances: Definition, genetics, and clinical significance. *Clinical Genetics* 46:80-87.

8

Differences in Rates of Dementia Between Ethno-Racial Groups

Barry Gurland, David Wilder, Rafael Lantigua, Richard Mayeux, Yaakov Stern, Jiming Chen, Peter Cross, and Eloise Killeffer

EPIDEMIOLOGICAL BACKGROUND

Dementia Rates and Subtypes

Dementia is the most common major mental disorder of very old age. This condition is characterized by a global and progressive decline in cognitive functions such as memory for recent events, learning, orientation, calculation, verbal ability, spatial manipulations, reasoning, planning, and competence in other complex tasks. Most noticeably, there is advancing impairment in the performance of the tasks of everyday living including managing personal business, shopping, cooking, dressing, feeding, and toileting. Extreme dependency on family and other care givers eventually supervenes, insight is lost, wandering and other disturbing behaviors emerge, frailty increases, and life is shortened.

The most common form of dementia is Alzheimer's disease, a slowly developing degenerative process of uncertain cause, affecting neural pathways, especially those serving memory functions, over large areas of the brain. Multi-infarct dementia arises from interruption of the blood supply to numerous small areas of the brain, with a cumulative effect over long periods of time. Neither condition can be reliably prevented or halted by treatment, though experimental long- and short-term interventions are being actively studied (Berg et al., 1992). Taken together, these two subtypes account for the great majority of dementias found in elderly populations.

Dementia is among the leading causes of disability and death in old age. Costs of care in the formal long-term care sector, including personal assistance and residential services, are high for the individual and for Medicaid or other third-party payers; often dementia places a financial as well as an emotional burden on informal care givers (Brodaty and Hadzi, 1990; O'Connor et al., 1991a, 1991b). These are serious consequences of dementia for the victims, their families, and other care givers, and they raise concerns that can be informed by data on the frequency and distribution of rates of dementia, its precedents, and its outcomes.

For persons 65 years or older, community studies report prevalence rates of dementia generally around 4 percent to 6 percent, but as high as 10 percent; an additional 2 percent to 3 percent are found in surveys of nursing homes (Gurland and Cross, 1982; Gurland, 1996a, 1996b; Bland et al., 1988; Folstein et al., 1991; Livingston et al., 1990). The proportions of people with dementias who live in community dwellings rather than nursing homes will be influenced by the availability and affordability of nursing home residence and the willingness of care givers to continue supporting the person with dementia at home. In most nursing homes and in many home care programs, longer term clients are predominantly people with dementias.

Prevalence rates of dementia are low in the age group 65 to 74 but increase rapidly with age, roughly doubling with each decade and culminating in rates reported to be as high as 40 percent or more for those surviving beyond age 85. Incidence rates are below 1 percent for the young old (65 to 74 years) but rise to 4 percent or more for the very old, 85 years and older. Dementia can last 10 or more years, and duration averages around 5 to 7 years depending on the age of occurrence.

Subtypes of dementia in Western nations are mainly Alzheimer's disease (about 75%), with a modest proportion (about 15%) being purely multi-infarct dementia. Around 15 percent of people with dementia have both Alzheimer's and multi-infarct features. Some studies have found these proportions to be 50 percent, 40 percent and 10 percent, respectively (Folstein et al., 1991). A residual group of around 10 percent includes people with secondary dementias (e.g., stroke dementia, Parkinsonism, or Huntington's chorea) and potentially treatable causes such as increased intracranial pressure; metabolic, toxic, or anoxic conditions; and depression. Alcohol and drug dependence as possible causes of dementia are uncommon (1% to 2%) in most reports on community elders (Bland et al., 1988; Kramer et al., 1985; Weissman et al., 1985). Females are reported by some studies to have higher rates. Risk factors for Alzheimer's disease itself have been attributed to head injury, stroke, coronary artery disease, depression, age of mother at birth, Down's syndrome, family history, and (very recently) abnormalities of the apolipoprotein E genotype series.

In addition to the small proportion of people who present convincing signs of dementia but are found to have an initially reversible condition, there are people with such treatable conditions as major depressive disorder or delirium due to drug or other toxicity whose dementias are simply mislabeled as primary dementia because the symptoms are not correctly evaluated. However, for the vast majority of properly diagnosed dementias, treatments to reverse the disease process are still experimental; there is no proven method of halting the progress of the condition. Nevertheless, health and social care management can provide invaluable relief to the patient through symptomatic approaches and attention to control of complications. It can also assist the care givers in maintaining the sufferer at home through psychological support and personal care services and, where necessary, can ease admission to a dignified, engaging, and nurturing sheltered environment.

Estimating Rates of Dementia

Almost all studies of prevalence and incidence of dementia rely upon two stages of assessment. The first stage is directed at maximizing the chances of finding cases in the population by use of screening techniques. Because these screens are brief and are reliable in the hands of interviewers from a wide variety of professional and nonprofessional backgrounds, it is feasible to administer them in the private homes of large numbers of the population under study. Simple threshold scores separate likely from unlikely cases of dementia, with a sensitivity and specificity that can be adjusted by raising or lowering the threshold score to suit the needs of the study.

In the second stage, concerned mainly with ascertaining the diagnosis, the study design may allow for an attempt to fully evaluate all likely cases or a representative selection of them. Typically this evaluation is carried out in a clinic equipped for conduct of an inquiry into presenting symptoms and signs, a history of the onset and course of the illness, a battery of psychological tests, general and neurological physical examination, and general and specific special investigations including brain imaging. Clinical judgment and/or algorithms are then applied to the accumulated information to make a diagnosis of dementia with reference to operational diagnostic criteria. A sample of unlikely cases, referred blind to the clinic personnel, is usually also fully evaluated in order to check on the efficiency of the screening procedure.

In some studies by design, and in some others by default, a greater or lesser proportion of likely cases may not be fully evaluated. In those circumstances, the rates of dementia may be projected from the findings on the cases fully evaluated. The projections take into account the fraction of subjects above and below the threshold of the screen who are expected to have dementia on the basis of the findings for the subjects who were fully evaluated.

Uncertainties enter into the case-finding and case ascertainment stages for the well-known reasons that confront surveys: nonresponding subjects, attrition between stages of evaluation, and unreliability of measures. Of particular importance for ethno-racial comparisons of rates and associations of dementia are the confounding effects of socioeconomic status on the validity of the two classificatory stages.

Ethno-Racial Differences in Rates of Dementia

Rates for indicators of dementia (cognitive impairment scores or diagnosis) have been reported to vary between ethno-racial groups. Among community residents aged 65 years and older, African Americans have been found to have a higher prevalence of a diagnosis of dementia, especially vascular dementias, than non-Hispanic whites (Heyman et al., 1991). Researchers have found concordant results using cognitive scores as an indicator of dementia, validated by diagnosis of a subsample (Folstein et al., 1991). The converse has been reported by researchers (de la Monte et al., 1989) drawing upon autopsy results; their rates were higher among non-Hispanic whites than among African Americans; non-Hispanic whites had more dementia associated with Parkinson's disease, and African Americans had more dementia associated with multi-infarct disease and alcoholism. Several other studies have reported higher rates of cognitive impairment and dementia among African Americans and Hispanics than among non-Hispanic whites (Escobar et al., 1986; Murden et al., 1991; Weissman et al., 1985).

Putative Effects of Education

Elders who have had low education are consistently reported as having unusually high rates of dementia (Gurland, 1981; Li et al., 1991; Folstein et al., 1991; Stern et al., 1994; Gurland et al., 1995b). Groups with lower education have been found to have a relatively greater proportion of multi-infarct dementia (Folstein et al., 1991) or increased rates of alcoholic dementia and unspecified types of dementia (Fratiglioni et al., 1991). However, the possibility of ethno-racial bias in assessment and diagnosis introduces ambiguity about the interpretation of study results that is mainly but not entirely attributable to educational influences (Salmon et al., 1989; Li et al., 1989; Murden et al., 1991).

Any substantial differences in rates of dementia between ethno-racial groups merit serious attention, given the personal and societal consequences of dementia; the related need to plan, finance, and deliver appropriate services; and the call for research to advance understanding and effective treatment of dementia. Moreover, valuable clues to etiology and treatment might emerge from the study of such ethno-racial variation. However, the inferences and action that should flow from findings of ethno-racial differences in rates of dementia continue to be inhibited by a critical uncertainty: namely, the possibility that case-finding and case ascertainment techniques might be biased towards overestimating dementia rates in socially disadvantaged ethno-racial groups (O'Connor et al., 1991b).

This issue is often expressed in terms of uncertainty about the distortions of educational bias. Educational achievement is not equally distributed among the various ethno-racial groups. Poorly educated people may make errors on the screening measures because they have less experience than better educated people in answering these kinds of test questions. Furthermore, the questions are often directed at general knowledge (e.g., the name of the president of the United States), calculation, spelling, repetition of phrases, current dates, residential address, and the like. The same biases may enter the full evaluation through the psychological test battery. Furthermore, clinical judgments may be influenced to discount the profile of deficits of a poorly educated person or to add undue weight to deficits in a highly educated person.

One root source of these ambiguities is that information derived from screening and full evaluation is concentrated on a person's current status and little reliance can be placed on historical information. Yet dementia is essentially a longitudinal diagnosis; the diagnosis implies a progressive course of illness. Thus, a person who falls short of normal standards at the time of screening or full evaluation is assumed to be on a decline trajectory, whereas he or she might have been below standard throughout life.

Various corrections have been suggested for redressing ethno-racial bias in cognitive test items (Uhlmann and Larson, 1991; Teresi et al., 1995). However, a recent analysis of data (Gurland et al., 1995) from the reporting component of the North Manhattan Aging Project registry found the educational effects on rates of dementia were robust, persisting across 13 different methods of salient classifications, which ranged from criterion-based diagnosis to cognitive scores, stages of severity, and mathematical techniques for minimizing ethno-racial bias in assessment.

METHODOLOGICAL ISSUES

The North Manhattan Aging Project
and the Active Life Expectancy Study

The study presented here was designed to examine rates of dementia in three ethno-racial groups: Hispanics, African Americans, and non-Hispanic whites, with due regard for potential ethno-racial biases. Data in this paper have been generated from work still in progress in a collaboration between the Columbia University Stroud Center/Center for Geriatrics, Sergievsky Center, and Department of Medicine.

The North Manhattan Aging Project and the Active Life Expectancy Study have jointly established a registry of people with dementia, stroke, and Parkinson's disease. The registry draws from a network of key informants (reporting component) and a cohort (survey component) of randomly selected people 65 years or older within a clearly bounded geographic area of north Manhattan. The analyses in this report are restricted to the survey component and the part of the reporting component that covered nursing home residents whose present or last location was in the target area.

Our Methods for Minimizing Biases in Ethno-Racial
Comparisons of Dementia

We describe the strategies that we have developed or adopted for our ethno-racial comparisons of rates of dementia. The following description is abstracted and modified from three papers (Gurland, et al., 1992; Gurland et al., 1995b; Gurland, 1996a). Many of these strategies are shared with other studies in this field; some are innovative.

Case Findings

We adopted two contrasting routes for case finding: a network of key reporters and a house-to-house survey of a representative sample of elders. Both methods were aimed at the same target: a geographically delimited multicultural population. The target area is 13 adjacent census tracts in north Manhattan: census data indicated that there would be substantial numbers of elders in each of the groups: Hispanic, African American, and non-Hispanic white. Poverty, crime, and unemployment rates are high in the study target area. A single hospital (Columbia-Presbyterian Medical Center) provides almost all inpatient and emergency medical care and much of the ambulatory medical services to the study's target area. A large contingent of Hispanic physicians runs solo or small group practices in the neighborhood, supplemented by some multicultural large group practices. Social and community agencies are well organized and in close touch with each other.

In the reporting component, which began in 1989, study staff repeatedly scrutinize records of subjects reported to be living in or entering service sites that are known to have a high rate of dementia, such as nursing homes, home care programs, and certain neurological clinics; staff members also receive referrals according to specified criteria from key informants in a wide variety of health, social, and community sites. If a person is eligible by present or (in nursing homes) last location, the research team institutes a further examination, with a screen for cognitive impairment. A referral for a research diagnostic evaluation is made if the 90 percent sensitivity threshold on the cognitive screen is exceeded and in a subsample of the remainder of the subjects.

The survey component first interviewed people in 1993 and 1994; its sampling frame consists of all Medicare beneficiaries, 65 years or older, within the geographic target area. By the use of random methods in replicated subsamples, subjects in the survey are drawn equally from the three cultural groups until the number of elders in any group is exhausted or the total of elders interviewed exceeds 2,100. All who cooperate are given a subject interview. In selected representative survey subsamples, an informant, if one is available, is interviewed and a diagnostic evaluation is carried out on all subjects regardless of screen score. In all other subsamples, the subject interview is given to all subjects, but an informant interview and a referral for a research diagnostic evaluation are made only if the 90 percent sensitivity threshold on the cognitive screen is exceeded and in one in four of the rest of the subjects. Trained raters administer the interviews using laptop computers for face-to-face interviews in the subject's home. Informant interviews are conducted by telephone.

The advantage of this two-pronged approach is that since all cases come from the same target area, researchers can compare the distribution of cases of dementia lodged on the registry through the two routes: key reporters and survey. The reported cases give a more complete representation of people with advanced dementia and people who are receiving services for dementia, whereas the survey cases offer better representation of mild and moderate cases and of people who are normal. The extent to which ethno-racial differences are constant across the two methods increases confidence in the findings.

The delimited nature of the target area makes it possible to superimpose the two methods of case finding. It also makes it possible for the researchers to conduct reevaluation over a long period of time, to track service utilization, and to maintain the cooperation of the community by facilitating services for those found to be in need. The other side of the coin is that the geographic generalizability of the findings must be tested through other studies, either previous or planned. Of course, were a nationally representative study of this kind achievable without sacrifice of the methodological refinement, its results would not be generalizable to the target area chosen for this study or to any other multicultural community in the nation. In our opinion, robust hypotheses worthy of further testing, especially with regard to etiological leads, are just as likely to emerge from a delimited sample as from a national one. Similar views could be expressed with respect to the public health significance of the findings or their significance for planning for service delivery.

In assembling the sample of subjects to represent elders in the target community for purposes of the survey, we added a frame for elders in nursing homes to that obtained from the Medicare list. There is no overlap between these frames: only the Medicare list was used for elders at home, and only the nursing home list was used for elders in nursing homes. This sampling procedure is more accurate than the alternative of tracing elders not found at home to a location in a nursing home (although this was done as a mutual check on the completeness of the frames). Any nursing home known to admit residents from the target area was repeatedly surveyed to capture new admissions during the course of the study.

Since this is a study of elder populations, not of nursing homes, the number of subjects in nursing homes is restricted to their appropriate contribution to the total sample of elders. We accomplished this by taking the number of elders who completed in-home interviews as the numerator and the total of all elders in the target area as the denominator, and applying the proportion this produced to all elders from the target area who completed interviews in the nursing homes over the same period as the in-home survey.

For purposes of calculating prevalence rates, the denominators are the number of persons interviewed in the first 27 subsamples of the in-home survey cohort and in the nursing home segment of the reporting component during the same period. The denominator numbers in the survey cohort (but not in the nursing home sample) were adjusted to fit the census age profile of the study target area. We have already described the adjustment of the total size of the nursing home sample. The numerators are the number of cases of dementia identified in the same samples with corresponding adjustments. The criterion diagnosis for dementia was used for those subjects who received a diagnostic evaluation (by a team designated as the clinical core), and it was projected from those subjects onto persons screened, but not diagnosed, by the use of the screen score probability of a diagnosis of dementia.

Screening and Field Classification Techniques

In both components of the study (i.e., reporting and survey components), efforts were made to render screening and field classification techniques as culture fair as possible. We conduct interviews in the subject's language of preference (English or Spanish). We prepared a Spanish translation of each assessment technique and checked it for comparability with the English version; in a few items, we chose a cultural equivalent rather than a literal translation.

We determined which subjects would be referred for full evaluation by analyzing the alternatives to show which was most consistent in operational characteristics (i.e., specificity and sensitivity) across ethno-racial groups (Wilder et al., 1995). We assembled a compendium instrument incorporating five widely used screens for cognitive impairment and dementia and tested it in the reporting component of the North Manhattan Aging Project. We obtained the best operating characteristics on this population from the Comprehensive Assessment and Referral Evaluation cognitive screen (Golden et al., 1984; Teresi et al., 1984) and therefore selected it as the benchmark screen for the survey component.

During the study, when we accumulated sufficient data we applied item bias statistical methods to construct a new relatively culture-fair scale. Although this new scale was not used for screening purposes, it helped to confirm or rebut findings from the other scales.

Criterion Diagnosis

In both components of the study, a criterion diagnosis is made after full evaluation by a research team (the clinical core). It is assumed (but arguable) that the resulting diagnostic classification has shed much of the potential ethno-racial biases, since the information at this evaluation is wide ranging, involves numerous internal checks on the diagnostic relevance of the information, and is guided by algorithms and operational criteria for integration of information from psychometric tests (with educational norms) and from laboratory and clinical sources. This diagnosis is made independently of, and is blind to, the field assessments. Details of the diagnostic process are given elsewhere (Stern et al., 1992).

After all evaluations are completed, diagnoses are assigned at a diagnostic conference. The initial separation is between demented and nondemented patients. If a patient is demented, then the cause of dementia is specified further. The two main subtypes of dementia have suggestive clinical and brain imaging indicators, but neuropathology must ultimately be combined with the in vivo signs in order to reach a definitive diagnosis.

All subjects who screen positive and a proportion of subjects who fall below the critical threshold score on the screen, in both the reporting and the survey components of the registry, are referred blind for diagnostic evaluation by the research teams. In addition, in selected subsamples of the survey, all subjects are referred for diagnostic evaluation.

Biological Indicators

Indicators of biological status, in the form of brain imaging, molecular genetics (especially the role of apolipoprotein E genotypes), and autopsy material, are obtained where subjects permit it. There are established relationships between these objective indices and measures of cognitive impairment or diagnoses of dementia subtypes (Maestre et al., 1995; Mayeux et al., 1993). Consistency of these relationships among ethno-racial groups adds confidence to the ethno-racial comparisons of cognitive and diagnostic data. Inconsistencies raise questions about bias in screening techniques or diagnosis or suggest the need for reconsideration of the biological underpinnings of the dementing conditions in the various ethno-racial groups.

Longitudinal and Outcome Information

We follow subjects annually, in both components of the study, in order to gather longitudinal and outcome information. Diagnoses of dementia of the two common subtypes (which account for the great majority of cases in a population) carry with them a prediction that a progressive decline will be detectable at annual intervals. Diagnosis may have to be revised when a case does not follow the expected course. Concurrent corrections of this kind incrementally reduce misclassifications due to ethno-racial biases, since ethno-racial membership does not convey immunity from deterioration over a year or more.

Dementia and Quality of Life

Examining the impact of dementia on the quality of life is an innovative strategy (Gurland et al., 1992, 1993). It is an attempt to go beyond comparing conditions that merely meet diagnostic criteria to comparing conditions with defined consequences for the patient, the family, and society (Katz and Gurland, 1991). We use this strategy only in the survey component.

It would be tautological to accept as unbiased only results that showed no differences in rates of dementia between ethno-racial groups, yet it is difficult to be certain that emergent differences do not reflect some hidden biases, despite our efforts to find and eradicate them. There may also be a differing pattern of biological processes that account for dementia in the various ethno-racial groups. Therefore, an appeal to culture-fair methods and biological indices may still leave lingering doubts as to the meaning of ethno-racial differences in rates of dementia. To cut this Gordian knot, we examine the extent to which dementia, as classified by our methods, has comparable consequences for quality of life in the ethno-racial groups. We look for the quality-of-life consequences that are characteristic of dementia: decreases in functioning in the higher level, cognitively controlled tasks of daily living, such as using the telephone, handling cash, managing personal business, and following a medication regime (Reed et al., 1989; Reisberg et al., 1985). We also look for subjective complaints of memory lapses (O'Connor et al., 1990) and nonspecific impairments of quality of life such as affective suffering (Wands et al., 1990).

Introducing observations on the impact of dementia, as diagnosed, on quality of life moves the focus from a medical model, in which diagnosis carries an implicit association with disease, its prognosis, and its treatment, to a more holistic model, in which diagnosis is viewed as a means of connecting causes to an explicit set of consequences for the person. The assumption that real differences in rates are accompanied by real causes and real consequences drives concern about whether ethno-racial variation in these rates is real or an artifact of diagnostic bias. The holistic model reverses this line of reasoning: diagnosis is real if it has real consequences; real consequences have real causes. Ethno-racial differences in rates of diagnosis are important if they are accompanied by corresponding differences in real consequences for quality of life. A corollary of this premise is that diagnosis, or some surrogate category, can be usefully modified to act as a marker of a distinctive pattern of consequences.

The subject interview in the survey component includes a wide range of self-reported functioning in daily tasks of living and in acts of memory. The informant interview (again, in the survey component only) covers a similar range of information on the subject's current functioning and historical information on the course of the subject's symptoms; it is obtained independently and blind to the subject interview. In addition, at the time of the interview with the subject, a performance test, the Medication Management Test, is administered (Gurland et al., 1994). Items from several standard measures of functioning have been imbedded in the subject and the informant interviews: Katz Index of Activities of Daily Living (Katz et al., 1963), Lawton Instrumental Activities of Daily Living (Lawton and Brody, 1969), and Comprehensive Assessment and Referral Evaluation (CARE) scales of activity limitation and mobility (Gurland et al., 1977; Golden et al., 1984). The items are directed at distinctive perspectives on functioning: self-report, informant report, and performance testing; cognitively and physically driven functions; and positive as well as negative functioning.

The full picture of quality of life includes at least these many aspects of functioning. For simplicity, we have selected a few important aspects, which will be sufficient for illustrative purposes. Each of these aspects has salience to quality of life. In this respect, it is worth noting that the self-perceptions reported by the subject with dementia (e.g., complaints about memory) are central to quality-of-life consequences and are not vitiated by presumed loss of insight. In fact, the subject's report correlates highly with the other measures of functioning, such as informant reports or performance testing, until late in the course of dementia (Chen, 1995).

Complaints of Memory Lapses. Subjective complaints of memory lapses are included because they are increased by the presence of dementia, although these complaints also occur at a lower rate in elders without dementia and may be missing in a substantial proportion of persons who do have dementia (O'Connor et al., 1990). This cluster of complaints is presented as a reflection of quality of life, not as a diagnostic indicator.

Affective Suffering. Items from a scale of depression in elders, the CARE Homogeneous Scale of Depression (Golden et al., 1984; Gurland et al., 1977; Teresi et al., 1984), have been reorganized to fit a quality-of-life perspective. Twenty of these items form a modified scale of affective suffering, which has a reliability coefficient alpha of .818. The content of the modified scale is free of items confounding mental and physical problems. Seven levels of severity of affective suffering are derived from references to intensity and extensity of distress. The extremes of intensity are defined at one pole by such expressions as "life not worth living" and at the other pole by an absence of negative symptoms together with claims of being "very happy." The corresponding extremes of extensity bear upon the persistence of affective distress at one pole and the absence of symptoms at the other. The size and severity of the worst level were set to make possible useful comparisons with major depression (the most severe diagnostic category of clinical depression in the standard nomenclature), and the combined size and severity of the two worst levels (intolerable and desperate affective suffering) were designed to be comparable to the combined diagnostic categories of major depressions and dysthymia (a form of chronic depression) (American Psychiatric Association, 1994).

Dementia and Service Utilization

An examination of the impact of dementia on service utilization (in the survey component only) is in part justified for reasons analogous to those put forward on behalf of the quality-of-life consequences of dementia. If ethnoracial differences in the rate of dementia are seen as bearing upon the relative needs of the different populations for therapeutic interventions, then the current use of relevant services by these populations is germane to an estimation of the extent to which these needs are being fulfilled.

Convergence of Conclusions

Information accumulated from the survey and the full diagnostic evaluation offers several ways of classifying and analyzing the rates and consequences of dementia. Where all sources and pathways of analyses converge on the same inference regarding relative rates of dementia among ethno-racial groups, we can have greatest confidence in the conclusions.

Border-Zone Dementias and Nondementias

It can be expected that diagnostic misclassifications due to ethno-racial biases will rarely occur for people who are obviously demented (advanced dementia) or clearly normal. Rather, misclassifications will occur mainly for people who have early or ambiguous signs of dementia, whom we have designated as border-zone dementias, and for those who are not diagnosably demented but have evidence of cognitive impairment, whom we call border-zone nondementias. Thus, the designation of a border-zone range is expedient for the study of ethnoracial influences on the validity of diagnoses of dementia and for testing methods of reducing bias (Gurland et al., 1995a, 1995b; Wilder et al., 1994, 1995). For operational purposes, the border-zone range of cognitive impairment (including border-zone dementias and nondementias) is defined as impairment that, in the reporting component of the registry, predicted criterion diagnosis in about half the instances overall, with a probability between about 30 percent and 70 percent for the scores within this range.

Since rates depend in part on how broad a concept of dementia is used, we refer to both advanced dementias and border-zone dementias when comparing ethno-racial groups. Advanced dementia represents a narrow (conservative) view of dementia; a broad concept is represented by expanding the definition of a case to include the border-zone dementias.

Designation of Ethno-Racial Membership

Ethno-racial classification is recorded (in both components of the study) from self-designation of ethno-racial membership. Our comparison groups are

Hispanics, African Americans, and non-Hispanic whites. Study procedures were modeled on those adopted by the U.S. Census Bureau for self-identification of racial and ethnic membership. Elders were assigned to the three ethno-racial groups on the basis of their self-description as to whether they came from Spanish/Hispanic origin or descent and if they did not, whether they were white or "black/Negro." In cases of doubt about the validity of the information obtained from the subject, an informant was consulted.

This typology is not synonymous with race, ethnicity or culture.[1] Nevertheless, the typology we used has the merit of replicating the census classification and contributing to informed decisions on allocation of health care resources based on census data. Moreover, this method of classification is the same as that usually underlying published reports on variation in rates of dementia among populations.

The study classification differed from the one that was initially available in the sampling frame, as Table 8-1 shows. Medicare lists made a distinction between black and white self-identification only. A match with 5,000 Spanish surnames was then superimposed. Table 8-1 shows discrepancies between the initial sampling frame and the ultimate study classifications. As many as 26 percent of the initial non-Hispanic white groups were reclassified as Hispanic; the other two groups were more stable. The study classification is validated by the preferred language of the interviewee: of those who preferred to be interviewed in Spanish, 98 percent were Hispanic in the final classification.

For purposes of collecting adequate numbers of the three ethno-racial groups in a community with unequal ethno-racial proportions, we stratified people by ethno-racial membership according to information on Medicare lists and the superimposed surname match. The result was a smaller non-Hispanic white group than we had intended in the ultimate study classification.

Most classifications of ethno-racial populations are reasonable entry points in the search for leads that might help us discover sociocultural, psychological, behavioral, or biological influences on the variation of rates of mental disorder. Refinement of the classification would have to be part and parcel of pursuing any such emergent leads. For example, variation tied to genetic differences might require subgroups with more homogeneous gene pools. Knowledge of the relationship of etiologies to styles of living (e.g., diet, smoking) would be advanced by analyses keyed to cultural subgroups. Service utilization and outcome differences might be best understood by issues of language, church affiliations, family constellations, neighborhood structures, and the matching ethno-racial health care arrangements.

---

[1]Definitions taken from the Random House Dictionary of the English Language (Random House, 1966), are as follows: *Ethnicity*: a group of people of the same race or nationality who share a common and distinctive culture. *Culture*: the sum total of ways of living built up by a group of human beings and transferred from one generation to another. *Race*: a group of persons related by common descent, blood, or heredity.

TABLE 8-1   Ethno-Racial Classification: Contrasts Between Initial and Final
Identification

Final Self-Identification at Interview	Initial: Medicare "Black/White" plus Spanish Surnames						
	Spanish surnames: Hispanic		Other Black: African American		Other White: Non-Hispanic		Total
	%	N	%	N	%	N	N
"Spanish/Hispanic origin":							
Hispanic	98	562	5	29	26	85	676
Dominican		304		10		28	
Puerto Rican		102		4		17	
Cuban		112		3		28	
Other		44		12		12	
"Black/Negro":							
African American	1	5	93	511	3	10	526
"White":							
Non-Hispanic white	1	5	2	13	71	229	247
Total	100	572	100	553	100	324	1,449

Note: The sample consisted of community-residing elders (65 years and older), $N = 1,449$, from the
North Manhattan Aging Project target area.

Other Socioeconomic Information

We recorded this information (collected in both components of the study)
from the most reliable informant; if the subject was judged unreliable, then a
family member was consulted.

We gathered a history of educational achievement and condensed it into
categories of 0 to 4 years, 5 to 11 years, and 12 or more years of education. The
category of less than 5 years of schooling is of special interest in studies of
dementia. Illiterate or marginally literate persons are disproportionately encountered in minority groups, but because they perform poorly on standardized screening instruments, they have been excluded from some studies or inadvisably combined with the next higher educational group.

We documented income by having the subject (or an informant) review a
card displaying monthly income brackets. The card specifically mentioned all
sources of income, including wages, salaries, Social Security or retirement benefits, help from relatives, and rent from property.

RESULTS

General Results

Yields from the Survey Component

The response rates for completed survey interviews vary among subsamples but are 62 percent overall. Comparison of the age and gender distributions of the responders and nonresponders for each ethno-racial group shows no significant differences for gender. However, responders in all ethno-racial groups are younger than nonresponders, and the differences rise to statistical significance for Hispanics ($p = .001$) and non-Hispanic whites ($p = .01$). The proportions 75 years and over for nonresponders and responders, respectively, are for Hispanics, 51.5 percent versus 39.6 percent; for African Americans, 49.7 percent versus 44.1 percent; and for non-Hispanic whites, 51.9 percent versus 42.9 percent.

As Table 8-2 shows, 1,449 subjects in the community setting received a field interview in the first 27 representative subsamples. The proportionate number selected for nursing home residents is 40. This total is greater than the number with an informant interview or the number referred to diagnostic evaluation in the clinical core. Eighty-one percent of subjects referred to the clinical core completed the full diagnostic evaluation.

Overrepresentation

Sampling strategies led to overrepresentation of certain subgroups, those 75 years of age or older, non-Hispanic whites, and persons in nursing homes. Wherever appropriate, we have weighted the numbers in the cells formed by ethno-

TABLE 8-2 Sizes of Samples of Subjects Interviewed by Age and Ethno-Racial Groups

Age	Hispanic		African American		Non-Hispanic White	
	Community ($N = 676$)	Nursing Home ($N = 9$)	Community ($N = 526$)	Nursing Home ($N = 14$)	Community ($N = 247$)	Nursing Home ($N = 17$)
65–74	347	2	224	3	107	1
74–85	259	3	221	5	86	6
85+	70	4	81	6	54	10

Note: The sample was restricted to 27 community subsamples ($N = 1,449$) and a proportionate ($N = 40$) group in nursing homes from the target area.

racial membership and age to match either the corresponding profile of characteristics evident in the original Medicare sampling frame or the census profile for the target area. The total number of nursing home subjects in the combined nursing home and in-home survey cohort has been adjusted to the proportion of target area elders who are in nursing homes. Stratification of ethno-racial groups in comparisons makes it unnecessary to adjust for this characteristic.

Differences in Prevalence Rates of Dementia

Rates of criterion dementias for the ethno-racial groups are found to be higher in Hispanics and African Americans and lowest in non-Hispanic whites as Figure 8-1 shows. The comparisons are made separately for age groups 65 to 74, 75 to 84, and 85 and older. In all age categories, Hispanic and African-American groups are comparable: if anything, the Hispanics have slightly higher rates, but

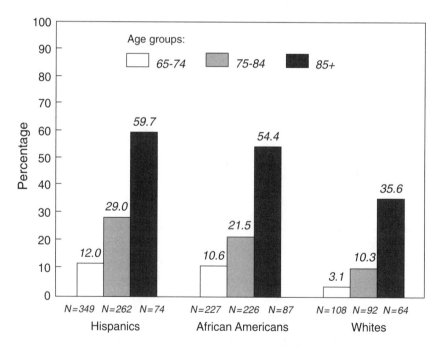

FIGURE 8-1 Rates of dementia by age and ethno-racial group. NOTE: The sample was restricted to 27 subsamples of community-residing elders, 65 years and older, $N = 1,449$, from the North Manhattan Aging Project target area; there was a proportionate group in nursing homes, $N = 40$. Diagnosis was made by research clinical evaluation or was generated from the probability of a diagnosis based on screen scores, which could be a decimal number.

there are no significant differences in any of the paired comparisons of these two ethno-racial groups within age categories. However, the non-Hispanic white group has dramatically lower rates of dementia in all age brackets compared with either of the other two ethnic groups. All of these paired comparisons are statistically significant: significance levels for the age groups 65 to 74, 75 to 84, and 85 and older are $p < .01$, $p < .001$, and $p < .001$, respectively, for Hispanics, and $p < 0.05$ for African Americans in all three comparisons.

All ethnic groups show a steep rise of rates of dementia with age. The graphic shape of the relationship between age and prevalence rates of dementia is close to linear for Hispanics and quadratic in non-Hispanic whites, with African Americans being intermediate in form.

Mislabeling

We compared the people with and without dementias in each ethno-racial group with an eye to the possibility that severe depression, presenting as a dementia-like syndrome (Larson et al. 1985; O'Connor and Roth, 1990), might be open to ethno-racial bias in assessment and classification of dementia. Depression rates are also raised in true dementia, especially in certain subtypes of dementia, such as those associated with multi-infarction or Parkinson's disease. Further complicating the meaning of concurrent depression and dementia is that more than half of the group with this combination later deteriorates cognitively (Kral 1983; Reding et al., 1985; McAllister and Price, 1982; O'Connor and Roth, 1990). As seen in Figure 8-2, severe depression is strikingly high among non-Hispanic whites with dementia, lower in Hispanics with dementia, and extremely low in the African-American dementia group. These findings are exactly opposite to what would be expected to support mislabeling of depression as an explanation for the excesses of dementia in the Hispanic and African-American groups.

Prevalence and Other Indices of Rates

Variation in prevalence rates among the ethno-racial or educational groups could be due to differences in incidence, duration, mortality, age of onset, or any combination of these. The incidence phase of our study began in the fall of 1994; neither new cases nor mortality rates are yet known. We have collected retrospective information from the informant on the duration and age of onset of functional and memory impairments of the subject, but we regard these data as unreliable. The age of onset was alleged to be earlier for Hispanic and African-American groups than for non-Hispanic whites: the onset of impairments after age 84 was 8 percent, 20 percent, and 40 percent, respectively. If this information is accurate, it might in part account for the relatively lower rates of dementia among the non-Hispanic whites since a later onset leaves a shorter duration of time for the condition to exist.

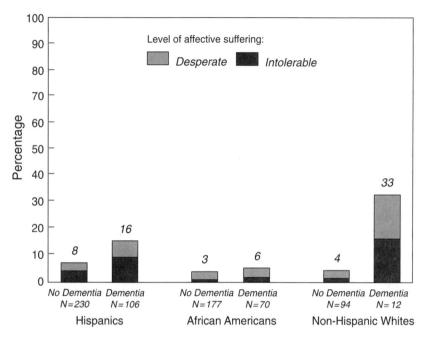

FIGURE 8-2   Affective suffering in subjects with and without dementia. NOTE: The sample was restricted to 27 subsamples of community-residing elders, 65 years and older, $N = 1,449$, from the North Manhattan Aging Project target area. Only those elders who have a research clinical evaluation are included.

Effect of the Breadth of the Concept of Dementia

The relatively higher rates of dementia among Hispanics and African Americans compared with non-Hispanic whites are consistently evident for concepts of dementia of varying breadth, as Figure 8-3 shows. For advanced dementias, rates for the Hispanics 10.0%) and African Americans (7.1%) are higher than for non-Hispanic whites (4.0%): compared with non-Hispanic whites, the Hispanic rates are significantly higher ($p < .003$), but not the African-American rates ($p < .10$, nonsignificant).   The relative ethno-racial rates are similar if border-zone dementias are added: Hispanics, 20.8 percent; African Americans, 18.2 percent: and non-Hispanic whites, 7.2 percent.   Now, however, compared with non-Hispanic whites, the Hispanic rates are significantly higher at the $p < .001$ level, and the African-American rates are also significantly higher ($p < .001$).   Hispanic and African-American rates remain not significantly different.   Even if people with-

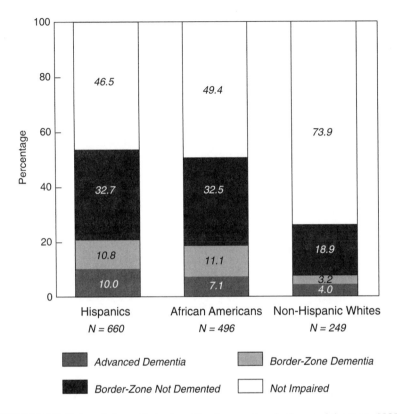

FIGURE 8-3 Rates of dementia by breadth of concept and ethno-racial group. NOTE:
The sample was restricted to 27 subsamples of community-residing elders, 65 years and
older, $N = 1,449$, from the North Manhattan Aging Project target area; there was a proportionate group in nursing homes, $N = 40$. Diagnosis was made by research clinical evaluation or was generated from the probability of a diagnosis based on screen scores. This
excludes persons with paradoxical classifications: those who had normal cognitive levels
but were diagnosed as demented, or who had severe cognitive impairment but were not
diagnosed as demented, and 44 persons who were projected to be paradoxical.

out dementias but with cognitive impairment are taken into account, non-Hispanic whites have substantially lower prevalence rates (26%) than Hispanics
(53.5%) or African Americans (50.6%), and the significance levels of differences
are unchanged. The ethno-racial differences in the prevalence rate of dementia
are apparently robust enough to withstand changes in the breadth of the concept
of dementia.

Risk Factors

Some of the possible causes of variations of rates in dementia between subgroups within ethno-racial groups were mentioned in the introductory section; these causes include age, gender, education, head injury, hypertension, coronary artery disease, alcohol, malnutrition, and genetic predisposition. However, our current principal interest is in variation of rates of dementia *between* ethno-racial groups; previous studies (mentioned in the introduction) led us to expect that education might be a main association of this variation. Since educational achievement is related to level of income, immigration patterns, and age cohort, we also included reference to these characteristics in our examination of the associations between education and rates of dementia.

Educational Associations

There are pronounced distribution differences by education, age, income, and immigration among the three ethno-racial groups. Only 48.8 percent of Hispanics are aged 75 years or older, of whom 10.4 percent are 85 years or older, while African Americans have 57.6 percent aged 75 or older, including 15.5 percent who are 85 or older. The non-Hispanic whites are the oldest of the three groups, with 57.5 percent who are 75 years or older, including 23.0 percent aged 85 years or older. Differences between educational distributions among the three ethno-racial groups are even more marked. Over 40 percent of the Hispanics have completed less than 5 years of schooling, but almost 90 percent of African Americans and virtually all non-Hispanic whites have gone beyond this level. Just 12.3 percent of the Hispanics have completed 12 or more years of schooling, but over one-third of the African Americans and almost three-quarters of the non-Hispanic whites have reached this educational level. Income differences are equally striking: 59.3 percent of Hispanics, 34.1 percent of African Americans, and 16.7 percent of non-Hispanic whites have monthly income of less than $551. Respective percentages for income over $1,000 are 9.5 percent, 25.2 percent, and 46.0 percent.

A multivariate regression analysis of education on rates of dementia, with age, income, gender, and ethno-racial membership taken into account is shown in Table 8-3. In this regression analysis, income for certain nursing home residents could not be reliably ascertained. Uncertainty was encountered particularly because of the custom of spending down financial reserves and divesting oneself of assets and income prior to admission in order to qualify for Medicaid reimbursement. In order to include all subjects with missing information on income, mean values were substituted.

Age and education are the most significant and strongest associations of rates of dementia, with odds ratios of 6.1 and 4.3, respectively. With age and education controlled, ethno-racial membership loses its association with rates of

TABLE 8-3   Regression of Age, Education, Income, Gender, and Ethno-Racial Groups on Rates of Dementia

Variable	Beta	p	Odds Ratio	95% Confidence Interval
Age	1.81	.000	6.1	5.47, 6.82
Education	−1.46	.000	4.3	3.42, 5.42
Income	−0.35	N.S.[a]	—	—
Sex (male = 1)	−3.02	N.S.	—	—
Ethnicity/race	−2.56	N.S.	—	—

[a]N.S. = nonsignificant.
Note: The sample was restricted to 27 subsamples of community residents (65 year and older), N = 1,449, from the North Manhattan Aging Project target area. Diagnosis was made by research clinical evaluation or generated from the probability of a diagnosis on the basis of the screen score. Forty nursing home residents are included in this analysis. All missing values of income are substituted by mean values. Each ethno-racial group is treated as an individual category.

dementia, and neither income nor gender is significantly associated with rates of dementia. The variance in rates of dementia accounted for by age and education is 19.6 percent, and the variance accounted for by all these demographic variables taken together, 20.3 percent. Even when the regression is repeated combining the two disadvantaged groups (namely Hispanics and African Americans) for comparison with non-Hispanic whites, ethno-racial membership still does not attain a statistically significant level.

Subtypes of Dementia Among Ethno-Racial Groups

Nonspecific risk factors for dementia should affect rates regardless of subtypes, but there may be ethno-racial risks specific to subtypes. The distributions of subtypes of dementia (border-zone and advanced stages combined) are shown in Table 8-4 for each ethno-racial group. The great majority of dementias are diagnosed as Alzheimer's disease in Hispanics and African Americans, and this is the exclusive diagnosis in non-Hispanic whites.

Alzheimer's disease with stroke is particularly high among African Americans. However, if the subcategory of stroke-related Alzheimer's disease is combined with the category of Alzheimer's disease with stroke, then the ethno-racial rates are fairly similar: 18.2 percent for Hispanics, 28 percent for African-Americans, and 20 percent for non-Hispanic whites. Alcohol-related dementia is not prominent in any group. We note that although there are ethno-racial differences in subtypes, overall rates are accounted for largely by age and educational controls. This supports a view that the risks attached to age and education are for increased rates of dementia in general, rather than for specific subtypes of dementia, and is also in keeping with the possibility that Alzheimer's disease is

TABLE 8-4   Distributions of Subtypes of Dementia by Ethno-Racial Group

Subtypes of Dementia	Hispanic (%)	African American (%)	Non-Hispanic White (%)
Alzheimer's disease	87.9	93.3	100
Uncomplicated	66.7	50.7	80
With Parkinson's	3.0	0	0
With stroke	12.1	25.3	20
With other complications	6.1	17.3	0
Stroke related	6.1	2.7	0
Focal	2.0	0	0
Other or unknown	4.0	4.0	0
	100 (N = 99)	100 (*N* = 75)	100 (*N* = 10)

Note: The sample consisted of people evaluated by research clinical diagnostic criteria, $N = 184$, from 27 subsamples of community-residing elders (65 years and older) from the North Manhattan Aging Project target area.

often the underlying disorder even when manifestations suggest diagnosis of another subtype.

Other Risk Factors: Income and Immigration

Income was shown in the regression analysis not to be a significant influence on rates of dementia when education and age are controlled, although this finding does not fully disentangle the effects of income and education. It is also difficult to separate the effects of immigration from those of ethno-racial membership and education. While Hispanics were almost never born in the United States, African Americans were almost never born in a foreign country. The percentages of foreign-born in these two subsamples are 98.2 and 9.6, respectively. Non-Hispanic whites are evenly divided between domestic and foreign birth, but have low rates of dementia.

Quality-of-Life Impairments

As long as a discussion about ethno-racial differences in rates of dementia does not go beyond counting the frequencies of diagnostic categories of dementia or cognitive scores, there is a risk that the clinical and policy implications of the findings will be obscured. Uncertainty about the appropriate techniques for assessment and classification that are unbiased by ethno-racial characteristics may inhibit the drawing of conclusions from findings. Therefore, the following series of analyses details the impact on the quality of life of people with dementia in the three ethno-racial groups.

Memory Complaints

Complaints about memory are greatly increased in dementia within each ethno-racial group, as Figure 8-4 shows. Among Hispanics and non-Hispanic whites, there is a clear step-up of memory complaints in people with and without dementia, with people in the two dementia categories (border zone and advanced) being decidedly worse than those in the two nondementia groups (normal and border zone). This is also evident, although less consistently, for the African Americans. Among non-Hispanic whites, people with advanced dementias show fewer complaints than those with border-zone dementias, possibly as loss of insight supervenes.

These findings confirm that the condition of dementia is troubling to all three ethno-racial groups and support the value of employing the broader concept of dementia (i.e., including border-zone as well as advanced stages) for understanding the elder's sense of the difficulties accompanying dementia. Specifically, the border-zone dementia that occurs in relatively high rates in the Hispanic and African-American groups is as serious in the consequences for subjective distress, expressed by memory complaints, as is the advanced dementia that is more prevalent in the non-Hispanic white group.

The type of memory problem most prominently noticed by the sufferer varies among the ethno-racial groups. Certain tasks served by memory are probably either more important, or more of a challenge, for one ethno-racial group than another and are thus more likely to be singled out as problematic when memory fails. However, some complaints about memory are also offered by normal people, and those complaints are therefore weaker indicators of the effects of dementia.

Tasks of Daily Living

Dementias typically undermine independence in carrying out the tasks of daily living from an early stage onwards (Edwards et al., 1991; Davis et al., 1990; Warren et al., 1989), although factors other than dementia also govern the level of functioning observed (Reed et al., 1989). The relative distribution of functional impairments, reported by an informant, between people with and without dementia and the rank order of the frequencies of task impairments are similar among the ethno-racial groups, as Figure 8-5 shows. For all ethno-racial groups, the level of impairment increases regularly from people who are normal to those with border-zone nondementias to those with border-zone dementias. In Hispanic and African-American groups, people with advanced dementia continue this progression. In non-Hispanic whites with advanced dementia, the impairments decrease

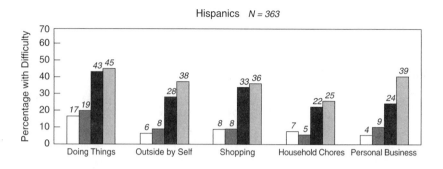

Hispanics *N = 363*

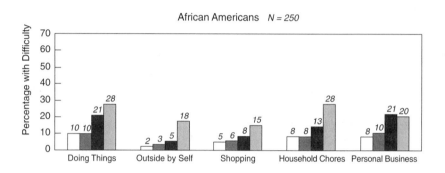

African Americans *N = 250*

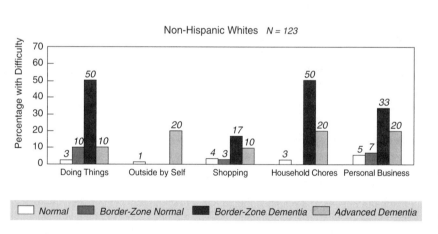

Non-Hispanic Whites *N = 123*

☐ *Normal* ■ *Border-Zone Normal* ■ *Border-Zone Dementia* ☐ *Advanced Dementia*

FIGURE 8-4 Memory complaints as reported by subject. NOTE: The sample was re-stricted to 27 subsamples of community-residing elders, 65 years and older, *N = 1,449*, from the North Manhattan Aging Project target area; there was a proportionate group in nursing homes, *N = 40*. Only the elderly who have a research clinical evaluation are included. This excludes 40 persons who had normal cognitive levels but were diagnosed as demented or who had severe cognitive impairment but were not diagnosed as demented.

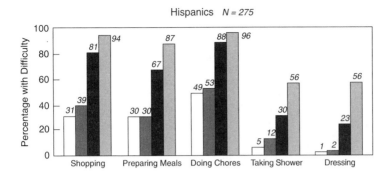

Hispanics *N = 275*

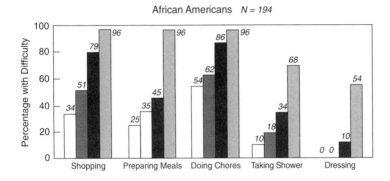

African Americans *N = 194*

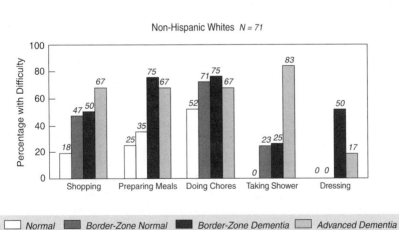

Non-Hispanic Whites *N = 71*

☐ *Normal* ■ *Border-Zone Normal* ■ *Border-Zone Dementia* ☐ *Advanced Dementia*

FIGURE 8-5 Task performance as reported by informant. NOTE: The sample was restricted to 27 subsamples of community-residing elders, 65 years and older, *N* = 1,449, from the North Manhattan Aging Project target area. Only the elderly who have a research clinical evaluation are included. This excludes 40 persons who had normal cognitive levels but were diagnosed as demented or who had severe cognitive impairment but were not diagnosed as demented.

somewhat; since these reports come from the informant, failure of insight due to dementia will not explain this finding.

Dementia appears to impair functioning to such an extent in the three ethno-racial groups as to overshadow reservations about the importance of the observed variation in rates among the ethno-racial groups, notwithstanding any possibility of ethno-racial bias in the assessment of cognitive status and in the criteria for diagnosis. These data again point to the pertinence, from the perspective of the dementia sufferer's quality of life, of including the broader concept of dementia (border-zone *and* advanced cases) in population studies. From these data, an argument might also be made for giving due attention to cases of border-zone nondementia on the grounds of their impact upon function in all three of the ethno-racial groups.

Affective Suffering

The relative distributions of affective suffering between people with and without dementia suggest that a shift to the intolerable and desperate levels of affective suffering takes place between the border-zone nondementia and the border-zone dementia stages. The longitudinal phase of the North Manhattan Aging Project is needed to confirm this inference. The frequency of the worst levels of affective suffering in dementia is much greater in the non-Hispanic whites and is least in the African Americans, as Figure 8-6 shows. Nevertheless, the increase of suffering appears to be marked for each ethno-racial group. These data strengthen the case for including the broader as well as the narrower definition of dementia in ethno-racial population studies.

Service Utilization

Among the more expensive long-term care services delivered to the elder population are nursing home placement, home health care, and hospitalization for acute episodes in chronic conditions. Use of these services is in part conditioned by type of health insurance coverage, as Table 8-5 shows. Since the frame for the sampling was drawn from Medicare lists, all subjects in the North Manhattan Aging Project and the Active Life Expectancy Study samples have Medicare insurance. It is estimated that more than 95 percent of the population 65 years or older resident in the target area, and more than 90 percent of any of the ethno-racial groups, are enrolled in Medicare. Among all three ethno-racial groups, the majority of people have either Medicaid or other health insurance in addition to Medicare. In general, people with dementia have an increased chance of being on Medicaid as opposed to other insurance coverage. However, while the majority of Hispanics and of African Americans with dementia have Medicaid and only a small minority of each group have other insurance, over 60 percent of the non-

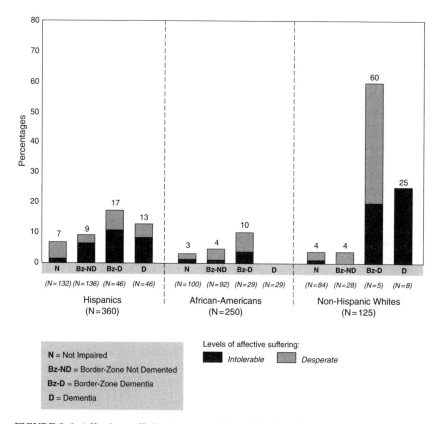

FIGURE 8-6 Affective suffering in stages of cognitive impairment. NOTE: The sample was restricted to 27 subsamples of community-residing elders, 65 years and older, N = 1,449, from the North Manhattan Aging Project target area. Only the elderly who have a research clinical evaluation are included here. This excludes 40 persons who had normal cognitive levels but were diagnosed as demented or who had severe cognitive impairment but were not diagnosed as demented.

Hispanic whites with dementia have other insurance, but less than 20 percent are covered by Medicaid.

Nursing Homes

Dementias account for the great majority of the use of nursing homes by residents from this target area. Utilization rates of nursing homes by people with dementia are vastly different between ethno-racial groups. Use by people with dementia among Hispanics (4.6%) and African Americans (9.9%) is very low compared with non-Hispanic whites (36.4%).

TABLE 8-5   Use of Health Insurance Coverage in Addition to Medicare (Part A) by Dementia in the Community

Population and Type of Coverage	Proportion with Coverage		
	Dementia	Nondementia	Total
Hispanic			
(Number)	(55)	(541)	(696)
Medicaid (%)	83.8	62.5	67.2
Other (%)	4.8	18.5	15.4
African-American			
(Number)	(96)	(401)	(497)
Medicaid (%)	57.6	38.1	41.9
Other (%)	22.8	45.7	41.3
Non-Hispanic White			
(Number)	(20)	(231)	(251)
Medicaid (%)	18.8	12.6	13.1
Other (%)	63.2	66.9	66.6
Total			
(Number)	(271)	(1,173)	(1,444)
Medicaid (%)	69.7	44.3	49.1
Other (%)	15.5	37.3	33.2

Note: The sample was restricted to 27 subsamples of community-residing elders (65 years and older), N = 1,449, from the North Manhattan Aging Project target area. Diagnosis was made by research clinical evaluation or was generated from the probability of diagnosis based on screen scores.

Home Care

To some extent, the neglect of nursing home admission as a resource for care of people with dementia in the African-American and Hispanic groups is made up for by a high volume of home care provision. This is particularly evident for African Americans with dementia in the community, who have a home care utilization rate of 45.7 percent. The corresponding rate for Hispanics is 31.6 percent, and for non-Hispanic whites 30 percent.

Emergency Clinics

Primary medical care is available in the target area in hospital-based, hospital-linked, and group and solo private practice. Emergency clinic visits can be taken as a rough guide to the degree to which a person is inadequately connected to the primary care system. Overall, emergency clinic attendance is reported for 37.7 percent of Hispanics with dementia and 38.8 percent of African Americans with dementia; for non-Hispanic whites with dementia it is 25 percent. Regardless of health insurance arrangements, there is a remarkably high use of emergency clinic services by people with dementia in the Hispanic and African-American groups. The utilization rate by non-Hispanic whites appears to be lower than for the other two ethno-racial groups, but the small size of the non-Hispanic white sample makes interpretation of this comparison uncertain.

Hospitalization

Admission to hospital inpatient status is increased by dementia for African Americans and non-Hispanic whites but not for Hispanics. Admissions are highest among African Americans with dementia (29.4%), next highest among non-Hispanic whites with dementia (23.5%), and lowest (19.6%) among Hispanics with dementia.

DISCUSSION

Limitations of the Findings and Potential of the Methods

The methods of this study provide further opportunities for testing the robustness of the findings on ethno-racial variation in rates of dementia. Additional representative subsamples, amounting to almost 700 elders from the target area, have been surveyed; these supplementary data will be especially useful for checking those findings so far reported here on the relatively small sample of non-Hispanic whites with dementia. Enlargement of the database will also allow analyses to be linked to more homogeneous ethno-racial groups, such as Hispanic groups of distinctive national origin.

Epidemiological studies of ethno-racial variation in health conditions benefit from the collection of stratification of sampling to equalize sizes of ethno-racial groups. In this study, equalization was attempted through "gerrymandering" of the target area on the basis of 1985 census data and stratification of recruitment based on the Medicare ethno-racial designation. However, non-Hispanic whites proved to have moved out of area more rapidly than expected; moreover, 26 percent of those designated non-Hispanic whites on Medicare lists were reassigned to the Hispanic group after interview. These situations resulted in a smaller group of non-Hispanic whites with dementia than planned.

In this presentation, the reporting component of the registry for Alzheimer's disease and related disorders has been combined with the survey component in order to amass a representative sample of elders from both community settings and nursing homes. Moreover, insight into possible selection biases can be pursued through the process of contrasting findings from the survey component and the reporting component. In economically disadvantaged neighborhoods, surveys typically fall short of desirable levels of response rates: resorting to information from a network of key informants can be a useful window into selective biases arising from the loss of information on nonresponders. Analysis of response bias, so far, shows that there is a skewing of age distributions; this is further discussed later.

Study methods incorporate molecular genetics, neuroimaging, and autopsy material. These methods have not yet been applied to the interpretation of the observed ethno-racial variations in rates of dementia. Of key importance will be the relationships within each ethno-racial group between, on the one hand, these markers of the biological processes of dementia and, on the other hand, the classifications of dementia employed to compare rates of dementia in ethno-racial groups. Biological markers will assist in the evaluation of the ethno-racial consistency in diagnosis of dementia and can either support or conflict with the relative rates of dementia diagnosed in the three ethno-racial groups.

Also yet to be exploited is the longitudinal element of this study's methods, which will clarify the contribution of incidence, duration, and mortality to the relative prevalence rates in ethno-racial groups. Course and outcome data will also better define the extent and causal pathways of the impact of dementia on function and quality of life in the various ethno-racial groups and will allow distinctive patterns of service use to be discerned.

Self-designation of ethno-racial membership was found to be a satisfactory method of classification for purposes of making ethno-racial comparisons of rates of dementia and was found to be better than reliance on assignments based on surnames. We do not at this stage have a hypothesis that would require a more refined classification of ethno-racial groups, but it is likely that more demanding hypotheses will arise.

Ethno-Racial Variation in Prevalence Rates

Non-Hispanic whites have dramatically lower rates of dementia than the other two ethno-racial groups. These relative rates remain consistent for concepts of dementia of varying breadth: for advanced dementia taken alone, when border-zone dementia is also included, and even if nondementia with cognitive impairment is taken into account. Age and education are the most significant and strongest demographic associations of rates of dementia.

Skewing of the responding sample of elders towards a younger age would lead to an underestimate of the absolute prevalence rates of dementia, especially among Hispanics and non-Hispanic whites. However, the analyses of this paper are directed at relative (not absolute) rates of dementia among the ethno-racial groups: in this respect, rates in the African-American group would be overestimated relative to the other two ethno-racial groups. This bias is controlled by the regression analysis, by age stratification of comparisons groups, by adjustment of age profiles of all the ethno-racial groups to that found in the non-Hispanic white group, and by weighting ethno-racial age categories to match the original Medicare sampling frame or that of the census profile.

With age and education controlled, there appears to be little influence on variation among ethno-racial groups that is explained by reference to the selected other potential associations. Differences in subtypes of dementia do not account for the ethno-racial variation in dementia. Neither could income or immigration status be shown to contribute to this ethno-racial variation. Mislabeling of depression as dementia also could not be implicated. A later age of onset could produce a tendency towards the relatively lower rates of dementia noted among the non-Hispanic whites, but the evidence in favor of this hypothesis is built on an informant's retrospective report which is viewed with reservations about reliability and which must defer to the relevant data that the longitudinal phase of the study will generate. Nevertheless, if the Hispanic and African-American groups are adjusted to match the age-education profile of the non-Hispanic whites, significant differences in the rate of dementia remain between non-Hispanic whites and each of the other two ethno-racial groups.

Note that in referring to the results of analyses of relationships between dementia and education or income, we use the neutral term *associations* rather than terms suggesting causality. Nevertheless, it is clear that the processes that result in educational level are completed many decades before the onset of evidence of dementia resulting from either Alzheimer's disease or multi-infarctions. Moreover, the great majority of cases of dementia have an onset at 75 years or older, 10 or more years after the average age of retirement, making it unlikely that the level of income could be influenced by the dementia. There does remain the possibility of the existence of a pre-dementia condition (e.g., prodrome or state of vulnerability), so far undetected, that could intervene in the educational and income-producing years of life.

Ethno-Racial Consistency in the Associations of Dementia

For all ethno-racial groups, the level of independently (i.e., informant) reported functional impairment increases regularly from normal people to those with border-zone nondementia to those with border-zone dementia. Correspondingly, memory complaints are greatly increased in the two dementia categories (border-zone and advanced) within each ethno-racial group, although more clearly among Hispanics and non-Hispanic whites than for African Americans. Although there are ethno-racial differences in the types of memory problems that are the content of complaints, the increase of memory complaints in dementia is consistent for all ethno-racial groups. An excess frequency of intolerable and desperate levels of affective suffering was also found in the two dementia categories: this excess is much greater in the non-Hispanic whites and is least in the African Americans.

It appears that the concepts of dementia applied in this study are associated with considerable impairment of subjective and objective aspects of functioning and qualities of life in the three ethno-racial groups. For these reasons, the findings on ethno-racial variation warrant attention. These findings also strengthen the argument for applying the broader concept (i.e., border-zone and advanced cases) of dementia in the investigation of ethno-racial variation in rates and effects of dementia. By extension, an argument can be made for investigating also the border-zone nondementias. All these categories have associations with impairments in the quality of life.

Working Hypotheses for the Effects of Education

Evidence is mounting that the educational effects on rates of dementia are real and not a methodological artifact, although it is supposed that education acts on a biologically predisposed substrate. Added to other brain insults and vulnerabilities, these educational factors raise the rates of Alzheimer's disease, multi-infarct dementia, and other subtypes of dementia. An account of the pathways by which education could appear to affect, or could actually affect, rates of dementia has been addressed in a recent paper (Gurland et al., 1995a, 1995b) by these investigators. The following summary is adapted from that paper:

1. Selective hypothesis: Persons who will develop dementia in late life already have reduced cognitive reserve from early childhood. They therefore have difficulty in coping with the challenges of the schooling process. Consequently, they drop out of school and thus produce a relationship between lower educational achievement and later development of dementia. Barriers to continuing schooling come at distinctive educational levels depending on the inadequacies of a particular educational system.

2. Associational hypothesis: Poor education goes hand in hand with many other potential mechanisms for inducing or precipitating dementia, including malnutrition, exposure to trauma, alcohol abuse, and inadequate health care.

3. Educational hypothesis: Good, lifelong education builds and maintains a robust neurobiological structure and cognitive reserves that compensate for any deteriorative forces that might come to bear upon the brain. Beneficial effects earlier in life might be extended through continuing intellectual stimulation.

Ethno-Racial Differences in Service Utilization

Given the ethno-racial equivalencies in the quality-of-life associations of dementia, the inequalities in service utilization take on added importance. Hispanics and African Americans with dementia are much less likely than non-Hispanic whites with dementia to be admitted to a nursing home. Preference for, and reliance on, home care of people with dementia rather than nursing home admission is stronger for Hispanics and African Americans than for non-Hispanic whites. The high use of emergency clinic services by Hispanics and

African Americans could indicate that their preference for home care is not supported by the adequate availability of primary medical care. Less consistent with this pattern of service use are that admissions to hospitals are highest among African Americans and non-Hispanic whites with dementia and lowest among Hispanics with dementia. Analyses of the service impacts have been presented elsewhere, with suggestions for policy and planning efforts (Chen and Gurland, 1995).

CONCLUSION

Age and education account for a substantial part of the variance in rates of dementia among the three ethno-racial groups under study. Other demographic variables that were tested do not appear to make a significant contribution to this variance. The methods of the study were directed at reducing ethno-racial (including educational) bias in making diagnostic comparison and support the inference that the findings are related to a process of dementia and not to mislabeling.

Given the profiles of demographic and other variables occurring in these ethno-racial groups, rates of dementia in Hispanic and African-American groups are dramatically in excess of that found in non-Hispanic whites. In all ethno-racial groups the presence of dementia is accompanied by a deterioration in the quality of life: functional limitations in the tasks of daily living, self-report of memory problems, and affective suffering. This reinforces the view that the diagnosis of dementia reflects a process that carries serious consequences for each of the ethno-racial groups.

The findings identify several useful lines of inquiry. Further investigation of the associations between education and rates of dementia could lead to preventive interventions: three working hypotheses have been proposed here. Distinctive ethno-racial service utilization patterns by people with dementia point to the value of examining the needs and need fulfillment of people with dementia in these groups more closely, with special reference to the impact these needs and their fulfillment have on the quality of life of people with dementia and of their family.

Methodological advances demonstrated in this study could allow the issues in ethno-racial variation in dementia to be approached with some confidence that ethno-racial bias will not confound the interpretation of findings unduly. Perhaps, the most important contribution of these methods is to clarify the associations of this health disorder with impairments in the quality of life. This step changes the focus of inquiry from diagnostic labels to conditions with serious consequences for those afflicted and their families.

ACKNOWLEDGMENT

This work was supported by the following grants: (1) North Manhattan Aging Project, National Institute on Aging (principal investigator Barry Gurland, co-principal investigator David Wilder), Project 5 P01 AG7232-04. (2) Epidemiology of Dementia in an Urban Community, National Institute on Aging (principal investigator Richard Mayeux, co-principal investigator Barry Gurland, and Yaakov Stern), Project P01 AG07232. (3) Active Life Expectancy Among Urban Minority Elderly, National Institute on Aging (principal investigator Rafael Lantigua, co-principal investigator David Wilder, co-investigators Barry Gurland, Sidney Katz) Project 5 R01AG10489-02. (4) A Transcultural Screen for Alzheimer's Disease and Related Disorders, New York Community Trust Foundation (principal investigator Barry Gurland), Project *NYCT CU 50404701. (5) The Morris W. Stroud, III, Program on Scientific Approaches to Quality of Life in Health and Aging, Endowment Fund (co-directors Barry Gurland and Sidney Katz).

Other staff members of the North Manhattan Aging Project were Virginia Barrett, Betty Barsa, Mabel Bolivar, Harold Browne, Jean Denaro, Priscilla Encarnacion, Maria Gonzalez, Lucia McBee, and Jeanne Teresi. Interviewers who completed over 100 interviews were Raul Almanzar, Carlomagno Baldi, Carlos Garcia, Consuelo McLaughlin, Annie Nuñez, Argentina Peralta, and Joseph Romero.

W. Edwards Deming designed the sampling plan for the North Manhattan Aging Project.

We thank the Bureau of Data Management and Strategy of the Health Care Financing Administration for providing the tape files of Medicare beneficiaries.

Assistants in formatting, illustrating, and compiling the bibliography for this paper were María Fernández and Aline Ratau.

REFERENCES

American Psychiatric Association
    1994   *Diagnostic and Statistical Manual of Mental Disorders*, 4th ed. Washington, DC: American Psychiatric Association.
Berg, L., J.P. Miller, J. Baty, and E.H. Rubin
    1992   Mild senile dementia of the Alzheimer type: IV. Evaluation of intervention. *Annals of Neurology* 31:242 (abstract).
Bland, R.C., S.C. Newman, and H. Om
    1988   Prevalence of psychiatric disorders in the elderly in Edmonton. *Acta Psychiatrica Scandinavica* 77(suppl. 338):57-63.
Brodaty, H., and P.D. Hadzi
    1990   Psychosocial effects on carers of living with persons with dementia. *Australian and New Zealand Journal of Psychiatry* 24:351-361.
Chen, J.
    1995   Insight in dementia: Increasing cognitive impairment and the strength of the relationship between self-report of function, informant report, and depression. Stroud Center publications 120. New York: Columbia University.
Chen, J., and B. Gurland
    1995   *Bird's Eye Reports*. Issues 1-7. Stroud Center publications 110-117. New York: Columbia University.
Davis, P.B., J.C. Morris, and E. Grant
    1990   Brief screening tests versus clinical staging in senile dementia of the Alzheimer type. *Journal of the American Geriatrics Society* 38:129-135.

de la Monte, S.M., G.M. Hutchins, and G.W. Moore
    1989   Racial differences in the etiology of dementia and frequency of Alzheimer lesions in the brain. *Journal of the National Medical Association* 81:644-652.

Edwards, D.F., C.M. Baum, and R.K. Deuel
    1991   Constructional apraxia in Alzheimer's disease: Contributions to functional loss. *Physical and Occupational Therapy in Geriatrics* 9(3-4):53-68.

Escobar, J.I., A. Burnam, M. Karno, A. Forsythe, J. Landsverk, and J.M. Golding
    1986   Use of the Mini-Mental State Examination (MMSE) in a community population of mixed ethnicity. *Journal of Nervous and Mental Disease* 174:607-614.

Folstein, M.F., S.S. Bassett, J.C. Anthony, A.J. Romanoski, and G.R. Nestadt
    1991   Dementia: Case ascertainment in a community survey. *Journal of Gerontology* 46:132-138.

Fratiglioni, L., M. Grut, Y. Forsell, M. Viitanen, M. Grafstrom, K. Holmen, K. Ericsson, L. Backman, and A. Ahlbom
    1991   Prevalence of Alzheimer's disease and other dementias in an elderly urban population: Relationship with age, sex, and education. *Neurology* 41:1886-1892.

Golden, R.R., J.A. Teresi, and B.J. Gurland
    1984   Development of indicator scales for the Comprehensive Assessment and Referral Evaluation (CARE) interview schedule. *Journal of Gerontology* 39(2):138-146.

Gurland, B.J.
    1981   The borderlands of dementia: The influence of sociocultural characteristics on rates of dementia occurring in the senium. Pp. 61-84 in *Clinical Aspects of Alzheimer's Disease and Senile Dementia*, N.E. Miller and G.D. Cohen, eds. New York: Raven Press.

    1996a   Epidemiology of psychiatric disorders among elders. In *Comprehensive Review of Geriatric Psychiatry (CRGP- II)*, J. Sadavoy, J. Foster, et al., eds. Washington, DC: American Psychiatric Press.

    1996b   Methods of screening for survey research on Alzheimer's disease and related dementias. In *Alzheimer's Disease*, Z.S. Khachaturian and T.S. Radebaugh, eds. Boca Raton, FL: CRC Press.

Gurland, B.J., and P.S. Cross
    1982   Epidemiology of psychopathology in old age: Some clinical implications. *Psychiatric Clinics of North America* 5(1):11-26.

Gurland, B.J., P. Cross, J. Chen, D.E. Wilder, Z.M. Pine, R.A. Lantigua, and R. Fulmer
    1994   A new performance test of adaptive cognitive functioning: The Medication Management (MM) Test. *International Journal of Geriatric Psychiatry* 9:875-885.

Gurland, B.J., S. Katz, R.A. Lantigua, and D. Wilder
    1993   Cognitive function and the elderly. Pp. 21-26 in *Proceedings of the 1991 International Symposium on Data on Aging, National Center for Health Statistics*. Series 5(7). Washington, DC: U.S. Department of Health and Human Services.

Gurland, B., J. Kuriansky, L. Sharpe, R. Simon, P. Stiller, and P. Birkett
    1977   The Comprehensive Assessment and Referral Evaluation (CARE): Rationale, development and reliability. *International Journal of Aging and Human Development* 8(1):9-14.

Gurland, B.J., D.E. Wilder, J. Chen, R. Lantigua, R. Mayeux, and J. Van Nostrand
    1995a   A flexible system of detection for Alzheimer's disease and related dementias. *Aging: Clinical and Experiential Research* 7:165-172.

Gurland, B.J., D.E. Wilder, P. Cross, R.A. Lantigua, J. Teresi, V. Barrett, Y. Stern, and R. Mayeux
    1995b   Relative rates of dementia by multiple case definitions, over two prevalence periods, in three cultural groups. *American Journal of Geriatric Psychiatry* 3:6-20.

Gurland, B.J., D.E. Wilder, P. Cross, J. Teresi, and V.W. Barrett
    1992   Screening scales for dementia: Toward reconciliation of conflicting cross-cultural findings. *International Journal of Geriatric Psychiatry* 7:105-113.

Heyman, A., G. Fillenbaum, B. Prosnitz, and K. Raiford
  1991   Estimated prevalence of dementia among elderly black and white community residents.
         Archives of Neurology 48:594 (abstract).
Katz, S., A.B. Ford, R.W. Moskowitz, B.A. Jackson, and M.W. Jaffe
  1963   Studies of illness in the aged. The index of ADL: A standardized measure of biological
         and psychosocial function. *Journal of the American Medical Association* 185:914-919.
Katz, S., and B.J. Gurland
  1991   Science of quality of life of elders: Challenges and opportunity. Pp. 335-343 in *The
         Concept and Measurement of Quality of Life in the Frail Elderly*, J. Birren, J.E. Lubben,
         J.C. Rowe, and D.E. Deutchman, eds. Los Angeles: Academic Press.
Kral, V.
  1983   The relationship between senile dementia (Alzheimer type) and depression. *Canadian
         Journal of Psychiatry* 28:304-306.
Kramer, M., P.S. German, J.C. Anthony, M. Von-Korff, and E.A. Skinner
  1985   Patterns of mental disorders among the elderly residents of eastern Baltimore. *Journal of
         the American Geriatric Society* 33:236-245.
Larson, E., B. Reifler, S.M. Sumi, C.G. Canfield, and N.M. Chinn
  1985   Diagnostic evaluation of 200 elderly outpatients with suspected dementia. *Journal of
         Gerontology* 40:536-543.
Lawton, M.P., and E.M. Brody
  1969   Assessment of older people: Self-maintaining and instrumental activities of daily living.
         Gerontologist 9:179-186.
Li, G., Y.C. Shen, C.H. Chen, Y.W. Zhau, S.R. Li, and M. Lu
  1989   An epidemiological survey of age-related dementia in an urban area of Beijing. *Acta
         Psychiatrica Scandinavica* 79:557-563.
  1991   A three-year follow-up study of age-related dementia in an urban area of Beijing. *Acta
         Psychiatrica Scandinavica* 83:99-104.
Livingston, G., A. Hawkins, N. Graham, B. Blizard, and A. Mann
  1990   The Gospel Oak Study: Prevalence rates of dementia, depression and activity limitation
         among elderly residents in inner London. *Psychological Medicine* 20:137-146.
Maestre, G., R. Ottman, Y. Stern, B. Gurland, M. Chun, M.X. Tang, M. Shelanski, B. Tycko, and R.
         Mayeux
  1995   Apolipoprotein E and Alzheimer's disease: Ethnic variation in genotypic risks. *Annals of
         Neurology* 37:254-259.
Mayeux, R., R. Ottman, M.X. Tang, L. Noboa-Bauza, K. Marder, B. Gurland, and Y. Stern
  1993   Genetic susceptibility and head injury as risk factors for Alzheimer's disease among
         community-dwelling elderly persons and their first-degree relatives. *Annals of Neurology*
         33(5):494-501.
McAllister, T.W., and T.R. Price
  1982   Severe depressive pseudodementia with and without dementia. *American Journal of Psy-
         chiatry* 139:626-629.
Murden, R.A., T.D. McRae, S. Kaner, and M.E. Bucknam
  1991   Mini-Mental State Exam scores vary with education in blacks and whites. *Journal of the
         American Geriatric Society* 39(2):149-155.
O'Connor, D.W., P.A. Pollitt, M. Roth, P.B. Brook, and B.B. Reiss
  1990   Memory complaints and impairment in normal, depressed, and demented elderly persons
         identified in a community survey. *Archives of General Psychiatry* 47(3):224-227.
O'Connor, D.W., P.A. Pollitt, M. Roth, C.P. Brook, and B.B. Reiss
  1991a Problems reported by relatives in a community study of dementia. *British Journal of
         Psychiatry* 156:835-841.

O'Connor, D.W., P.A. Pollitt, and F.P. Treasure
   1991b   The influence of education and social class on the diagnosis of dementia in a community population. *Psychological Medicine* 21(1):219-224.

O'Connor, D.W., and M. Roth
   1990   Coexisting depression and dementia in a community survey of the elderly. *International Psychogeriatrics* 2:45-53.

Reding, M., J. Haycox, and J. Blass
   1985   Depression in patients referred to a dementia clinic: A three year prospective study. *Archives of Neurology* 42:894-896.

Reed, B.R., W.J. Jagust, and J.P. Seab
   1989   Mental status as a predictor of daily function in progressive dementia. *Gerontologist* 29:804-807.

Reisberg, B., S.H. Ferris, and E. Franssen
   1985   An ordinal functional assessment tool for Alzheimer's-type dementia. *Hospital Community Psychiatry* 36(6):593-595.

Salmon, D.P., P.J. Riekkinen, R. Katzman, M.Y. Zhang, H. Jin, and E. Yu
   1989   Cross-cultural studies of dementia: A comparison of Mini-Mental State Examination performance in Finland and China. *Archives of Neurology* 46(7):769-772.

Stern, Y., H. Andrews, J. Pittman, M. Sano, T. Tatemichi, R. Lantigua, and R. Mayeux
   1992   Diagnosis of dementia in a heterogeneous population: Development of a neurophysiological paradigm-based diagnosis of dementia and quantified correction for the effects of education. *Archives of Neurology* 49:453-460.

Stern, Y., B. Gurland, T.T. Tatemichi, M. Xin Tan, D. Wilder, and R. Mayeux
   1994   Influence of education and occupation on the incidence of Alzheimer's disease. *Journal of the American Medical Association.*

Teresi, J., R. Golden, P. Cross, B. Gurland, M. Kleinman, and D. Wilder
   1995   Item bias in cognitive screening measures: Comparisons of elderly white, Afro-American, Hispanic and high and low educational subgroups. *Journal of Clinical Epidemiology* 48:473-483.

Teresi, J.A., R.R. Golden, B.J. Gurland, D.E. Wilder, and R.G. Bennett
   1984   Construct validity of indicator-scales developed from the Comprehensive Assessment and Referral Evaluation interview schedule. *Journal of Gerontology* 39(2):147-157.

Uhlmann, R.F., and E.B. Larson
   1991   Effect of education on the Mini-Mental State Examination as a screening test for dementia. *Journal of the American Geriatrics Society* 39(9):876-880.

Wands, K., H. Merskey, V.C. Hachinski, M. Fisman, H. Fox, M. Boniferro
   1990   A questionnaire investigation of anxiety and depression in early dementia. *Journal of the American Geriatrics Society* 38:535-538.

Warren, E.J., A. Grek, D. Conn, N. Herrmann, E. Icyk, J. Kohl, and M. Silberfeld
   1989   A correlation between cognitive performance and daily functioning in elderly people. *Journal of Geriatric Psychiatry and Neurology* 2(2):96-100.

Weissmann, N.M., J.K. Myers, G.L. Tischler, C.E. Holzer III, P.J. Leaf, H. Orvaschel, and J.A. Brody
   1985   Psychiatric disorders (DSM-III) and cognitive impairment among the elderly in a U.S. urban community. *Acta Psychiatrica Scandinavica* 71:366-379.

Wilder, D.E., P. Cross, J. Chen, B.J. Gurland, R.A. Lantigua, J. Teresi, M. Bolivar, and P. Encarnación
   1995   Operating characteristics of brief screens for dementia in a multicultural population. *American Journal of Geriatric Psychiatry* 3(2):96-107.

Wilder, D.E., B.J. Gurland, J. Chen, R.A. Lantigua, E.H.P. Killeffer, S. Katz, and P. Encarnación
   1994   Interpreting subject and informant reports of function in screening for dementia. *International Journal of Geriatric Psychiatry* 9:887-896.

9

Cardiovascular Disease Among Elderly Asian Americans

Dwayne Reed and Katsukiko Yano

INTRODUCTION

Migration of people from one environment to another provides an unusual opportunity to observe a natural experiment, for while the genetic characteristics of the people remain relatively unchanged, the new place is different from the place of origin in many physical, biological, and social ways. Such contrasts are important to our interest in ethnic differences in chronic disease in the elderly as they allow for the examination of the risk of disease among migrants and non-migrants in both places, and between migrants and their offspring at the place of destination.

The migration of Japanese to Hawaii and California between 1885 and 1923 provided the basis for one of the most extensively studied examples of this kind of process. Stimulated by the heavy demand for agricultural labor, many Japanese men from the southern prefectures of Honshu, the main island of Japan, responded to advertisements for work in the United States. Most of them prospered, sent for wives, and established permanent residences. The importance of this situation became apparent in the late 1950s when international comparisons of mortality rates from coronary heart disease showed that Japanese in Japan had among the lowest rates in the world and that Japanese in Hawaii and California had rates that were two and three times higher (Gordon, 1957) (Figure 9-1).

In order to examine the validity of these data, a collaborative epidemiological investigation using the acronym Ni-Hon-San was initiated in Japan, Hawaii, and California in 1965; a standardized protocol was used to minimize methodological differences. After a baseline study, follow-up examinations and surveillance of the incidence of coronary heart disease and all causes of death have been

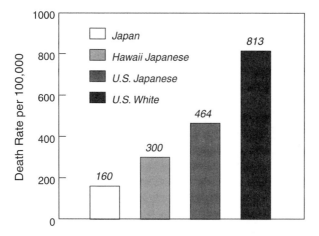

FIGURE 9-1 Atherosclerotic heart disease mortality rates for Japanese men aged 55-64 by geographic area, 1950. SOURCE: Gordon, 1957.

maintained to date in Japan and Hawaii but not in California. The main objectives of this prospective study were (1) to verify the reported differences among Japanese men in the three geographic locations by comparing prevalence of, incidence of, and mortality from coronary heart disease measured the same way, and (2) to search for the factors that could explain the observed differences. In this report, we review the findings concerning the cultural, lifestyle, and biological differences among the different population and nativity groups, and provide data on the effect of these characteristics on the incidence of cardiovascular disease. We will place special emphasis on the generational subgroups within the Honolulu Heart Program cohort, which has been followed for more than 25 years.

METHODS

Study Population

Details of the recruiting methods, population characteristics, and examination procedures for the cohorts have been published elsewhere (Kato et al., 1973; Kagan et al., 1974; Nichaman et al., 1975; Marmot et al., 1975; Worth et al., 1975). A brief summary follows (Table 9-1). In Japan, the target population included approximately 2,400 Japanese men who were born between January 1, 1900, and December 31, 1919, selected from the Adult Health Study population of the Radiation Effects Research Foundation in Hiroshima and Nagasaki. These men have been examined biennially since 1958 to study the late effects of indirect exposure to atomic bomb radiation. Among these men, 2,141 participated in the initial examination of the Ni-Hon-San Study in 1965-1966.

TABLE 9-1   The Ni-Hon-San Study Design

Characteristic	Japan	Hawaii	California
Residence	Hiroshima, Nagasaki	Honolulu	San Francisco
Initial exam date	1965-1966	1965-1968	1969-1970
Number examined	2,141	8,006	1,844
Response rate (%)	80	72	68
Mean age (years)	56.2	54.4	52.8

In Hawaii, over 11,000 men of Japanese ancestry who were born between 1900 and 1919 and were residing on Oahu Island as of January 1, 1965, were identified and located through an updated record of the World War II Selective Service registration. Among these men, 8,006 participated in the initial examination from 1965 to 1968.

In California, a special census was conducted in 1967 to locate Japanese Americans living in the eight counties of the San Francisco Bay area. Of more than 2,700 men born between 1900 and 1919, 1,844 were examined in 1969 and 1970.

In all geographic areas, all four grandparents had to be Japanese for a participant to be included in the study.

Baseline Examination

All participants were interviewed to obtain information on sociodemographic variables, past medical history, family medical history, smoking habits, alcohol consumption, and dietary intake. Anthropometric measurements, three blood pressure determinations, tests of lung function, a resting 12-lead electrocardiogram, and measurements of hematocrit, serum cholesterol, triglycerides, uric acid, and glucose were performed 1 hour after ingestion of 50 grams of glucose on nonfasting blood specimens. Physical examinations focusing on the cardiovascular system were also performed. The values recorded at this baseline examination were used as risk factor levels throughout the present report unless otherwise noted.

Measures of Acculturation for the Hawaii Cohort

The variables used in this study as measures of the degree of exposure to Japanese culture include birthplace (mainly Japan or Hawaii), total number of years lived in Japan, ability to read and write Japanese, ability to speak Japanese, and an index of preference for a Japanese over a Western diet. This information was obtained from each subject at the baseline examination.

Those men who were born in Japan and migrated to the United States are called Issei (first generation), and those born in other areas are called Nisei (second generation). About 10 percent of the Hawaiian Nisei went to Japan for education and returned after living in Japan 10 years or longer. These men were called Kibei (literally, "returned to America"). For all of these men, most of the time spent in Japan was during childhood and early adult life. About three-fourths of the Issei migrated to Hawaii after age 12, and most of the Kibei went to Japan before age 10.

Special skill in the use of the Japanese language was acquired during childhood either by formal education in Japan or by attending special language schools run by Japanese communities in Hawaii. These language schools were attended by most Nisei after regular school hours, but the duration and frequency of attendance varied. Evaluation of the language skill was made on the basis of self-assessment.

The Japanese diet score (Japanese foods/sum of Japanese and American foods) was calculated, by asking each subject the frequency of eating typical Japanese and typical American food items during the previous day. A higher score indicates preference for a more traditional Japanese diet.

Additional cultural information was available for a subset of 4,653 men in the Hawaii cohort who completed a sociocultural questionnaire in 1971. The questionnaire contained a variety of questions relating to acculturation, theoretically stressful life situations, and social networks that are thought to be protective against the stressful aspects of cultural changes.

Follow-up Examinations and Surveillance

In Japan, follow-up information was obtained by reexamination every 2 years and by surveillance of death certificates. In Hawaii, follow-up examinations were done 2 and 6 years after the baseline examination, and routine surveillance of hospital discharge records and death certificates has been maintained to date. In California, surveillance of death certificates was maintained for 2 years.

Definition of Cases

The prevalence of coronary heart disease at the initial Ni-Hon-San examination included definite and probable myocardial infarction diagnosed by electrocardiogram findings and angina pectoris diagnosed by the World Health Organization standard questionnaire. The incidence of cases among men without any clinical coronary heart disease at baseline was classified by the worst level of disease. Fatal cases of coronary heart disease were defined as deaths due to acute coronary heart disease (including myocardial infarction, coronary insufficiency, and sudden death with coronary-type chest pain) or to chronic coronary heart disease (including congestive heart failure and severe arrhythmia with a prior history of coronary heart disease).

Sudden deaths within 1 hour after the onset of symptoms without clear evidence of coronary heart disease (by electrocardiogram, cardiac enzyme, or chest pain), and in the absence of other attributable causes, are usually regarded in the United States as fatal coronary heart disease and were included in studies of the Hawaii cohort. Because of inconsistencies, however, it was decided to exclude this category for comparisons of U.S. and Japanese cases. Old myocardial infarctions found incidentally at autopsy without a clinical history of coronary heart disease were also excluded because it was difficult to determine whether the myocardial infarction occurred before or after the baseline examination. Another category of exclusion was coronary heart disease death diagnosed only by death certificate without supportive evidence from either clinical or autopsy findings. In the original study protocol, a comparison of the incidence of nonfatal myocardial infarction was also planned. However, different methods of case ascertainment made a valid comparison difficult.

In order to ensure the comparability of case ascertainment, one of the staff physicians from each study group visited the other study site and independently reviewed all potential cases in each cohort. Only those cases with a diagnosis agreed upon by physicians of both groups were accepted for the study.

For analyses of the association of risk factors upon the incidence of coronary heart disease within the Hawaii cohort, total coronary heart disease, subgroups of fatal coronary heart disease, nonfatal myocardial infarction, and angina pectoris were used. Ascertainment was based on both temporal changes of electrocardiograms at follow-up examinations and hospital surveillance records of diagnostic electrocardiograms and cardiac enzyme values.

Comparison data on incidence cases were available for a 2-year follow-up period in Hawaii and California and for a 12-year period in Hawaii and Japan. Incidence case data for risk factor analyses were available for a 23-year follow-up period in Hawaii.

Age Categories

The men in the Ni-Hon-San baseline examination were born between 1900 and 1919 and ranged from 45 to 70 years of age at that examination. The statistical models used follow-up duration and person-years at risk during 5-year age intervals. Thus, for the Hawaii-Japan 12-year follow-up comparisons, it was possible to examine rates from ages 45 to 79.

Within the Hawaii cohort, special attention has been given to comparison of coronary heart disease risk factors in elderly and middle-aged men. Data for these studies used the measurements of risk factors made in the third follow-up exam for 1,419 elderly men aged 65 to 74 and 3,440 middle-aged men aged 51 to 59. Among the generational subgroups in Hawaii, nearly all of the Issei were 55 or older at the baseline examination, so comparisons of risk factors were made only for men aged 55 to 68 at baseline.

RESULTS

Ni-Hon-San Comparisons

Table 9-2 presents age-adjusted means and percentages of selected variables measured at the initial examination for the three study cohorts. Both the Hawaii and the California cohorts were more obese (greater body mass index) and had higher mean values of serum cholesterol and glucose 1 hour after ingestion of 50 grams of glucose than the members of the Japan cohort. Systolic blood pressure was highest in California and similar in both Japan and Hawaii. Diastolic blood pressures were highest in California, intermediate in Japan, and lowest in Hawaii. The percentage of men currently smoking cigarettes was highest in Japan, intermediate in Hawaii, and lowest in California. Most of these differences between the Japan cohort and the two migrant cohorts were statistically significant.

Table 9-3 shows age-adjusted means of nutrient intake for the three cohorts. The assessment of dietary intake was carried out using the 24-hour recall method in all study sites (Kato et al., 1973). Both the Hawaii and the California cohorts had substantially higher percentages of total calories derived from animal protein and fat, as well as a higher intake of dietary cholesterol than the Japan cohort. Animal protein accounted for 50 percent of total protein in Japan and 75 percent in both Hawaii and California. Similarly, saturated fat accounted for only 40 percent of total fat in Japan and 70 percent in both Hawaii and California. In contrast, percentages of total calories derived from carbohydrates, especially complex carbohydrates, and alcohol were significantly greater in Japan than in Hawaii and California.

Table 9-4 shows age-adjusted prevalence rates per 1,000 men of definite or

TABLE 9-2   Age-Adjusted Means and Percentages of Selected Variables at Baseline Examination for the Ni-Hon-San Study

Variable	Japan	Hawaii	California
Body mass index (kg/m^2)	21	24[a]	24[a]
Systolic blood pressure (mm Hg)	134	134	138[a]
Diastolic blood pressure (mm Hg)	84	82	88[a]
Serum cholesterol (mg/dL)	186	218[a]	225[a]
Serum glucose (mg/dL)	145	162[a]	160[a]
Current smokers (%)	76	44[a]	35[a]

[a]Significantly different from Japan ($p < .05$).

TABLE 9-3 Age-Adjusted Mean Intake of Nutrients at Baseline Examination for the Ni-Hon-San Study

Variable	Japan	Hawaii	California
Total calories	2,190	2,267	2,262
Total protein (% of calories)	14	17	16
Animal protein (% of calories)	7	12	12
Total fat (% of calories)	15	33	38
Total carbohydrate (% of calories)	63	46	44
Complex carbohydrate (% of calories)	51	30	27
Alcohol (% of calories)	9	4	3
Cholesterol (mg)	468	544	533

possible myocardial infarction diagnosed at the baseline exam, 2-year incidence rates of definite coronary heart disease (nonfatal myocardial infarction and fatal coronary heart disease), and 12-year incidence rates of fatal coronary heart disease per 1,000 person-years by place. These rates follow the same stepwise increase from Japan to Hawaii to California as was shown in the earlier reported mortality rates and indicate that this pattern was not due to statistical or diagnostic differences in the three areas.

Studies comparing the incidence of coronary heart disease among the Ni-Hon-San Study cohorts found that the major risk factors predicted the risk of coronary heart disease in a generally consistent way in all cohorts, and that the differences in the incidence of or mortality from coronary heart disease could be largely explained by the differences in the levels of known risk factors among indigenous Japanese men and among men of Japanese ancestry living in the United States (Robertson et al., 1977; Yano et al., 1988). For example, in regression of the incidence of coronary heart disease, the effects on baseline serum cholesterol were the same in Japan and Hawaii, but the distribution of serum cholesterol was much higher in Hawaii. Thus, we can infer that there can be a twofold to threefold difference in the risk of coronary heart disease among men of the same Japanese ancestry living in difference places and that the increased risks

TABLE 9-4 Age-Adjusted Prevalence and Incidence of Coronary Heart Disease Among Japanese Men by Place

Disease Measure	Japan	Hawaii	California
Prevalence of myocardial infarction by ECG/1,000	25.0	35.0	45.0
2-year incidence of definite CHD/1,000 person-years	1.4	3.0	4.3
12-year incidence of fatal CHD/1,000 person-years	1.0	1.4	—

Note: ECG = electrocardiogram; CHD = coronary heart disease.

were due to social and behavioral influences of the place, which are manifested in differences in blood pressure, serum cholesterol, cigarette smoking, and obesity.

Cultural Pathways to Coronary Heart Disease in the Elderly

The first stage of understanding how the social and cultural environment of the United States affected the risk of coronary heart disease among the different generational subgroups was to verify whether the known biological risk factors were the major predictors of the incidence of the disease among the elderly men of Japanese ancestry in the Hawaii cohort.

At the third examination of the Hawaii cohort (1971-1973), 1,419 men were between ages 65 and 74 and were free of cardiovascular disease. Risk factor measures made at that time were used to predict the incidence of coronary heart disease during a 12-year follow-up period. Figure 9-2 shows the age-adjusted relative risks for developing coronary heart disease from Cox regression models with all variables included simultaneously. All of these risk factors were statistically significant for these older men, and the strength of the associations were similar to those found for middle-aged men (Benfante et al., 1989; Benfante and Reed, 1990; Reed and Benfante, 1992).

Having verified the importance of the biological risk factors for coronary heart disease among these Japanese men, we proceeded to examine the cultural experiences that might further our understanding of the international differences.

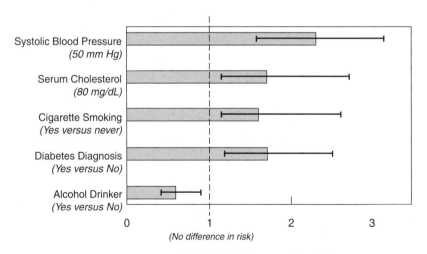

Relative Risk of Coronary Heart Disease

FIGURE 9-2 Age-adjusted multivariate relative risks (with 95% confidence limits) for developing coronary heart disease among elderly Japanese-American males during a 12-year follow-up period. Note: BP = blood pressure; Hx = diagnosis.

TABLE 9-5   Age-Adjusted 6-Year Incidence Rates of Total CHD/1,000 by
Birthplace and Years in Japan for Men Aged 60 to 68 at Baseline[a]

Birthplace and Years in Japan	Number at Risk	CHD Incidence
Japan (Issei)		
1-40	729	46
Hawaii-U.S. (Nisei)		
10+	108	46
1-9	136	73
0	179	75

[a]$p < .01$ from logistic regression models.
Note: CHD = coronary heart disease.

One of our first efforts was to focus on childhood experiences in terms of birth-place and the number of years spent in Japan.

Table 9-5 shows age-adjusted 6-year incidence rates of total coronary heart disease for men aged 60 to 68 at the initial examination, by place of birth and number of years in Japan. The rates were lowest for Issei men born in Japan and for the Nisei who were sent to Japan for 10 or more years of schooling. The rates were over 60 percent higher for Nisei who never went to Japan, and for those who spent less than 10 years in Japan. These differences were statistically significant in logistic regression models that included age (Yano et al., 1979).

Another approach was to analyze the baseline risk factor levels for the two groups. Risk factor levels were compared for 823 Issei and 2,070 Nisei (with less than 10 years in Japan), all aged 55 to 68 at the initial examination. As Table 9-6 shows, the Issei men born in Japan had significantly lower levels of all major risk factors for coronary heart disease except for serum glucose and cigarette-pack years. Additional analyses indicated that the Issei usually ate a more tradi-

TABLE 9-6   Age-Adjusted Levels of Selected CHD Risk Factors at Baseline
Exam by Generation Subgroup for Men Aged 55 to 68

Variable	Issei ($N = 823$)	Nisei ($N = 2,070$)
Systolic blood pressure (mm Hg)	136	138[a]
Diastolic blood pressure (mm Hg)	81	83[a]
Serum cholesterol (mg/dL)	214	218[a]
Serum triglyceride (mg/dL)	193	229[a]
Serum glucose (mg/dL)	171	170
Physical activity index	34	32[a]
Body mass index (kg/m^2)	23.2	23.6[a]
Cigarette-pack years	26	24

[a]$p < .05$ for age-adjusted group mean differences.
Note: CHD = coronary heart disease.

tional Japanese diet, with significantly lower levels of total fat and saturated fatty acids. When incidence rates of definite coronary heart disease over a 23-year follow-up period were adjusted for the major risk factors, there were no statistically significant differences between the generational subgroups. This finding indicates that the difference in risk for coronary heart disease can be accounted for by the differences in known risk factors.

More detailed studies of acculturation, that is, cultural change from Japanese to Western lifestyle, were made on a subset of 4,653 men in the Hawaii cohort who completed a sociocultural questionnaire in 1971 and were followed for the incidence of definite coronary heart disease for 7 years (Reed et al., 1982, 1983, 1984). Acculturation items were grouped as follows:

1. Culture of upbringing: these items measured exposure to Japanese influences during childhood, including years of Japanese language school, years in Japan, childhood religion, and ethnicity of childhood friends.

2. Cultural assimilation: these items measured the degree to which an individual maintained Japanese cultural forms during adult life, including language use and religion.

3. Social assimilation: these items measured the degree to which an individual had maintained contact with Japanese ethnic groups and customs in the community.

4. Total acculturation: this was a summary score of all items.

When the men were grouped into quartiles of acculturation scores, there was a statistically significant inverse association between the total acculturation score and the incidence of coronary heart disease of all kinds as shown in Table 9-7.

Age-adjusted baseline risk factor levels were then calculated for men in quartiles of the total acculturation score. Table 9-8 shows that men in the most Western groups consistently had levels indicating higher risk. They were more obese, were less physically active, smoked more cigarettes, had higher serum cholesterol levels, ate less complex carbohydrate, and drank less alcohol than men in the more traditional Japanese groups. There were no differences in socioeconomic status among these groups.

When each acculturation score was included in multiple logistic models that also included the major biological risk factors, none of the acculturation scores were associated with any clinical measure of coronary heart disease (Reed et al., 1982). In separate analyses, we also looked at individual questions used in the scores. The frequency of speaking or reading Japanese was the only item that was significantly inversely associated with the incidence of coronary heart disease of all kinds in the presence of the other risk factors.

Rates of coronary heart disease have been linked to a variety of theoretically stressful psychosocial factors, including rapid culture change, social alienation, and value conflicts. Social support networks theoretically provide protection

TABLE 9-7   Age-Adjusted 7-year CHD Incidence Rates/1,000 by Quartiles of
Total Acculturation Scores

Quartiles	Total CHD[a]	Fatal Myocardial Infarction	Nonfatal Myocardial Infarction[b]	Angina
1, most Western	62	15	32	15
2	43	16	19	8
3	50	21	15	14
4, most Japanese	35	16	14	5

[a]$p = .02$.
[b]$p = .06$.
Note: CHD = coronary heart disease.
The probability level was obtained from bivariate logistic regression of acculturation score and age
on CHD incidence.

against such forms of social stress. We were able to examine these hypotheses
within the Hawaii cohort, using the 4,653 men who completed the detailed questionnaire in 1971 and who were followed for 7-year incidence of coronary heart
disease (Reed et al., 1983, 1984).

The general pattern of results indicated that such psychosocial processes as
geographic mobility, generational mobility, sociocultural inconsistency, and occupational stress were not associated with the incidence of coronary heart disease
or with other chronic diseases of the elderly men in this cohort. Measures of
social support networks were inversely associated in bivariate analyses with age,
but in multivariate models that included the main risk factors, the associations
were not statistically significant (Reed et al., 1983). Furthermore, there were no

TABLE 9-8   Age-Adjusted Mean Values of Selected Risk Factors by
Quartiles of the Total Acculturation Score

Risk Factors	Quartiles[a]			
	1	2	3	4
Systolic blood pressure (mm Hg)	133	134	134	134
Serum cholesterol (mg/dL)	221	220	218	215[b]
Serum glucose (mg/dL)	160	161	159	157
Body mass index (kg/m^2)	26	24	24	23[b]
Physical activity index	31	33	34	35[b]
Cigarettes/day	11	9	9	7[b]
Alcohol (ounces/month)	10	12	13	15[b]
Complex carbohydrate (grams/24 hr.)	161	167	171	176[b]
Socioeconomic status	2.0	1.9	2.1	2.0

[a]Quartiles reflect a scale based on the most Western or non-Japanese response quartile to the most
traditional Japanese response quartile.

[b]$p < .05$ from bivariate multiple regression of risk factor and age on acculturation score.

significant interactions indicating that social support networks were especially protective for men in stressful social or occupational situations.

DISCUSSION

The major inferences from the Ni-Hon-San studies can be summarized as follows: (1) there is a twofold to threefold higher risk of coronary heart disease among Japanese men in the United States compared with Japanese men in Japan, and (2) this difference can be accounted for largely by differences in the major risk factors, especially serum cholesterol, serum glucose, blood pressure, smoking, and alcohol intake. Thus, while we know of genetic determinants of some of these risk factors, the behavioral influences appear to play an overwhelming role. These behavioral influences can affect all groups migrating from low-risk to high-risk areas; our recognition of the significance of these influences points out the importance of prevention efforts to lower the risk of coronary heart disease. The path, however, is two way; we can predict that the rapid westernization taking place in Japan will result in an appreciable increase in the occurrence of coronary heart disease within the next few decades unless preventive measures are taken.

The studies of groups by birthplace and acculturation within the Hawaii cohort confirmed that the major risk factors for coronary heart disease in middle-aged U.S. males also predicted the incidence of coronary heart disease in elderly Japanese Americans in Hawaii. In addition, it was clear that the experiences of early life, in terms of exposure to traditional Japanese culture and lifestyle, profoundly influence the risk of coronary heart disease in late life by affecting the known biological and behavioral risk factors. The most common pattern was a change from a traditional Japanese lifestyle involving high physical activity to a sedentary lifestyle along with a change from an Asian diet low in animal fat and protein to a high-calorie, high-fat Western diet; these changes lead to obesity, hypertension, diabetes, and high serum cholesterol.

We found no independent association between sociocultural measures and the risk of coronary heart disease, with the single exception of Japanese language ability, which could also be an indirect measure of exposure to Japanese diet during childhood. This does not mean that cultural influences are unimportant. On the contrary, they are among the most important determinants of health behavior. Our goal should be to understand which cultural characteristics, such as a Japanese diet, are healthy and to support their continuation while at the same time focusing on decreasing such unhealthy characteristics as cigarette smoking. We should also be aware that some risk factors may help protect against developing one disease and increase the likelihood of developing another. It is therefore important to concentrate on risk factors that are common denominators for numerous diseases. Cigarette smoking, a high-fat diet, obesity, and hypertension are good examples.

There was no evidence from these studies that psychosocial measures of theoretically stressful life situations were predictive of the incidence of coronary heart disease. Since this field of study is complicated and the Japanese Americans under study were unique in many characteristics, it would be a mistake to extrapolate these findings to other cultures. We would, however, put a low priority on this type of research.

We had no information on access to and use of health care for the Hawaii cohort. Socioeconomic status as measured by education, type of housing, and occupation had no independent association with the risk of coronary heart disease in this cohort, but it should be noted that the range was narrow and that health care in Hawaii has been available to nearly everyone.

To our knowledge, there are no other prospective studies of cardiovascular disease among Asians living in the United States. There are, however, several cross-sectional surveys of risk factors for cardiovascular disease that provide some interesting comparisons. A study of risk factors among 346 elderly Chinese immigrants in Boston showed that they had lower levels of obesity, blood pressure, and serum cholesterol and that they ate less fat and more carbohydrate than elderly whites (Choi et al., 1990).

A 1979 study of hypertension among four Asian and Pacific Island groups in California showed great variation among the different Asian ethnic groups (Stavig et al., 1984). Filipinos had the highest rates of hypertension and Japanese the lowest. The authors implied that change in dietary patterns involving adoption of American foods resulted in increased obesity and hypertension.

A more recent study of risk factors for cardiovascular disease among over 13,000 Asian Americans in California confirmed the existence of important differences among the different Asian subgroups (Klatsky and Armstrong, 1991). Of interest was the finding that obesity was higher among U.S.-born Asian-American men than among men born in Asia. Cigarette smoking, however, was higher among U.S.-born women than among their Asian-born counterparts. These findings indicated that cultural influences differ by sex.

FUTURE RESEARCH

The findings from the Ni-Hon-San studies are consistent with those of studies of other populations that have migrated from areas of low to high risk of coronary heart disease. All support the concept that differences in the occurrence of coronary heart disease are due mainly to specific behavioral and lifestyle characteristics that are influenced by social and cultural standards. Modification of high-risk behavior offers the clearest and most effective way to prevent cardiovascular disease and the resulting physical disability in the elderly. Because it is also well established that the underlying disease process of atherosclerosis begins in childhood and progresses through adult life (Wissler, 1991), major efforts need to be directed towards children and young adults.

We would therefore suggest two levels of activities for future research. The first would focus on children and young adults. There is a need to determine current levels of the risk factors that are common denominators for the major chronic diseases of late life among different ethnic subgroups. As noted earlier, cigarette smoking, obesity, physical inactivity, and a high-fat diet are open to modification. Once high- and low-risk groups are identified, there is a need to determine which cultural characteristics promote healthy and unhealthy behaviors, and which are open to influence.

The second focus would be on communities. What elements within a community promote healthy and unhealthy behaviors? A growing body of literature indicates that it is possible to alter risk factor levels through intervention at the community rather than the individual level (Farquhar et al., 1990). Food preparation in school lunch programs and community efforts to reduce cigarette smoking are examples of this kind of intervention.

In summary, we believe that a major part of the differences in the risk of coronary heart disease among ethnic groups can be accounted for by a small number of known biological and behavioral factors. Studies of migrants and native-born groups show that these risk factors can be modified by cultural influences. These findings also provide us with a realistic goal. If we cannot completely prevent a disease, we can attempt to reduce its occurrence to the level experienced by the group with the lowest risk.

REFERENCES

Benfante, R., and D. Reed
    1990   Is elevated serum cholesterol level a risk factor for coronary heart disease in the elderly? *Journal of the American Medical Association* 263:393-396.
Benfante, R.J., D.M. Reed, C.J. MacLean, and K. Yano
    1989   Risk factors in middle age that predict early and late onset of coronary heart disease. *Journal of Clinical Epidemiology* 42:95-104.
Choi, E.S., R.B. McGandy, G.E. Dallal, M.D. Russell, R.A. Jacob, E.J. Schaefer, and J.A. Sadowski
    1990   The prevalence of cardiovascular risk factors among elderly Chinese Americans. *Archives of Internal Medicine* 150:413-418.
Farquhar, J.W., S.P. Fortmann, J.A. Flora, C.B. Taylor, W.L. Haskell, P.T. Williams, N. Maccoby, and P.D. Wood
    1990   Effects of community wide education on cardiovascular disease risk factors. The Stanford Five-City Project. *Journal of the American Medical Association* 264:359-365.
Gordon, T.
    1957   Mortality experience among the Japanese in the United States, Hawaii, and California. *Public Health Reports* 72:543-553.
Kagan, A., B.R. Harris, W. Winkelstein Jr., K.G. Johnson, H. Kato, S.L. Syme, G.G. Rhoads, M.L. Gay, M.Z. Nichaman, and H.B. Hamilton
    1974   Epidemiologic studies of coronary heart disease and stroke in Japanese men living in Japan, Hawaii, and California: Demographic, physical, dietary, and biochemical characteristics. *Journal of Chronic Disease* 27:345-364.

Kato, H., J. Tillotson, M.Z. Nichaman, G.G. Rhoads, and H.B. Hamilton
  1973   Epidemiologic studies of coronary heart disease and stroke in Japanese men living in
          Japan, Hawaii, and California: Serum lipids and diet. *American Journal of Epidemiology*
          97:372-385.
Klatsky, A.L., and M.A. Armstrong
  1991   Cardiovascular risk factors among Asian Americans living in northern California. *American Journal of Public Health* 81:1423-1428.
Marmot, M.G., S.L. Syme, A. Kagan, H. Kato, J.B. Cohen, and J. Belsky
  1975   Epidemiologic studies of coronary heart disease and stroke in Japanese men living in
          Japan, Hawaii, and California: Prevalence of coronary and hypertensive heart disease
          and associated risk factors. *American Journal of Epidemiology* 102:514-525.
Nichaman, M.Z., H.B. Hamilton, A. Kagan, T. Grier, S.T. Sacks, and S.L. Syme
  1975   Epidemiologic studies of coronary heart disease and stroke in Japanese men living in
          Japan, Hawaii, and California: Distribution of biochemical risk factors. *American Journal of Epidemiology* 102:491-501.
Reed, D., and R. Benfante
  1992   Lipid and lipoprotein predictors of coronary heart disease in elderly men in the Honolulu
          Heart Program. *Annals of Epidemiology* 2:29-34.
Reed, D., D. McGee, J. Cohen, K. Yano, S. Syme, and M. Feinleib
  1982   Acculturation and coronary heart disease among Japanese men in Hawaii. *American Journal of Epidemiology* 115:894-905.
Reed, D., D. McGee, and K. Yano
  1984   Psychosocial processes and general susceptibility to chronic disease. *American Journal of Epidemiology* 119:356-370.
Reed, D., D. McGee, K. Yano, and M. Feinleib
  1983   Social networks and coronary heart disease among Japanese men in Hawaii. *American Journal of Epidemiology* 117:384-396.
Robertson, T.L., H. Kato, G.G. Rhoads, A. Kagan, M.G. Marmot, S.L. Syme, T. Gordon, R.M.
Worth, J.L. Belsky, D.S. Dock, M. Miyanishi, and S. Kawamoto
  1977   Epidemiologic studies of coronary heart disease and stroke in Japanese men living in
          Japan, Hawaii, and California. Incidence of myocardial infarction and death from coronary heart disease. *American Journal of Cardiology* 39:239-243.
Stavig, G.R., A. Igda, and A.R. Leonard
  1984   Hypertension among Asian and Pacific Islanders in California. *American Journal of Epidemiology* 119:677-691.
Wissler, R.W.
  1991   USA multicenter study of the pathobiology of atherosclerosis in youth. *Annals of the New York Academy of Science* 623:26-39.
Worth, R.M., H. Kato, C.G. Rhoads, A. Kagan, and S.L. Syme
  1975   Epidemiologic studies of coronary heart disease and stroke in Japanese men living in
          Japan, Hawaii, and California: Mortality. *American Journal of Epidemiology* 102:481-490.
Yano, K., W.C. Blackwelder, A. Kagan, G.G. Rhoads, J.B. Cohen, and M.G. Marmot
  1979   Childhood cultural experience and the incidence of coronary heart disease in Hawaii
          Japanese men. *American Journal of Epidemiology* 109:440-450.
Yano, K., C.J. MacLean, D.M. Reed, Y. Shimizu, H. Sasaki, K. Kodama, H. Kato, and A. Kagan
  1988   A comparison of the 12-year mortality and predictive factors of coronary heart disease
          among Japanese men in Japan and Hawaii. *American Journal of Epidemiology* 127:476-487.

10

Health Status of Hispanic Elderly

Kyriakos S. Markides, Laura Rudkin, Ronald J. Angel, and David V. Espino

INTRODUCTION

Hispanics represent one of the fastest growing segments of America's elderly population. Although Hispanics accounted for only 3.7 percent of the 65 and older population in 1990, their share is projected to increase to 15.5 percent by the middle of the next century (Bureau of the Census, 1993). The future increases in the numbers and proportions of elderly Hispanics will be fueled by the recent rapid growth in the total number of U.S. Hispanics. Persons of Hispanic origin numbered 22.4 million in the 1990 census; this makes them the second largest minority population in the nation (Bureau of the Census, 1991). During the 1980s, this population increased by 53 percent, considerably faster than the general population.

By far the largest segment of the Hispanic population (61.2%) is of Mexican origin and resides primarily in the southwestern states of California, Texas, Arizona, Colorado, and New Mexico; they are followed by Puerto Ricans (12.1%), who live mainly in Puerto Rico and the New York City area, and by Cuban Americans (4.8%), who are concentrated in south Florida (Bureau of the Census, 1991). A variety of other Hispanic populations originating in various Central and South American countries live principally in the Northeast. The elderly Hispanic population in the United States reflects this diversity, although the distribution across subgroups differs in the older population. In 1990, roughly half (49%) of Hispanic elders were of Mexican origin, 15 percent were of Cuban origin, and 12 percent were of Puerto Rican origin. The relatively large proportion of Cuban-origin elders is due to the older age distribution of this subgroup. In general,

285

Hispanics are a relatively youthful population, with only 5 percent being 65 and older (Bureau of the Census, 1993), but that proportion varies markedly across the ethnic subgroups. Less than 5 percent of Mexican Americans and Puerto Ricans are in the elderly age group, whereas 17 percent of Cuban Americans are elderly (Bureau of the Census, 1990).

The limited gerontological research on older Hispanics has tended to focus on the importance of the strength of family ties and how these might be changing with greater industrialization, urbanization, and the acculturation of younger generations into the larger society (Angel and Hogan, 1991; Bastida, 1984; Lacayo, 1992; Markides and Martin, 1983; Paz, 1993; Sotomayor and Garcia, 1993). Despite increases in education and acculturation across generations, the elderly in various Hispanic groups appear to enjoy good relationships with their children (Markides et al., 1986), experiencing closer proximity, more frequent contact, and stronger familial attitudes than Anglo elderly (Keefe and Padilla, 1987; Sabogal et al., 1987).

Other research has pointed out the needs of Hispanic elderly for health and social services, has emphasized the importance of linguistic and cultural barriers to adequate service provision, and has discussed the need for culturally sensitive health care and social services (e.g., Ginzberg, 1991; Ramirez de Arellano, 1994; Wolinsky et al., 1989). The literature on the non-Cuban Hispanic elderly has emphasized their low education, low incomes, and generally low political power and socioeconomic standing in society (e.g., Sotomayor and Garcia, 1993).

MORTALITY AND LIFE EXPECTANCY

Despite their disadvantaged socioeconomic status, Hispanics appear to have a generally favorable mortality profile (see reviews by Hayes-Bautista, 1992; Markides and Coreil, 1986; Rosenwaike, 1991; Vega and Amaro, 1994). As early as 1970, regional epidemiological evidence suggested that Spanish surnamed persons (largely Mexican Americans) had a life expectancy only slightly below that of Anglos and markedly higher than that of blacks (Bradshaw and Fonner, 1978; Schoen and Nelson, 1981; Siegel and Passel, 1979). Regional data for 1980 indicated that the already small Hispanic-Anglo gap in life expectancy had narrowed even further (California Center for Health Statistics, 1984; Gillespie and Sullivan, 1983). More recently, national data have provided more definitive evidence that older Hispanics appear to be advantaged relative to both Anglos and blacks in terms of mortality (Sorlie et al., 1993; National Center for Health Statistics, 1994).

For the period 1989-1991, Hispanics in the age group 65 to 74 experienced 1,975 deaths per 100,000 population. In comparison, non-Hispanic whites had a death rate of 2,575 and blacks a death rate of 3,735. The Hispanic advantage held for deaths due to heart disease, cancer, stroke, and all other causes combined. Middle-aged (45 to 64 years) Hispanics experienced a similar advantage in rates of death due to heart disease and cancer. Only Asian Americans experienced more favorable mortality conditions at the older ages (see National Center for Health Statistics, 1994).

A recent analysis of the National Longitudinal Mortality Study has added further evidence of a favorable mortality and health situation for Hispanics. This prospective study has found lower death rates for middle-aged (45 to 64) and older (65 and over) Hispanics than for non-Hispanic whites (Sorlie et al., 1993). The Hispanic advantage holds for both genders and for all Hispanic subgroups, although some of the differences were not statistically significant owing to the small number of deaths. Overall, for every 10 deaths among non-Hispanic white males and females aged 65 or older, Hispanic males experienced 7.2 deaths and Hispanic women 8.2 deaths. As might be expected, when adjustments for income were introduced, the relative Hispanic advantage was even greater for all causes of death (all causes, cardiovascular disease, cancer, and all other causes combined) for men of all ages and women younger than 65. Adjustments for income did not influence the relative mortality risks of older women.

The analysis by Sorlie et al. (1993) of mortality by specific cause, which combined all ages (25 and over) because of small numbers, showed Hispanic adults to have lower rates of death for most cancers and cardiovascular diseases when compared with non-Hispanic whites. Both Hispanic men and women experienced this advantage, a contradiction of earlier regional research that had suggested the advantage in cardiovascular disease was confined to males, at least among the Mexican-origin population (Mitchell et al., 1990). In contrast, one recent analysis did not reveal an advantage for Mexican-American males in mortality from ischemic coronary disease and myocardial infarction (Espino et al., 1994). These data, however, were confined to 1 year in one city, San Antonio. The national data on mortality from specific cancers are consistent with previous data suggesting that Hispanics have a relatively lower incidence of major cancers, such as lung, colon, breast, and prostate cancers. At the same time, it has been found that Hispanics have a higher incidence of stomach, liver, gallbladder, and cervical cancer, all generally low-incidence cancers not considered separately in the analysis by Sorlie and colleagues. (For discussions of cancer incidence in Hispanic populations, see Gutierrez-Ramirez et al., 1994; Markides and Coreil, 1986; Montes, 1989; Polednak, 1989; and Trapido et al., 1990.)

The analysis of the National Longitudinal Mortality Study did identify excess risk for Hispanics on two main causes of death. Consistent with past research, Sorlie et al. (1993) found that mortality rates from diabetes were roughly twice as high among Hispanic men and women than among non-Hispanics. Hispanics of both genders also experienced higher rates of death from liver disease/cirrhosis. Whereas this finding was expected for males, the female excess is a surprise because of the relatively low alcohol consumption rates among Hispanic women (Black and Markides, 1993).

The Hispanic mortality advantage appears to be shared by all of the major subgroups, although some diversity among the groups is evident. The advantage appears to be more marked for men than for women among older Mexican Americans and Puerto Ricans, and the largest advantage is observed for older Cuban Americans of both genders (Sorlie et al., 1993). Of the three major Hispanic groups, Puerto Ricans appear to have the highest age-adjusted mortality rates and Cuban Americans the lowest (Rosenwaike, 1991; Sorlie et al., 1993). Among Puerto Ricans, mortality rates are higher for residents of New York City than for those living in Puerto Rico or elsewhere in the United States. The excess mortality among New York City Puerto Ricans is primarily due to higher death rates from homicide and from cirrhosis of the liver (Rosenwaike and Hempstead, 1990). Comparisons among Hispanic groups also reveal that the Mexican-origin population has higher mortality from accidents, but lower suicide rates than the populations of Cuban and Puerto Rican origin. Puerto Ricans have the highest death rate from cirrhosis of the liver, and the populations of both Puerto Rican and Mexican origin have higher death rates from diabetes than do Cuban Americans. The mortality profile of Cuban Americans by cause of death is generally similar to that of the non-Hispanic white population (Rosenwaike, 1991).

The generally favorable mortality and health profile of Hispanics has been attributed both to possible protective cultural factors and to selective immigration. It is becoming increasingly evident that immigrants tend to be healthier than native-born persons at any age (Stephen et al., 1994), and large rates of Hispanic immigration in recent decades are no doubt a factor contributing to a favorable health profile. Foreign-born Hispanic males experience significantly lower death rates in middle and old age than do native-born Hispanic males, whereas among females, death rates are significantly lower for the foreign born only in middle age (Sorlie et al., 1993). These analyses suggest the operation of a "healthy-migrant" effect to explain the low mortality of Hispanics. However, even when place of birth is adjusted for, Hispanic rates remained lower for men and women in middle age and for men in old age.

EXPLAINING THE HISPANIC ADVANTAGE IN HEART DISEASE AND CANCER MORTALITY

Why Hispanics, especially men, appear to have an advantage in mortality from heart disease and cancer, remains a bit of a mystery. In addition to being socioeconomically disadvantaged, Hispanics tend to have risk profiles for chronic disease that are similar to or worse than the risk profiles of Anglos (e.g., Castro et al., 1985; Diehl and Stern, 1989; Mitchell et al., 1990; Samet et al., 1988). The development of chronic disease begins with health behaviors and conditions at younger ages. Therefore, most studies addressing risk factors, including those discussed in this section, focus on adults of all ages, not specifically elderly persons.

Studies have shown that compared with Anglos, Mexican Americans are more likely to have been diagnosed with diabetes (Samet et al., 1988), are more likely to be obese (Balcazar and Cobas, 1993; Mitchell et al., 1990; Samet et al., 1988; Winkleby et al., 1993), and are more likely to experience upper-body obesity (Haffner et al., 1986). Mixed results have been obtained regarding ethnic differences in hypertension. Some studies report that Hispanics have higher prevalence than Anglos (Mitchell et al., 1990; Stern et al., 1987; Kraus et al., 1980); other studies find Hispanics to have lower prevalence rates (Franco et al., 1985; Sorel et al., 1991; Pappas et al., 1990; Samet et al., 1988), and at least one study finds no ethnic differential in hypertension rates (Winkleby et al., 1993). Cholesterol levels among Hispanics have been reported to be lower than Anglos (Mitchell et al., 1990), higher than Anglos (Kraus et al., 1980; Winkelby et al., 1993), and not significantly different (Derenowski, 1990). Likewise, results regarding ethnic differentials in physical activity have been mixed (Haffner et al., 1986; Markides and Coreil, 1986; Winkleby et al., 1993).

Acculturation has been shown to be associated with risk factors for chronic disease. For example, recently analyzed data from the Hispanic Health and Nutrition Examination Survey (Hispanic HANES) found that acculturation was positively related to the presence of hypertension in Mexican Americans aged 55 to 74, suggesting that the prevalence of hypertension may very well increase as the population becomes more acculturated into the larger society (Espino and Maldonado, 1990). Acculturation has also been found to be negatively related to both diabetes and obesity (Hazuda et al., 1988), suggesting the possibility of some health benefits from becoming acculturated.

Unpublished data from the recently conducted Hispanic Established Populations for the Epidemiologic Study of the Elderly (EPESE) that covered 3,050 Mexican Americans aged 65 and over from the five southwestern states (conducted by the authors) do not support the notion that rates of hypertension are lower among Mexican Americans, at least among the elderly. Data from this representative sample indicate that approximately 44 percent of Mexican-American elderly report being hypertensive (having been told by a doctor) compared with approximately 39 percent in a national sample interviewed in 1985-1987 (National Center for Health Statistics, 1993). As in the general population, hypertension rates were significantly higher among females than among males. Moreover, the Mexican-American excess in hypertension is confined to females. Among Mexican-American males, as among males in the general population, the prevalence of hypertension declines somewhat from ages 65 to 74 to ages 75 and over. Female rates, in contrast, show a slight increase, suggesting the operation of greater selective survival among males at advanced ages.

Another factor that may be related to low rates of both heart disease and cancer mortality in Mexican Americans is the population's traditionally low cigarette smoking rates. Among males, however, these rates have gone up in recent years and are now equal to, if not higher than, other groups (Haynes et al., 1990). Hispanic females have relatively low smoking rates, but these increase with acculturation (Coreil et al., 1991). Data from the Hispanic HANES (Rogers, 1991) show that smoking rates among Puerto Ricans in the Northeast have increased substantially in recent years and may very well translate into higher rates of heart disease and smoking-related cancers. These data show high smoking rates among males in all three major Hispanic populations (Mexican Americans, mainland Puerto Ricans, and Cuban Americans). However, Mexican-American males smoke significantly fewer cigarettes compared with males in the general population and other Hispanic males. Cuban-American males smoke the most, which is consistent with their high lung cancer mortality rates.

Alcohol consumption is another important health behavior to consider. As mentioned earlier, Mexican-American and Puerto Rican men have high mortality from cirrhosis of the liver, which is probably related to heavy use of alcohol. Data for Mexican-American men indicate continued heavy use into late middle age, but rather low rates of consumption in old age (Markides et al, 1990; Rogers, 1991). Mexican-American women have low alcohol use, with alcohol consumption being positively associated with acculturation, at least among younger women (Black and Markides, 1993). Heavy drinking rates are also high among Puerto Rican males (Rogers, 1991), while Cuban American males exhibit more moderate consumption patterns similar to those in the general population (Black and Markides, 1994). Of the three Hispanic groups, Puerto Rican Americans exhibit the highest consumption of hard liquor at any age and in both genders (Rogers, 1991).

When all the above evidence is considered, any advantage in heart disease and cancer in Mexican Americans and Puerto Ricans is difficult to explain. However, this advantage appears to be narrowing and may very well disappear in the near future as more Hispanics adopt the lifestyle of the larger society. Why the advantage appears to be greater among men is not clear, except that older Hispanic males, especially Mexican Americans, may be survivors from cohorts experiencing high mortality in earlier years.

OTHER DISEASES

Whereas Hispanics may be advantaged in some major diseases, they are disadvantaged in others. For example, both Mexican Americans and Puerto Ricans have high rates of diabetes. Various research projects have shown that the prevalence rate of non-insulin-dependent diabetes mellitus is two to five times greater among Mexican Americans than among the general population. Higher prevalence is present in all age groups, with the risk being highest in older Mexican-American women (Stern and Haffner, 1990).

Factors related to the high prevalence of diabetes in Hispanics include high rates of obesity and high levels of poverty. However, even after these factors are controlled for, Mexican Americans have substantially higher rates of diabetes than non-Hispanic whites. There has been speculation that genetic factors are involved, related to the high degree of American Indian admixture found in Mexican Americans (Diehl and Stern, 1989; Stern and Haffner, 1990). Puerto Ricans also have significant rates of Indian admixture as well as a significant degree of African-American ancestry. Cuban Americans, on the other hand, do not appear to have substantially higher rates of diabetes than non-Hispanic whites (Rogers, 1991).

The high prevalence of diabetes among Mexican Americans is also present in persons 65 and over. Data from the Hispanic EPESE indicate that approximately 23 percent of elderly Mexican Americans report having been told by a doctor that they have diabetes compared with approximately 10 percent in the general population (National Center for Health Statistics, 1993). Moreover, both male and female rates among Mexican Americans decline significantly from ages 65 to 74 to ages 75 and older, a situation that does not occur in the general population. This finding underscores the much higher negative consequences of diabetes among Mexican Americans, including higher mortality rates. Previous literature has suggested that not only do Mexican Americans have higher diabetes prevalence and mortality, but they are also more likely to suffer severe complications of the disease than are diabetics in the general population (Stern and Haffner, 1990).

Other diseases of high prevalence in Hispanics, including the elderly, include infectious and parasitic diseases, influenza and pneumonia, tuberculosis, and gallstone disease, at least in Mexican Americans (Carter-Pokra, 1994; Vega and Amaro, 1994). Gallstone disease appears to be associated with the population's high degree of American-Indian admixture, much like the case with diabetes (Diehl and Stern, 1989; Mauer et al., 1990). Research by Mauer et al. (1990) shows that among Hispanics, Mexican Americans of both genders have a higher prevalence of gallstone disease than do Puerto Ricans or Cuban Americans.

Recent research in San Antonio has found that for Mexican Americans of both sexes the risk for hip fracture is lower than for other whites, but higher than for African Americans. Other research showed that Mexican-American women are at substantially lower risk for vertebral fracture. Both these findings have led to speculation about the need for different recommendations regarding prophylactic treatment for osteoporosis in Mexican-American women compared with other white women (Bauer and Deyo, 1987).

Data from Los Angeles, from San Antonio, and from the Hispanic HANES southwestern sample have also suggested that the prevalence of arthritis might be lower among middle-aged and older Mexican Americans (Espino et al., 1991). However, these data are based on small numbers of older people. Data from the Hispanic EPESE show that approximately 41 percent of Mexican-American elderly report having arthritis compared with over 50 percent in the general elderly population (Guralnik et al., 1989).

FUNCTIONAL LIMITATIONS

While data on mortality and disease prevalence are important in describing the health status of populations, functional health indicators also provide information that is particularly important among the elderly. Data on the functional limitations of Hispanic elderly have been lacking until recently. Limited information, mostly on Mexican Americans, has traditionally suggested that the functional health of Hispanic elderly is slightly worse than the functional health of other whites and better than that of African Americans (Markides et al., 1989). More recent data show the same: in 1986, for example, 19.2 percent of Hispanics 65 and older reported needing assistance with everyday activities, compared with 22.7 percent of African Americans and 15.4 of whites (Bureau of the Census, 1992). The recently conducted Hispanic EPESE makes it possible to compare data on specific functional limitations among Mexican-American elderly in the Southwest with national estimates for whites and African Americans. Table 10-1 presents such comparisons for five activities of daily living. The table shows that more Mexican Americans than whites and nonwhites report difficulty with eating, toileting, and dressing. On bathing and transferring (out of a bed), Mexican Americans report greater difficulty than whites but less than nonwhites. As Table 10-2 shows, with respect to four instrumental activities of daily living (meal preparation, shopping, using the telephone, and performing light housework), Mexican-American elderly are more dependent than both white and nonwhite elderly.

Data from a 1988 survey of elderly Hispanics permits comparisons across the ethnic subgroups on rates of difficulty with activities of daily living and instrumental activities of daily living. Regarding the activities of daily living (bathing, dressing, eating, etc.), Mexican-origin and Cuban-origin elders exhibit comparable rates of functional limitations, whereas Puerto Ricans report consistently higher rates of limitation. Older Puerto Ricans and Mexican Americans tend to report greater difficulty in performing instrumental activities of daily

TABLE 10-1   Percentage of Persons 65 and Older Reporting Difficulty Performing Selected Activities of Daily Living by Ethnicity

Activities of Daily Living	Whites (N = 24,753)	Nonwhites (N = 2,784)	Mexican Americans (N = 3,050)
Eating	1.9	1.3	5.4
Toileting	4.4	7.0	7.5
Dressing	5.7	8.6	9.6
Bathing	9.5	14.0	11.8
Transferring out of a bed	8.2	11.6	8.9

SOURCE: Data on whites and nonwhites are from the 1986 National Health Interview Survey (National Center for Health Statistics, 1993). Data on Mexican Americans are from the 1993-1994 Hispanic EPESE.

TABLE 10-2   Percentage of Persons 65 and Older Reporting Difficulty
Performing Instrumental Activities of Daily Living by Ethnicity

Instrumental Activities of Daily Living	Whites (N = 24,753)	Nonwhites (N = 2,784)	Mexican Americans (N = 3,050)
Meal preparation	6.6	12.8	14.0
Shopping	12.1	18.8	22.3
Using telephone	4.8	6.7	11.2
Light housework	11.2	12.8	15.6

SOURCE: Data on whites and nonwhites are from the 1986 National Health Interview Survey (National Center for Health Statistics, 1993). Data on Mexican Americans are from the 1993-1994 Hispanic EPESE.

living (preparing meals, managing money, shopping, housework, etc.) than do older Cuban Americans. The data also confirm that Hispanic elderly face higher rates of limitation on both categories of activities than does the general population of elderly persons (see Ramirez de Arellano, 1994).

SELF-ASSESSED HEALTH

Self-assessed health is frequently used as an indicator of global health status because it correlates with the entire range of health outcomes, including mortality and use of health care. Self-assessments are the result of complex subjective processes that are influenced by culture and temperament, as well as by actual health status (Angel and Guarnaccia, 1989; Angel and Thoits, 1987). Data from the Hispanic HANES corroborate other data showing that among Hispanics, Puerto Ricans rate their health as poorest and Cuban Americans rate their health as best, with Mexican Americans somewhere in between (Angel and Angel, 1992; Angel and Guarnaccia, 1989). Of course, factors besides group membership influence self-assessments of health. For example, findings from the Hispanic HANES show that although Puerto Ricans consistently rate their health as poorer than do Mexican Americans, for individuals in either group, depression lowers self-assessments of health independently of physician's evaluations. Among the elderly, social interaction, such as attending church, seeing friends, and engaging in group activities, is associated with better self-assessed health. In one study, social involvement of this sort largely accounts for the difference in self-assessed health between elderly Mexican Americans and Puerto Ricans (Angel and Angel, 1992).

Recent findings based on the Health and Retirement Survey show that Hispanics, especially Mexican Americans, are much more likely than non-Hispanic whites to rate their health as fair or poor, rather than as excellent, very good, or good (Angel and Angel, 1996). Speculation that this indicates that Hispanics are health pessimists may be premature since these same data show that a large fraction of African Americans also rate their health as fair or poor. In light of the occupational and health insurance disadvantages faced by poor and minority Americans, poorer self-assessments of health at all ages may be more a reflection of the real health risks they face than of a culturally based pessimistic outlook.

MENTAL HEALTH

More recently, however, there is increasing evidence of high rates of psychological distress among the elderly, particularly among women. One study of Mexican Americans yielded rates of depression that were very high among older women and very low among older men (Mendes de Leon and Markides, 1988); this parallels the findings on physical health discussed earlier and also suggests the potential presence of selective factors in the survival of males. Data from the Hispanic HANES yielded low rates of depressive symptoms among Mexican Americans aged 20 to 74 (Moscicki et al., 1989). Although no age differences were noted, rates were lower among the foreign born and the less acculturated, which is consistent with a healthy-migrant effect also suggested with respect to physical health. A similar finding was observed with the Los Angeles Epidemiologic Catchment Area Study (Burnam et al., 1987). These low rates compare with inconsistent findings of other literature comparing Mexican Americans and non-Hispanic whites (Vega and Rumbaut, 1991).

A different pattern has been observed among Puerto Ricans, who have been found to have higher rates of depression in New York than in Puerto Rico, and who also have higher rates than Mexican Americans, African Americans, and non-Hispanic whites. These patterns, along with relatively low rates among Cuban Americans in Miami, remain unexplained. However, they do provide useful insights for further research (Vega and Rumbaut, 1991). The numbers of older people in these studies were too small for meaningful analysis of age difference in depression (Moscicki et al., 1987).

At this point, we simply do not know what the prevalence of Alzheimer's disease and other dementias is among Hispanic elderly. Limited evidence, however, suggests that the typical Hispanic elderly person diagnosed with possible Alzheimer's disease is younger than is the case among the general population. Clearly, research utilizing appropriate instruments with large and representative samples is needed to give us a better picture of the mental health functioning of older Hispanics.

ISSUES IN MEDICAL CARE

There has been a long tradition of research with Hispanic populations that has suggested that the population underutilizes formal medical care, including psychiatric care. Suggested reasons for underutilization have included culturally inappropriate services and lack of adequate access to care because of low rates of insurance coverage and other factors. More recent data, however, suggest that elderly Hispanics utilize physicians at rates equal to or greater than those of Anglo elderly, leading to speculation that many Hispanics underutilize services until they turn 65, when most qualify for Medicare (Vega and Amaro, 1994). Data from the Hispanic EPESE suggest that the proportion of Mexican-American elderly in the Southwest who have Medicare is approximately 87 percent.

There is strong evidence that Hispanic elderly underutilize nursing homes, much as black elderly do. Possible factors behind these low rates include discrimination against members of minority groups and stronger family supports. Hispanic families may view the nursing home as a last resort; this is borne out by recent data from San Antonio suggesting that Hispanic nursing home residents are significantly more functionally impaired and have higher rates of mental impairment than Anglo residents (Chiodo et al., 1994; Espino and Burge, 1989).

Although elderly Hispanics may not underutilize physician services, there is evidence that they may delay seeking treatment for certain symptoms or conditions. This has been particularly noted in studies of cancer treatment in Texas and, more recently, New Mexico (Samet et al., 1988).

CONCLUSION

What does the available evidence tell us? With respect to mortality, there is accumulating evidence of a Hispanic advantage at least at ages 45 and above. This advantage is greater among men than women and results from lower cardiovascular and cancer mortality. However, the evidence on risk factors explaining such an advantage is mixed, and researchers have speculated about the protective effects of cultural factors such as strong family ties as well as selective immigration (Mitchell et al., 1990; Markides and Coreil, 1986). Recent data show that immigrant Hispanics have better health than native-born Hispanics (Stephen et al., 1994). Age-adjusted proportions of persons 18 years and older show that immigrant Hispanics were slightly less likely than native-born Hispanics to assess their health as fair or poor or to report activity limitation due to chronic conditions or impairments, and less likely to report 4 or more bed days in the previous year. These rates increased steadily with years since immigration (less than 5, 5 to 9, and 10 or more years), suggesting better health among recent immigrants.

Although these data were adjusted for age, they were not broken up by age group, so it is not clear that a healthy-migrant effect is present among the elderly. When we analyzed data on a variety of health indicators from the Hispanic EPESE, we found no consistent differences between foreign-born and native-born Mexican-American elderly. Since most foreign-born Mexican-American elderly have lived in the United States for many years, the absence of a healthy-migrant effect in old age is not surprising.

When all available evidence is considered, the mortality advantages of Hispanics do not translate into health advantages in the older years. The data suggest, if anything, more functional limitations among Hispanic than among other white elderly.

Until recently, research on elderly Hispanics has concentrated on the population's general needs relating to its poverty, linguistic and cultural barriers, and family relationships. An important matter to underscore is the great heterogeneity of the Hispanic population. Mexican-American and Puerto Rican elderly have a great deal in common by virtue of their lower socioeconomic status, whereas Cuban Americans are closer to the general population in socioeconomic status and prevalence of most conditions. All three groups share a common language. Furthermore, little is known about the increasing numbers of elderly in a variety of groups that have their origins in Central and South American countries. One thing is clear: Hispanic populations, including the elderly, are increasing at much more rapid rates than the general population. We need large and more systematic studies that identify the population's special problems and needs as well as the various socioeconomic, cultural, and genetic factors relevant to understanding the health and health care behavior of its members.

REFERENCES

Angel, J.L., and R.J. Angel
   1992   Age at migration, social connections, and well-being among elderly Hispanics. *Journal of Aging and Health* 4:480-499.
Angel, J.L., and D.P. Hogan
   1991   The demography of minority aging populations. Pp. 1-13 in *Minority Elders: Longevity, Economics, and Health.* Washington, DC: The Gerontological Society of America.
Angel, R.J., and J.L. Angel
   1996   The extent of private and public health insurance coverage among adult Hispanics. *The Gerontologist* 36:332-340.
Angel, R.J., and P.J. Guarnaccia
   1989   Mind, body, and culture: Somatization among Hispanics. *Social Science and Medicine* 28:1229-1238.
Angel, R.J., and P. Thoits
   1987   The impact of culture on the cognitive structure of illness. *Culture, Medicine, and Psychiatry* 11:23-52.
Balcazar, H., and J.A. Cobas
   1993   Overweight among Mexican Americans and its relationship to life style behavioral risk factors. *Journal of Community Health* 18:55-67.
Bastida, E.
   1984   Reconstructing the world at sixty: Older Cubans in the U.S.A. *The Gerontologist* 24:465-470.
Bauer, R.L., and R.A. Deyo
   1987   Low risk of vertebral fracture in Mexican American women. *Archives of Internal Medicine* 147:1437-1439.
Black, S.A., and K.S. Markides
   1993   Acculturation and alcohol consumption in Puerto Rican, Cuban American and Mexican American females in the United States. *American Journal of Public Health* 83:890-893.

1994   Aging and generational patterns of alcohol consumption among Mexican Americans, Cuban Americans, and mainland Puerto Ricans. *International Journal of Aging and Human Development* 39:97-103.

Bradshaw, B.S., and E. Fonner, Jr.

1978   The mortality of Spanish surnamed persons in Texas: 1969-1971. Pp. 261-282 in *The Demography of Racial and Ethnic Groups*, F.D. Bean and W.P. Frisbie, eds. New York: Academic Press.

Bureau of the Census

1990   *The Hispanic Population in the United States: March 1989.* Current Population Reports, Series P-20, No. 444. Washington, DC: U.S. Department of Commerce.

1991   *Race and Hispanic Origin.* 1990 census profile, no. 2 (June). Washington, DC: U.S. Department of Commerce.

1992   *Sixty-Five Plus in America.* Current Population Reports, Series pp. 23-178. Washington, DC: U.S. Department of Commerce.

1993   Racial and ethnic diversity of America's elderly population. *Profiles of America's Elderly.* POP/93-1. Washington, DC: U.S. Department of Commerce.

Burnam, A., R.L. Hough, M. Karno, J.L. Escobar, and C.A. Telles

1987   Acculturation and lifetime prevalence of psychiatric disorders among Mexican Americans in Los Angeles. *Journal of Health and Social Behavior* 28:89-102.

California Center for Health Statistics.

1984   *Health Status of Californians by Race/Ethnicity, 1970 and 1980.* Sacramento, CA: State of California Health and Welfare Agency.

Carter-Pokra, O.

1994   Health profile. In *Latino Health in the U.S.: A Growing Challenge*, C.W. Molina and M. Aguirre-Molina, eds. Washington, DC: American Public Health Association.

Castro, F.G., L. Baezconde-Garbanati, and H. Beltran

1985   Risk factors for coronary heart disease in Hispanic populations: A review. *Hispanic Journal of Behavioral Sciences* 7(2):153-175.

Chiodo, L.K., D.N. Kanten, M.B. Gerety, C.D. Mulrow, and J.E. Coreil

1994   Functional status of Mexican American nursing home residents. *Journal of the American Geriatrics Society* 42:293-296.

Coreil, J., K.S. Markides, and L.A. Ray

1991   Predictors of smoking among Mexican Americans: Findings from the Hispanic HANES. *Preventive Medicine* 20:508-517.

Derenowski, J.

1990   Coronary artery disease in Hispanics. *Journal of Cardiovascular Nursing* 4:13-21.

Diehl, A.K., and M.P. Stern

1989   Special health problems of Mexican-Americans: Obesity, gallbladder disease, diabetes mellitus, and cardiovascular disease. *Advances in Internal Medicine* 34:73-96.

Espino, D.V., and S.K. Burge

1989   Comparisons of age of Mexican American and non-Hispanic white nursing home residents. *Family Medicine* 21:191-194.

Espino, D.V., S.K. Burge, and C.A. Moreno

1991   The prevalence of selected chronic diseases among the Mexican American elderly: Data from the 1982-1984 Hispanic Health and Nutrition Examination Survey. *Journal of the American Board of Family Practice* 4:217-222.

Espino, D.V., and D. Maldonado

1990   Hypertension and acculturation in elderly Mexican Americans: Results from the 1982-1984 Hispanic HANES. *The Journal of Gerontology: Medical Sciences* 45:M209-213.

Espino, D.V., E.O. Parra, and R. Kriebiel

1994   Mortality differences between elderly Mexican Americans and non-Hispanic whites in San Antonio, Texas: 1989. *Journal of the American Geriatrics Society* 42:604-608.

Franco, L.J., M.P. Stern, M. Rosenthal, S.M. Haffner, H.P. Hazuda, and P.J. Comeaux
    1985   Prevalence, detection, and control of hypertension in a biethnic community. *American Journal of Epidemiology* 121:684-696.
Gillespie, F.P., and T.A. Sullivan
    1983   What do current estimates of Hispanic mortality really tell us? Unpublished paper presented at the annual meeting of the Population Association of America.
Ginzberg, E.
    1991   Access to health care for Hispanics. *Journal of the American Medical Association* 265(2):238-241.
Guralnik. J.M., A.Z. LaCroix, D.F. Everett, and M.G. Kovar
    1989   Aging in the eighties: The prevalence of comorbidity and its association with disability. Advanced data. *Vital and Health Statistics* 70.
Gutierrez-Ramirez, A., R.B. Valdez, and O. Carter-Pokras
    1994   Cancer. In *Latino Health in the U.S.: A Growing Challenge*, C.W. Molina and M. Aguirre-Molina, eds. Washington, DC: American Public Health Association.
Haffner, S.M., M.P. Stern, H.P. Hazuda, M. Rosenthal, and J.A. Knapp
    1986   The role of behavioral variables and fat patterning in explaining ethnic differences in serum lipids and lipoproteins. *American Journal of Epidemiology* 123:830-839.
Hayes-Bautista, D.
    1992   Latino health indicators and the underclass model: From paradox to new policy models Pp. 32-47 in *Health Policy and the Hispanic*, A. Furino, ed. Boulder, CO: Westview Press.
Haynes, S.G., C. Harvey, H. Montes, H. Nicken, and B. Cohen
    1990   Patterns of cigarette smoking among Hispanics in the United States: Results from HHANES 1982-1984. *American Journal of Public Health* 80(suppl.):47-54.
Hazuda, H.P., S.M. Haffner, M.P. Stern, and C.W. Eifler
    1988   Effects of acculturation and socioeconomic status on obesity and diabetes in Mexican Americans. *American Journal of Epidemiology* 128:1289-1301.
Keefe, S.E., and A.M. Padilla
    1987   *Chicano Ethnicity*. Albuquerque, NM: University of New Mexico Press.
Kraus, J.F., N.O. Borhani, and C.E. Franti
    1980   Socioeconomic status, ethnicity, and risk of coronary heart disease. *American Journal of Epidemiology* 111:407-414.
Lacayo, C.G.
    1992   Current trends in living arrangements and social environment among ethnic minority elderly. Pp. 81-90 in *Diversity: New Approaches to Ethnic Minority Aging*, E.P. Stanford and F.M. Torres-Gil, eds. Amityville, NY: Baywood.
Markides, K.S., J.S. Boldt, and L.A. Ray
    1986   Sources of helping and intergenerational solidarity: A three-generations study of Mexican Americans. *Journal of Gerontology* 41:506-511.
Markides, K.S., and J. Coreil
    1986   The health of southwestern Hispanics: An epidemiologic paradox. *Public Health Reports* 101:253-265.
Markides, K.S., J. Coreil, and L.P. Rogers
    1989   Aging and health among southwestern Hispanics. Pp. 177-210 in *Aging and Health: Perspectives on Gender, Race, Ethnicity, and Class*, K.S. Markides, ed. Newbury Park, CA: Sage Publications.
Markides, K.S., and H.W. Martin, with Gomez, E.
    1983   *Older Mexican Americans: A Study in an Urban Barrio*. Monograph of the Center for Mexican American Studies. Austin: University of Texas Press.

Markides, K.S., L.A. Ray, C. Stroup-Benham, and F. Trevino
  1990   Acculturation and alcohol consumption in the Mexican American population of the south-western United States: Findings from the HHANES 1982-84. *American Journal of Public Health* 80(suppl.):42-46.

Mauer, K.R., J.E. Everhart, W.C. Knowler, T.H. Shawker, and H.P. Roth
  1990   Risk factors for gallstone disease in the Hispanic populations of the United States. *American Journal of Epidemiology* 131:836-844.

Mendes de Leon, C.F., and K.S. Markides
  1988   Depressive symptoms among Mexican Americans: A three-generations study. *American Journal of Epidemiology* 127:150-160.

Mitchell, B.D., H.P. Hazuda, S.M. Haffner, J.K. Patterson, and M.P. Stern
  1991   Myocardial infarction in Mexican-Americans and non-Hispanic whites. *Circulation* 83:45-51.

Mitchell, B.D., M.P. Stern, H.P. Hazuda, and J.K. Patterson
  1990   Risk factors for cardiovascular mortality in Mexican Americans and non-Hispanic whites. *American Journal of Epidemiology* 131:423-433.

Montes, J.H.
  1989   Specific cancers affecting Hispanics in the United States. Pp. 21-33 in *Minorities and Cancer*, L.A. Jones, ed. New York: Springer-Verlag.

Moscicki, E.K., B.Z. Locke, D.S. Rae, and J.H. Boyd
  1989   Depressive symptoms among Mexican Americans: The Hispanic Health and Nutrition Examination Survey. *American Journal of Epidemiology* 130:348-360.

Moscicki, E.K., D.S. Rae, D.A. Regier, and B.Z. Locke
  1987   The Hispanic Health and Nutrition Examination Survey: Depression among Mexican Americans, Cuban Americans and Puerto Ricans. Pp. 145-159 in *Health and Behavior: Research Agenda for Hispanics*, M. Gaviria and J.D. Arana, eds. Chicago: Simon Bolivar Hispanic-American Psychiatric Research and Training Program, University of Illinois at Chicago.

National Center for Health Statistics
  1993   Health data on Americans: United States, 1992. *Vital and Health Statistics* 3(27).
  1994   *Health, United States, 1993*. DHHS publication PHS 94-1232. Hyattsville, MD: Public Health Service.

Pappas, G., P.J. Gergen, and M. Carroll
  1990   Hypertension prevalence and the status of awareness, treatment, and control in the Hispanic Health and Nutrition Examination Survey (HHANES), 1982-1984. *American Journal of Public Health* 80:1431-1436.

Paz, J.J.
  1993   Support of Hispanic elderly. Pp. 177-183 in *Family Ethnicity: Strength in Diversity*, H.P. McAdoo, ed. Newbury Park, CA: Sage.

Polednak, A.P.
  1989   *Racial and Ethnic Differences in Disease*. New York: Oxford University Press.

Ramirez de Arellano, A.B.
  1994   The elderly. Pp. 189-208 in *Latino Health in the U.S.: A Growing Challenge*, C.W. Molina and M. Aguirre-Molina, eds. Washington, DC: American Public Health Association.

Rogers, R.G.
  1991   Health-related lifestyles among Mexican Americans, Puerto Ricans, and Cubans in the United States. Pp. 145-167 in *Mortality of Hispanic Populations*, I. Rosenwaike, ed. New York: Greenwood Press.

Rosenwaike, I., ed.
  1991   *Mortality of Hispanic Populations*. New York: Greenwood Press.

Rosenwaike, I., and K. Hempstead
  1990   Mortality among three Puerto Rican populations: Residents of Puerto Rico and migrants in New York City and in the balance of the United States, 1979-81. *International Migration Review* 24:684-702.
Sabogal, F., G. Marin, R. Otero-Sabogal, B.V. Marin, and E.J. Perez-Stable
  1987   Hispanic familism and acculturation: What changes and what doesn't? *Hispanic Journal of Behavioral Sciences* 9:397-412.
Samet, J.M., D.B. Coultas, C.A. Howard, B.J. Skipper, and C.L. Hanis
  1988   Diabetes, gallbladder disease, obesity, and hypertension among Hispanics in New Mexico. *American Journal of Epidemiology* 128:1302-1311.
Schoen, R., and V.F. Nelson
  1981   Mortality by cause among Spanish-surnamed Californians, 1969-1971. *Social Science Quarterly* 62:259-274.
Siegel, J.S., and J. Passel
  1979   Coverage of the Hispanic population of the United States in the 1970 census. Current Population Reports, Series P-23, No. 82. Washington, DC: U.S. Department of Commerce.
Sorel, J.E., D.R. Ragland, and S.L. Syme
  1991   Blood pressure in Mexican Americans, whites, and blacks. *American Journal of Epidemiology* 134:370-378.
Sorlie, P.D., M.S. Backlund, N.J. Johnson, and F. Rogat
  1993   Mortality by Hispanic status in the United States. *Journal of the American Medical Association* 270:2466-2468.
Sotomayor, M., and A. Garcia, eds.
  1993   *Elderly Latinos: Issues and Solutions for the 21st Century*. Washington, DC: National Hispanic Council on Aging.
Stephen, E.H., K. Foote, G.E. Hendershot, and C.A. Schoenborn
  1994   Health of the foreign-born population: United States, 1989-90. Advance data. *Vital and Health Statistics* 241.
Stern, M.P., B.S. Bradshaw, C.W. Eifler, D.S. Fong, H.P. Hazuda, and M. Rosenthal
  1987   Secular decline in death rates due to ischemic heart disease in Mexican Americans and non-Hispanic whites in Texas, 1970-1980. *Circulation* 76(6):1245-1250.
Stern, M.P., and S.M. Haffner
  1990   Type II diabetes and its complications in Mexican Americans. *Diabetes Metabolism Review* 6:1437-1439.
Trapido, E.J., C.B. McCoy, N. Strickman-Stein, S. Engel, H.V. McCoy, and S. Olejniczak
  1990   The epidemiology of cancer among Hispanic women: The experience in Florida. *Cancer* 66:2435-2441.
Vega, W.A., and H. Amaro
  1994   Latino outlook: Good health, uncertain prognosis. *Annual Review of Public Health* 15:39-67.
Vega, W.A., and R.G. Rumbaut
  1991   Ethnic minorities and mental health. *Annual Review of Sociology* 17:351-383.
Winkleby, M.A., S.P. Fortmann, and B. Rockhill
  1993   Health-related risks in a sample of Hispanics and whites matched on sociodemographic characteristics. *American Journal of Epidemiology* 137:1365-1375.
Wolinsky, F.D., B.E. Aguirre, L.J. Fann, V.M. Keith, C.L. Arnold, J.C. Niederhauer, and K. Dietrich
  1989   Ethnic differences in the demand for physician and hospital utilization among older adults in major American cities: Conspicuous evidence of considerable inequalities. *Milbank Quarterly* 67:412-449.